Organizing for Quality

Organizing for Quality

The improvement journeys of leading hospitals in Europe and the United States

PAUL BATE BA, PhD
Professor of Health Services Management
Royal Free & University College Medical School
University College London

PETER MENDEL BS, MA, PhD
Associate Social Scientist
RAND Corporation
Santa Monica, CA

and

GLENN ROBERT BA, MSc, PhD
Principal Research Fellow
Royal Free & University College Medical School
University College London

Foreword by
DONALD M BERWICK

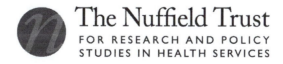

The Nuffield Trust
FOR RESEARCH AND POLICY
STUDIES IN HEALTH SERVICES

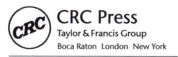

CRC Press
Taylor & Francis Group
Boca Raton London New York

CRC Press is an imprint of the
Taylor & Francis Group, an **informa** business

CRC Press
Taylor & Francis Group
6000 Broken Sound Parkway NW, Suite 300
Boca Raton, FL 33487-2742

Printed on acid-free paper
Version Date: 20150921

International Standard Book Number-13: 978-1-84619-151-0 (Paperback)

Visit the Taylor & Francis Web site at
http://www.taylorandfrancis.com

and the CRC Press Web site at
http://www.crcpress.com

Contents

Foreword

On a bright, warm April day this year, I joined two friends for a walk through an Audubon sanctuary on the Ipswich River, an hour's drive from my Massachusetts home. At the beginning of the path we followed was a gift shop, with dozens of books and pamphlets on the many species of birds in our region. I leafed through a few, but not being a 'birder' of any sort, bought none. I'd just see the birds myself. It was a lovely walk – silent. Within a few minutes, however, my friends and I were commenting on *how* silent it was. We saw no birds, and heard none. After a mile or so we encountered a man, maybe 65 years old, peculiarly dressed in camouflage, a many-pocketed vest, and a Raiders-of-the-Lost-Ark fedora. He smiled and greeted us. 'Nice day,' he said. We agreed. 'But,' we asked, 'where are the birds?' He looked confused for an instant, then he smiled. 'All around you,' he said. 'Here, hold out your hands.' He reached into one of the pockets in his vest and withdrew a small fistful of birdseed. He poured a little from his hand into each of ours. And then he, also, held his hand out. 'Now shhhh,' he said.

Magic happened. Within seconds a bird alighted on his open hand to nibble at the seed. An instant later our own hands were occupied likewise. And, suddenly, the woods were teeming with birds. Our newfound guide pointed, high and low, to the right and the left, naming one species after another. Our 'empty' forest was, in fact, full of life and sound. It had been there; without the 'birdman', we had not seen it or heard it.

Looking is not seeing. Listening is not hearing. It is possible to miss so much that is right in front of us if we lack the categories and skills to notice. The greatest of these skills is, perhaps, to put aside our expectations, and to stay open to the actual. Paul Bate, Peter Mendel, and Glenn Robert are expert at noticing. For sociology novices like me, their exact methods and skills are elusive. The closest analogue in normal experience is, I suppose, story-telling. Their way of harvesting useful lessons and generalizations seems to me a high form of creativity, combining disciplined methods of enquiry with open minds, so that new categories and insights can form, stemming directly from their observations. A bird-watcher, I suppose, knows more about how to watch than about what will be seen. Most species will be familiar, but the expert is always open to the possibility that something quite new, quite unexpected, will come into view. In the words of these authors, '. . . our own journey has been very similar to that of the stories of QI we heard from the organizations that we studied: that is to say, emergent and unpredictable, and full of twists and turns.'

This humility in enquiry is not just generous, it is methodologically important, because neither these researchers nor their subjects in the complex world of organizational change and improvement can hope to escape '. . . the hazards and uncertainties lying in wait in the punishing contextual terrain that has to be crossed . . .'. I will long remember that phrase – 'the punishing contextual terrain' – since it so clearly labels the facts-on-the-ground for the ambitious, even courageous clinicians, managers, executives, and others in healthcare who seek to make care far better. They have discovered that almost nothing about effective action in improvement is 'installable' without constant, recursive adjustments to ever-changing local context. Researchers who wish to understand how improvement works, and why and when it fails, will never succeed if they regard context as experimental noise and the control of context as a useful design principle.

This humility – humility in the face of contextual determinants of effects – finds its strongest expression in this book in the wealth of direct quotations that the authors have chosen to include. As they write, '. . . no "journey to quality" story we heard could be too detailed, no anecdote too pithy or trivial'. This bias toward quotation lengthens this book, but the price is worth it; the words of the actors themselves embed experiences and insights that mere summary would miss. The extensive use of the subjects' own words, in my view, transforms this book from a history to an archive. These case studies will deserve reference and study for decades to come.

That the authors arrive at last at a model of their own – their 'Color Codebook' for Quality and Service Improvement – is a gift to the reader that will add efficiency to future case studies. Of enormous value as well are their stunningly comprehensive reviews of theories and studies of organizational change with a magisterial bibliography that will from here on simplify the work of many grateful students of the field. But, in my opinion, neither of these is their most valuable achievement here. Rather, their achievement is to have populated our literature on organizational change with a suite of accounts at a level of detail never before available. They are leading the field by example, showing in their honest, careful, thorough inquiry how important are an open mind and an attitude of respect. These can unite those who try to take effective action and those who study effective action as (if the reader–scholar will excuse the expression when science is at stake) soul mates.

May I indulge one final, personal, observation as I commend this book to the student of change? I have the pleasure of knowing personally one of the authors, Paul Bate, for a dozen years or so. I was a novice in improvement when we first met, and he, I believe, was a novice in the study of improvement. We met first on uncertain ground – me uncertain of the methods I was trying to learn and master, and he uncertain of whether, in a positivist sense, the methods 'worked'. Our nascent friendship was, I would say, tinged with tension – as perhaps between a movie director and the *Times* movie critic. I am less sure today that my level of skill has changed since than that Paul's has. I believe I have seen in the years that followed our first meeting that scholarship of the authentic form, not the showy form, guides Paul's dialogues, writings, and enquiries. As 'open-mindedness' and 'respect' characterize the best of social research, so did these two qualities appear to me again and again as Paul's trademarks as a student of organizations trying to improve their work. In his work and in this book, this important thinker shows that humility need not be mistaken for confusion, and that learning depends far more on recognizing what we do not yet know than on displaying what we do. I have not had the pleasure yet of getting to know Peter Mendel and Glenn Robert personally. But, I will wager, based on this book, that they share with Paul Bate curiosity in its most genuine form. With their guidance, dear reader, get ready to see things you do not yet know how to see, and to hear what you do not yet know to listen for.

Donald M Berwick MD KBE
President and CEO, Institute of Healthcare Improvement;
Clinical Professor of Pediatrics and Health Care Policy, Harvard Medical School
September 2007

Preface and acknowledgements

The story we tell in this book begins around the end of 2002, when our small, but doughty and determined, team set off on its quest to discover the 'secrets' of high-performing, high-quality organizations within the healthcare domain. This naïve, almost romantic, endeavour was seeking answers to how it was that these organizations had managed to achieve and, more impressively, to spread and sustain exemplary levels of care for their patients. It was a quest that would eventually take us to a number of healthcare organizations that enjoy world-class reputations for the quality of care they provide.

Some four years on, older and hopefully a little wiser, we are now able to reflect upon and share the lessons and insights we gained on this journey, based on hundreds of conversations we had with people on our travels – front-line clinicians, managers and nurses, and other healthcare professionals. This book is therefore a 'story within a story', its aim being to bring together the many tales of quality that we heard on our travels while at the same time giving an account of our own parallel journey of discovery as change and quality improvement (QI) researchers. The richness and diversity of these tales from the field are striking, but, paradoxically, so too are their similarities. The aim of this book is to reveal both aspects to the reader.

Our quest has inevitably taken us many thousands of miles, over many different kinds of terrain and across two major continents (Figure A, *see* color plate section): first to the United Kingdom (UK) itself, from the rolling meadows around the Royal Devon and Exeter NHS Foundation Trust in the south-west of England, to the Peterborough and Stamford Hospitals NHS Foundation Trust on the edge of the atmospheric East Anglian fenlands; and then back to King's College Hospital NHS Foundation Trust, a large inner-London hospital on the south side of the River Thames. All three are very different from each other but enjoy the same reputation for the high quality of services they provide for their diverse patient populations.

Then, on to the United States (US) and SSM Healthcare, based in St Louis, Missouri, but comprising 20 acute hospitals spread across four states, and the first healthcare organization to win the prestigious Baldridge award for quality; and from there across to the west coast and San Diego Children's Hospital, rising like a mirage from the parched ground of southern California, before heading north to Cedars-Sinai hospital a few miles south of the Hollywood hills in Los Angeles and healthcare provider to some of the richest and poorest people in the world. Then, back east again, this time to Wisconsin and Luther Midelfort in Eau Claire, an affiliate of the world-renowned Mayo Health System; and, as winter began to close in, to the snows of the upstate capital of New York and the Albany Medical Center, one of the first HIV centers in the US, and a pioneer in AIDS treatment and care.

Finally, we headed to mainland Europe and the Reinier de Graaf hospital in Delft in the Netherlands, one of six European organizations (including two of our UK sites, Royal Devon and Exeter and Kings) selected to participate in Pursuing Perfection, a pioneering international learning collaborative sponsored by the Institute for Healthcare Improvement (IHI). Unfortunately, only a selection of these cases can be included in a single volume like this, although we have drawn on them all in terms of both data and conceptual development.*

For those already raising a suspicious eyebrow, we should point out that we are all too well aware of the dangers that lie in 'jet plane ethnography', where the researchers act as little more than academic tourists, stopping briefly before jetting off to somewhere else even more exotic than their last stopover.[1] In our defence, we chose to linger, practising what we like to call 'organizational loitering', leaning against doorposts and water coolers, watching and observing, talking with staff, and above all listening to and recording the stories and insights they had to offer about their QI endeavours. We were anxious to hear from members of these world-class healthcare organizations – people from all types of professional backgrounds – what, in their view, made their organizations special as regards having achieved high levels of care, and the factors and processes that had allowed them to attain, and then remain, at such heights.

We wanted to hear and document their stories in their words, not ours, and then, with them, begin to retrace the steps they had taken on their various journeys, the wrong ones and the right ones, the highs and the lows, and the various forks in the road where crucial choices had to be made. Above all, we wanted to gather their first-hand *experiences* of sustaining high levels of quality within what we know to be complex, pluralistic and therefore highly challenging organizations. This involved getting to the heart of their 'theories of practice' as opposed to the academic theories that are in plentiful supply – their own theories and practices that helped them to deal with the three major 'change challenges' that will face any QI team embarked on such a journey:

❐ the challenge of implementation (making it happen)
❐ the challenge of diffusion or spread (making it reach across a whole organization)
❐ the challenge of sustainability (making it last).

Our underpinning philosophy and logic was simple, but pervasive: hindsight (the process of looking backwards – reflection) gives insight (appreciation and understanding – sensemaking), which gives foresight (a view of how to get better at what we do in future – prescription and direction). In this regard, no 'journey to quality' story we heard could be too detailed, no anecdote too pithy or trivial. We wanted to take a 'deep dive' into the practical world of quality and service improvement to see it as the participants saw it, and to tell it how they told it, complicating ourselves to the degree that the subject matter warranted it, but realizing that it is all too easy for both us and readers to end up lost or drowning in the detail. Here we took heart from the philosopher and social scientist Alfred Schutz, who once said that understanding evolves through three phases: simplistic, complex and profoundly simple. We would like to think that during this study we have moved through all three stages, ending with simplicity, which, of course, is very different from starting with it.

Our core team, the three authors of this book, has remained the same throughout this journey, but there have been many others who have joined us on various legs

---

* The choice of which to include and which to exclude was a difficult one. King's and SSM were finally left out because we felt that the two core themes that emerged there, namely organizational citizenship and spiritual capital, almost needed a book in their own right to do them full justice, and also because having spent a little longer at these two sites, with wider and deeper access to staff, we felt the final write-up would be better suited to a free-standing extended ethnographic case study rather than a, necessarily, shorter chapter of a book.

of our tour whom we now wish to thank on record, and without whom we would never have made it, there or back: Jim Zazzali, from RAND, who accompanied us on most of the UK and US legs and took the lead on the first draft of the original Luther Midelfort case (Chapter 6); Keith McInnes, from Harvard Medical School, who acted as lead researcher and author on the original Albany case (Chapter 8); Tony Riley, from UCL, who did much of the early scouting work at King's, Reinier de Graaf (Chapter 5) and Albany (Chapter 8); Louise Locock, who co-researched the Peterborough chapter (Chapter 7); and Mirjam van het Loo of RAND Europe, who joined us briefly, but impressively, for the Dutch leg (Chapter 5).

We have indicated the contributors to each of the original seven organizational case studies included in this book at the beginning of Chapters 2 to 8. Each of the initial narratives for the case studies presented in these chapters has been extensively edited by one of us (PM) so that they can be included here. Others far more experienced than us in the jungle craft of quality expeditions have also given freely of their time, advice and encouragement en route, most notably Paul Cleary (Harvard) and Steve Shortell (University of California, Berkeley), and we thank them deeply for that.

Financial backers obviously need to be found for such trips, and in this regard we are deeply grateful to The Nuffield Trust in the UK, who generously sponsored the work for the 18 months of the formal project, before we – realizing it was then too late to turn back, and massively overcommitted and under-equipped – were compelled to fall back on other meagre resources in order to survive and complete the final legs of the journey. Some key figures at The Nuffield Trust became more like mentors than sponsors, and we would like to put on record our thanks to John Wyn Owen, Sir Denis Pereira Gray, Kim Beazor and Helena Scott. Their support was especially welcome early on in the face of stiff opposition from certain academic high priests of medicine sitting around the table who insisted that gathering primary accounts and observations from the field – no matter how rigorously recorded or expertly analyzed – if lacking the hallowed method of the randomized controlled trial, was neither 'real research' nor 'serious science' (they were right and wrong: 'science', in their narrow terms, no; serious and real, most definitely yes).

These, fortunately rare but nevertheless bruising, encounters with fellow members of the research community brought to mind Ramachandran's amusing allegory,[2] cited recently by Siggelkow[3] to describe a similar bias in neurobiology against close examination of limited cases, which, ironically, has led to many of the signature advances in that discipline. In this tale (slightly embellished here for our purposes), Ramachandran tells of a team of researchers who go out into the field and find a talking pig. They cart the pig into a room of academic peers, snap their fingers, and the pig starts talking, from time to time even quoting Shakespeare, its favorite writer. What will be the response? Will there at last be recognition of the value of (by the researchers' own admission) an unrepresentative, small-sample case study? Unfortunately not. Their response is: 'Interesting, but that's just one pig. Show us a few more and we might believe you,' adding, 'And why on earth show us a pig that is clearly so untypical of the rest of the pig population?'

During these early days and encounters, Bob Brook from RAND was also highly effective in defending the value of our approach, and as director of the RAND Health Research Unit provided highly valuable supplemental support when needed for the field work at two US sites. Another RAND colleague, Shan Cretin, played an influential role in the formative days of the project as well, helping to give it both voice and direction. We are similarly grateful to Anne Marie Weggelaar-Jansen for introducing us to the 'color code for change', and to Hans Vermaak from the Twynstra Group in the Netherlands for granting us permission to cite and develop his original 'color code' work in Chapter 9. Gillian Nineham, our commissioning editor at Radcliffe Publishing, also proved to be a firm but generous guide throughout the preparation of this manuscript, which has benefited greatly from her own deep commitment to quality.

Gaining access to outstanding healthcare organizations is never an easy task, and we would like to express special thanks to Don Berwick of IHI and Helen Bevan of the NHS Institute for Innovation and Improvement, who helped to broker many of the initial links and connections on our behalf, and who were sufficiently trusting to allow their names to support our requests for research access and entry. At the other end of our journey, we also owe a debt of gratitude to the three anonymous peer reviewers who appraised the text. Their comments were extremely helpful in clarifying and refocusing parts of the manuscript to serve both practitioner and research audiences.

However, we reserve our biggest thanks till last, and that is to the hundreds of people in the organizations themselves, senior leaders and front-line doctors, managers and nurses, and the variety of clinical professionals and other dedicated staff in different levels and positions who gave so freely and generously of their time, and granted us the privilege of hearing their stories and accounts first hand.

A preface such as this often concludes with the words 'all final responsibility for the text rests with the authors'. On this occasion we are happy to report that this will not be the case, and although we accept full responsibility for any errors in reporting and interpretation, the responsibility – but also credit – for the stories themselves remains with their original tellers. And this, we believe, is how it should be.

In his wonderful book *Invisible Cities*, Italo Calvino writes, 'Journeys to relive your past are journeys to recover your future.'[4] This book is dedicated to all those who took this journey backwards so that others may learn to live theirs forwards.

Paul Bate, Peter Mendel, Glenn Robert
September 2007

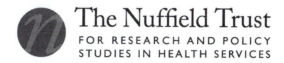

The Nuffield Trust
FOR RESEARCH AND POLICY STUDIES IN HEALTH SERVICES

The Nuffield Trust is proud to publish, in association with Radcliffe Publishing, this important contribution to the debate about quality in healthcare. The Nuffield Trust is one of the leading independent health policy charitable trusts in the UK. It was established as the Nuffield Provincial Hospitals Trust in 1940 by Viscount Nuffield (William Morris), the founder of Morris Motors. In 1998 the name The Nuffield Trust for Research and Policy Studies in Health Services was adopted, retaining 'The Nuffield Trust' as its working name.

The Nuffield Trust mission is to promote independent analysis and informed debate on UK healthcare policy. The Nuffield Trust's purpose is to communicate evidence and encourage an exchange around developed or developing knowledge, in order to illuminate recognized and emerging issues.

It achieves this through its principal activities:
- Bringing together a wide national and international network of people involved in UK healthcare through a series of meetings, workshops and seminars.
- Commissioning research through its publications and grants program, to inform policy debate.
- Encouraging interdisciplinary exchange between clinicians, legislators, academics, healthcare professionals and management, policy makers, industrialists and consumer groups.
- Supporting evidence-based health policy and practice.
- Sharing its knowledge in the home countries and internationally through partnerships and alliances.

The Trust's work is steered by a board of governing trustees, chaired by Professor Dame Carol Black CBE. To find out more please refer to our website www.nuffieldtrust.org.uk or contact:

The Nuffield Trust
59 New Cavendish St
London W1G 7LP
United Kingdom

Tel: +44 (0)20 7631 8450
Fax: +44 (0)20 7631 8451
Website: www.nuffieldtrust.org.uk
Email: info@nuffieldtrust.org.uk
Charity number: 209201

About the authors

Paul Bate holds the Chair of Health Services Management within the Medical School, University College London. A social anthropologist and organization theorist by background, Paul works with clinicians, managers and staff at all levels of the National Health Service (NHS) to help bring about major improvements in health services. He is the author of six books (two of them nominated for international awards) and numerous journal articles on quality, service improvement and change.

Peter Mendel is an Associate Social Scientist at the RAND Corporation, a non-profit policy research institute based in Santa Monica, California. As a sociologist specializing in organizations and globalization, Peter's research has focused on the dynamics of healthcare systems, healthcare reform, and quality improvement. His co-authored study of institutional change and healthcare organizations in the US over the past half-century[1] received best scholarly book awards in organizational sociology (2001) and medical sociology (2002) from the American Sociological Association.

Glenn Robert is Principal Research Fellow within the Medical School, University College London. A sociologist by background, Glenn's research centers on quality and service improvement in healthcare, with a focus on the policy implementation process at the local level and securing sustained change within healthcare organizations. A recent book with his co-author Paul Bate and others[2] was the 2006 winner of the Baxter Award for the most outstanding contribution to healthcare management in Europe.

List of figures, tables and boxes

Figures

Tables

Boxes

Glossary

ACE	Annual Comprehensive Examination
AMC	Albany Medical Center
AMCAP	Albany Medical Center AIDS Program
ATC	AIDS Treatment Center
BPR	Business Process Re-engineering
CCM	Chronic Care Model
CCU	Critical Care Unit
CEO	Chief Executive Officer
CFO	Chief Financial Officer
COPD	Chronic Obstructive Pulmonary Disease
CQI	Continuous Quality Improvement
CT	Computed Tomography
DAC(s)	Designated AIDS Center(s)
ED	Emergency Department
ENT	Ear, nose and throat
GP(s)	General Practitioner(s)
HR	Human Resources
HRM	Human Resources Management
HRSA	Health Resources and Services Administration (US)
ICT	Information and Communication Technology
IHI	Institute for Healthcare Improvement (US)
IOM	Institute of Medicine (US)
IT	Information technology
JCAHO	Joint Commission for Accreditation of Healthcare Organizations (US)
MRI	Magnetic resonance imaging
NHS	National Health Service (UK)
NP	Nurse practitioner
OD	Organizational Development
OMT	Organization and management theory
PA	Physician assistants
PCT(s)	Primary Care Trusts (UK)
PDH	Peterborough District Hospital
PDSA	Plan-Do-Study-Act
PEOC	Princess Elizabeth Orthopaedic Centre (Royal Devon and Exeter NHS Foundation Trust)
PIC	Performance Improvement Committee
PP	'Pursuing Perfection'
QI	Quality Improvement
QIC	Quality Improvement Committee

RdGG	Reinier de Graaf Groep
RD&E	Royal Devon and Exeter NHS Foundation Trust
SI	Service improvement
STS	Socio-technical systems theory
TQM	Total Quality Management
UK	United Kingdom
US	United States

Reader's guide

Before we set off and begin relating the stories from our travels, we invite our readers, whom we anticipate to be a fairly eclectic group of both practitioners (including health service managers, clinical leaders and improvement specialists) and researchers, to take a moment to orient themselves by means of this brief guide.

Like any good tale, or rather collection of tales, it seems sensible to start at the beginning, and so we suggest that all readers take a few moments to review our introduction (Chapter 1) and become familiar with the type of terrain we intend to cover. We then retrace our steps back to seven of the nine high-performing healthcare organizations we stopped at en route (Chapters 2 to 8). In the final leg, we map out some possible future directions for those who may wish to embark on, revisit or think further about organizational journeys to quality in the healthcare context (Chapters 9 to 11).

Chapters 2 to 8 are the stories from seven of our nine ports of call. On first encountering these, some readers might prefer to pause only briefly before hurrying to take in the view from the higher ground of Chapters 9 and 10; others may prefer to dive straight into the detail before pulling back to reflect, with our help, on what they have read. Whichever route you choose, Chapter 9 aims to assist (mainly) practitioners by:

- ❏ providing a checklist of the challenges any QI effort will face
- ❏ giving improvement activists a method for identifying any 'gaps' in their own QI activities (by means of a self-administered checklist)
- ❏ allowing implicit assumptions about the theory and practice of QI to surface and be exposed to conscious thought and challenge, perhaps for the first time
- ❏ providing people with a common framework and language to think, talk about and debate the issues and challenges associated with QI, and together be able to come up with a set of hypotheses or solutions.

Chapter 10 then explores in more detail the similarities and differences among our case study sites in terms of the dynamic nature of their efforts to solve each of these challenges.

This division is not a parting of the ways. Although Chapter 9 is largely written for practitioners and Chapter 10 for researchers and theorists, we believe researchers will benefit from reading Chapter 9 so that they can understand the basic components of our model, and many practitioners will want, we hope, to go the extra step and delve further into the dynamics of the change processes explained in Chapter 10.

Our journey concludes with a backward glance over the territory covered and suggests some implications for both practitioners and researchers (Chapter 11).

Introduction

Organizing for quality

Mapping out the terrain for our journey

It is an axiomatic and now almost constant assertion in health services research, policy and practice that the healthcare systems in many developed societies, despite their relative affluence, are plagued with dysfunction and under-achievement in the effectiveness and quality of the care they provide.[1–8] This conclusion has become ever more evident and difficult to ignore as health services research grows more adept at measuring health outcomes and quality. For example, a recently acclaimed national study in the US by McGlynn *et al.*[9] which looked across 439 quality indicators for 30 acute and chronic conditions, documented that only 54.9% of patients receive what is considered the recommended level of care – an astounding finding given the resources and sophistication associated with modern medicine.

Contemporary research into initiatives to improve the outcomes and quality of healthcare processes also reveals striking variation in terms of their impact and overall levels of success, both between and within countries[10–13] and organizations.[14–16] Just imagine for a moment that we could look down on the global healthcare terrain from high above. We would see huge differences in quality and patient and staff experiences, a topography of high peaks and low valleys with infinite colors and shades. From this vantage point one of the first things we would notice would be the marked differences between countries.[4,17–21] For instance, we could not fail to notice how woefully poor five-year cancer survival rates are for UK patients relative to many other European countries. A recent report has revealed that British cancer patients are substantially more likely to die of the disease than those in other western European countries (mainly because of poor access to the latest drugs).[22]

Move in closer and we would also begin to notice the large variation between organizations, even within a single country. For instance, Jarman's work[23] has revealed that a patient is many times more likely to die in some US hospitals than in others. His analysis of hospital-standardized mortality rates for US hospitals plotted against the charge per admission (standardized for age and diagnosis) shows a 450% variation in a patient's chance of dying depending on which hospital he or she enters, as well as an 800% variation in standardized reimbursement.

Zoom in yet closer and even sharper differences would come into view, this time between clinical departments (micro-systems) within the same healthcare organization, a mixed terrain of oases and deserts of quality where one wrong turn to the left or right could make the difference between superb and substandard care. Adler *et al.* have termed this the 'Six West Problem':[24] patients receive fabulous care on ward 6 West that should be spread and be the norm hospital-wide, but when they cross the corridor to ward 6 East or 5 North they experience something altogether different. The contrast is stark and disturbing. As novelist Ian McEwan put it in a recent book, 'the difference between good and bad care is near-infinite'.[25]

Stark and revealing though they are, cold statistics like those quoted above, and neutral, almost aseptic, words like 'variation', can easily disguise or downplay the serious human consequences of such differences in healthcare quality. Replace, for example, the word 'variation' with 'inequality' and these differences begin to acquire darker and more troubling undertones, which echo throughout healthcare systems in many developed countries.[26,27] In anyone's book, 'inequalities' of this nature and extent must be unacceptable. Why, for example, Children's Commissioner Al Aynsley-Green asks, should 'an inner city child live fifteen years less than someone in the leafy suburbs five miles down the road?'[28] Why, for that matter (referring back to Jarman's work), should a person have a much greater chance of dying in one hospital than in another? Put this way, a journey like ours to understand how to narrow this variation – inequality – becomes more relevant and purposeful.

While being quite good at measuring these variations (or inequalities if you prefer), we are, unfortunately, much further behind in our understanding of what causes them, and even further behind in knowing how to reduce or remove them altogether: 'Despite the stepped-up collection of information, experts know little about why variations in patient care persist'.[9]

At the same time, many of our leading voices on healthcare quality point increasingly to understanding organizational issues in health service delivery as central to explaining variations in care and making progress towards improvement. The Institute of Medicine's watershed *To Err is Human*[1] and *Crossing the Quality Chasm*[2] reports specifically identified organizational failings as one of the root causes of poor quality, with the latter devoting an entire chapter to analyzing healthcare organizations as complex, adaptive systems and the implications of this perspective for implementing change. As elaborated by others, this perspective includes recognizing the multiple levels of the healthcare system, and that high-level influences such as policy, payment rules, regulation and accreditation are strongly mediated by dynamics and responses at the levels of healthcare organizations, and the smaller units of healthcare providers they support in delivering services to the level that matters most – patients.[29]

The general consensus is that our healthcare systems, in their current state of organization, are incapable of providing the quality of healthcare that most developed countries expect (and pay for).[1,2,29] Reviewing assessments of quality of care across numerous countries yields a similar conclusion that 'fundamental changes in the way medical care is organized, managed, and delivered will be necessary' in order to seriously address the presently intractable quality deficiencies of our healthcare systems.[6] One should not underestimate the size of the task this presents. This type of roll-up-the-sleeves organizational transformation is hard work and requires investment and effort from many different types of stakeholders throughout the healthcare system.[30]

Yet in trying to come to grips with the organizational dimension to healthcare quality, most of these same voices can only point vaguely to the 'complexity' and 'diversity' of the healthcare system, and the lack of sophisticated and integrated information systems that would provide data necessary for implementing improvements and for proper accountability of services. In its typical form, this suggestion implies that if only healthcare providers and other stakeholders had access to data they would be able to overcome everything, and figure out the way of delivering higher levels of care. Would it were that simple.

Although access to information is certainly one piece of the quality puzzle, on further inspection this appears a somewhat naïve view of organizational and individual behavior in terms of the non-trivial processes of how information systems are implemented and the way information is put to use and acted upon. It also seems to us that terms such as 'complexity' and 'diversity' are less explanations than placeholders for an explanation, joining other all-time favorites such as 'culture',[31] terms that are often deployed as a vague catch-all for any unexplained variance in an organization's performance.

A rigorous, if relatively small, body of research does exist in the health services literature which specifically attempts to unravel this 'black box' of organization in healthcare delivery. Informed by organization and management theory (OMT), the better-accepted branches of this work focus on identifying organizational predictors of successful implementation of quality improvement (QI), typically using multivariate statistical methods and quasi-experimental data (see, for example,[32,33]). This research has been able to highlight a number of factors – such as leadership support, particular dimensions of organizational culture and climate, and team-based structures and composition – that appear to be associated with successfully implementing change in healthcare organizations. Unfortunately it has been less adept at shedding light on why these factors relate to one another, how they are related, and how in practice organizations go about influencing and setting these 'key success factors' in motion.

Juxtaposed to this work is a large body of descriptive accounts of improvement initiatives in healthcare organizations (see, for example,[34–38]). It is too simple to criticize much of this literature as self-reports, unmethodical, or otherwise non-reflective. Many of these accounts serve the highly useful purpose of illustrating the types and varieties of improvement activities taking place, what may be possible and, if nothing else, the intentions and mindsets of the authors who often themselves are involved in these endeavours.

There also happen to be a number of examples in this body of writing that do present systematic in-depth details and comparisons (see, for example,[39,40]). However, even these examinations tend to be overly descriptive, plagued by relative under-development of organizational concepts that would help to explain why some actions, strategies or initiatives worked and others did not, and in the end, frequently appear intent on regenerating the lists of factors common to the above literature rather than providing insight into how they interact and unfold.

As a result, we are left with a general literature on healthcare quality that, reflecting the wider field of health services research, for the most part remains atheoretical, aprocessual, acontextual and/or ahistorical.[41] This is a problem organization and organizational change research has worked hard to address during the past two decades, but which still impedes our ability to make the transition between research that is good on the descriptive 'what' to research that is also good on the explanatory 'why'? This is particularly true of QI, which we believe remains under-theorised and over-popularized as a field: one joke told by Micklethwait and Wooldridge[42] (cited by Weick and Quinn[43]) is that the reason people often talk of quality and change 'gurus' is that they can't spell the word 'charlatan'. The total quality management (TQM) and continuous quality improvement (CQI) field generally is tired and in need of new theories as well as new practices.

Perhaps it is overstating the case, but to us the overwhelming majority of studies in healthcare quality are descriptive rather than explanatory, and rarely take the time to construct theories or explanations for what they observe or find in their analyses. This is particularly true of the organizational or human dimensions of QI, which are the focus of this book. One of the fundamental notions we are keen to reveal is that although technical factors, such as information systems, do play a major role in accounting for the quality 'gap', many of these are themselves rooted in organizational and human failures at a deeper perceptual, attitudinal, structural, cultural or processual level. Better information systems may therefore help, but don't expect the problem to go away: such technical improvements are likely to be necessary but not sufficient to remove the inequalities discussed above.

Unfortunately, given the strong traditional focus on the technical aspects of quality, it has been all too easy to forget (or simply fail to acknowledge) the fact that every aspect of care is accomplished through organization – or more accurately, processes of organizing – and therefore that organizational and human processes can be expected to play a huge part in determining the level and quality of care patients receive. If this is the case, and we will show that it is, it becomes imperative that as quality researchers we begin to widen our remit and seek to give greater prominence to the distinct characteristics and dynamics of these processes, design (or redesign) healthcare systems with these processes more clearly and explicitly in mind, and actively manage and guide these processes, rather than treating them as an afterthought, or leaving them almost to take care of themselves.

It still never fails to surprise us just how little attention has been paid by theorists and practitioners alike to this issue of *organizing* for high-quality healthcare. This is an omission we shall be seeking to rectify in this book by mapping out what such an organizational perspective on quality looks like, and then 'populating' it with real data from the healthcare field. In this respect, our study is arguably one of the first to apply contemporary streams of organizational theory – relatively untapped by conventional research on healthcare quality – to detailed, multi-level accounts of QI experiences across a variety of healthcare organizations. Our hope and aim in doing this is that it will help to unravel some of the mysteries of how the *process* of improving quality works, both in the complex ways different organizational and human factors influence each other, and in how the different levels of an organization can contribute in distinctive ways to making this process effective (or not).

Actually, the word 'factors' is not right here, because we cannot simply substitute organizational or human factors for technical or clinical factors. As we discuss in the next section, organization research of the kind we shall be calling on has repeatedly drawn attention to the weaknesses and limitations of the 'variables paradigm' and its associated logical-analytical language.[44] It has shown that, while nice if it were true, there is rarely a single, or even dominant, set of factors that can explain why, say, only 55% of patients in McGlynn *et al.*'s study[9] received their recommended care; or, for that matter, why some healthcare systems do significantly better or worse than the average in this regard.

The explanation is much more likely to be systemic and multi-factorial, and no amount of correlation between selected independent and dependent variables is therefore likely to be able to come up with a satisfactory explanation. Rather, it is in the interactions between a multiplicity of factors and processes (rather than the factors or processes themselves) that the answer is to be found; for instance, in the interrelationships between the attitudes people, individually and collectively, bring to the care enterprise, the behavioral routines they create, and the aspects of their situation to which they choose to pay attention. This brings us naturally to a discussion of some of the main differences between this present study and previous ones.

Five differences between this quality research expedition and previous ones

The reasons why we still lack good explanations for the 'quality variation' between and within healthcare systems may be traced to the somewhat narrow tastes and preferences researchers have cultivated towards the quality issue over the years.

Gazing down from the sky rather than searching on the ground

First, there is the traditional preference for a high-level, in some cases positively stratospheric view of the subject matter far away from where the action takes place, accompanied by a taste for big picture statistics that favor sweeping trends rather than the nuances, the shades and the ups and downs of everyday improvement activity on the ground. Given this, it is hardly surprising that the minutiae of QI programs and processes remain shrouded in mystery. As Øvretveit and Staines[45] have recently pointed out:

> Apart from a few projects, the details of which interventions were actually made are often not presented, and there are few adequate or independent research descriptions of actual implementations of organizational and system wide programs over time.

In contrast, the research approach we have adopted could hardly have been further from such a high orbit one, which, we believe, inevitably runs the risk of turning a varied and interesting landscape into one that is flat and featureless. We favored a 'deep dive' groundwards in order to get closer to the action. So what, in broad terms, did we find? Interestingly – though probably not surprisingly – this deep dive revealed a rich variety of approaches to QI, some of them similar but others quite different to each other, all offering strong support for the 'equifinality principle' in systems thinking that there are 'many different paths up the mountain' and many different ways of getting to the top. Just why some approaches have been chosen and work in one situation, while other very different approaches seem to work just as well in another situation, is a major theme for our discussion in Chapter 10, following the presentation of our seven organizational case studies in Chapters 2 to 8.

Descriptions of the 'what' rather than explanations of the 'how' or 'why'

Second, the existing literature has traditionally focused on 'what' works rather than 'how' or 'why' it works, the dangerous and in our view doubtful[46] assumption being that once it is known what works the solution can simply be replicated anywhere, without ever needing to know the detail of how or why it works. Again, in contrast to this approach, our work has been more on the explanatory 'contingency' side than the descriptive 'universal' side, the guiding belief being that once we know why and how something works in one organization we can avoid the trap of (invariably) failed replication in another and begin to construct specific, targeted interventions and home-grown, context-specific solutions that stand a more reasonable chance of working.

A search for variables rather than processes

Third, the customary preference for single (and simple) cause–effect 'variable' explanations for the quality differences ('variance theory') rather than systems or process explanations ('process theory')[47] may be another reason why we lack good explanations for why some organizations perform better than others. Over the years, quality research in healthcare and beyond has come to be dominated by a kind of 'menu mentality', which loves to list and label all the key success factors that appear to correlate with quality healthcare (measurements and metrics, care pathways and evidence-based approaches being among the more popular). Our view is that menus like this are of limited value, especially to practitioners, because they:

❐ are mostly self-evident and already well known to all
❐ are usually couched in terms so broad as to be unusable in a practical setting (e.g. the 'leadership factor', 'team-working')
❐ only tell you about the list of dishes on offer but provide little sense of how they taste or are best combined for a successful meal
❐ make the cardinal error of assuming that the 'keys' to quality lie in individual factors or variables rather than, as we shall be proposing, the process and system interactions between them; that is to say, the chemistry or mix, the 'between-ness', and the flows and connections rather than specific factors themselves.

Conceptually, the root of the problem is that menus are fixed and static, whereas what we should be investigating (and will do so in what follows) are the interactions and dynamics over time, the positive 'thermals' or virtuous circles that may take an organization's improvement efforts skywards, or the negative downdraughts and vicious circles that take them downwards to mediocrity and disappointment. We believe there is an urgent need to find out how these system or constellation effects (what Pettigrew *et al.*[48] call 'complementarities') work, but unfortunately no amount of knowledge about the role of individual factors is likely to help in this regard. Pettigrew *et al.* define the task thus:

> Focusing on interaction moves away from the variables paradigm toward a form of holistic explanation. The intellectual task is to examine how and why constellations of forces shape the character of change processes rather than 'fixed entities' with variable qualities.

Such is the central task of this book, one that will require a major shift in language and perspective that frees us up to think and talk about quality in terms of:

❐ dynamics rather than variables (including situational dynamics) – Siggelkow's elegant phrase for this is trying 'to unravel the underlying dynamics of phenomena that play out over time'[49]
❐ an ongoing, emergent process (improv*ing* as opposed to improve*ment*, develop*ing* as opposed to develop*ment*), what Weick[50] once referred to as 'the innocent little i-n-g' that makes process research what it is
❐ bottom-up, exploratory learning and inquiry rather than the top-down implementation of a program or plan
❐ growth rather than structure.

These features are strongly in evidence in the work of the 'new OD' (organization development) theorists, which draws on a number of convergent intellectual streams such as sequence theory, spiral dynamics, generative theory, and action inquiry.[51–53] They may also be found in the work of a growing number of organization theorists who have been petitioning for a shift in organization and management theory (OMT) from 'variance' or 'variables' theory to 'process theory'.

One such theorist in the healthcare domain is Ann Langley, who describes in the following extract[54] what this is likely to involve, conveniently offering at the same time a near-perfect description of the way we went about the research for this book:

> Process research is concerned with understanding how things evolve over time and why they evolve in this way, and process data therefore consist largely of stories about what happened and who did what when – that is, events, activities, and choices ordered over time . . . Whereas variance theories provide explanations for phenomena in terms of relationships among dependent and independent *variables* (e.g. more of X and more of Y produce more of Z), process theories provide explanations in terms of the sequence of *events* leading to an outcome (e.g. do A and then B to get C). Temporal ordering and probabilistic interaction between entities are important here. Understanding patterns in *events* is thus key to developing 'process theory'.

The problem, as ever, is that this is all so much easier said than done. Although well-established methods do exist for identifying and measuring cause–effect relationships of the traditional kind, this is certainly not the case with 'systems' and process models. Having surveyed what little there was actually on offer we found ourselves with no option but to recognize that if we wanted to move from a 'variables' to a 'process' model of change and improvement, then we would have to develop our own, the main fruits of this endeavour being the network mapping technique described and applied to our cases in Chapter 10.

Macro- or micro-system research (but rarely both together)

Fourth, traditional QI research takes either a macro- or micro-system focus, but rarely (if ever) both together. We have already drawn attention to the strength (but also the weakness) of healthcare research at the macro-system level (Leatherman and Sutherland's often-cited quality of care chartbook[55] being a good example of one that is strong on descriptive statistics but characteristically weak on explanations). However, thanks to the pioneering micro-systems work of Dartmouth-Hitchcock researchers in the US over the past five years we now have considerable strength at the front-line caregiving level,[56–58] significant because if there had been any knowledge lacuna up to that point it would have been here. Unfortunately, while we also have a strong affinity for this micro-system locus of attention, it does not help resolve the original problem of the single-level focus; indeed, all that has happened is that the level in question has shifted from the macro to the micro.

In responding to this issue – and, in our view, shortcoming – of single-level explanations, we have been greatly influenced by the work of House *et al.*,[59] who have led us to the hypothesis that 'quality' is a *multi-level phenomenon* that requires a simultaneous 'both-and', multi-level analytical focus, what they describe as a 'meso' paradigm or approach. The 'key' to understanding, they propose, lies not in any one level of the organization, be it the macro or micro (strategic or operational), but in the various and complex ways the different levels combine (or not) and interact with each other:

> Meso research and theory are aimed at synthesizing micro and macro organizational processes. A synthesis is a co-ordination of elements into an integral whole – a new entity distinctly different from its parts . . . It is our argument that micro and macro processes cannot be treated separately and then added up to understand behavior in organizations

Drawing on their ideas, we shall describe how we developed and then applied a similar 'meso paradigm for quality' to our own organizational case studies, resisting the temptation to choose between studying quality at the macro *or* the micro level, and trying instead to look at both. What we could not have anticipated was just how different the perspectives, rationales and explanations for their success of staff working at these two levels would turn out to be. Not only this, but also how the success of these organizations is closely bound up in the multi-level interactions and interdependencies between these two levels.

A focus on clinical and technical factors and processes to the exclusion of human and organizational processes

Finally, a point already alluded to and perhaps the biggest and most significant difference between our work and others, is that it moves the spotlight from the 'science' of improvement (the systematic 'left brain' aspects) to the 'sociology' of improvement (the messy 'right brain' human or people aspects). In other words, we see quality as not just a method, technique, discipline or skill, but as a human and organizational accomplishment, something that is constructed by people in their everyday actions and interactions with and for each other – a social process. In our view this is a paradigm shift in the way we think about quality that uncovers themes and issues that have lain undiscovered because of researchers looking elsewhere.

The journeys to quality described in Chapters 2 to 8 of this book do indeed clearly demonstrate that 'quality' and QI is a human and organizational – not just a technical or mechanical systems – phenomenon. If, therefore, we are to truly understand why there is a 45% 'defect rate' in healthcare[9] and what needs to be done to reduce or eliminate it, then we have no choice but to look to the myriad of human and organizational causes that lie behind it (*see* Figure 1.1).

To date, the hard left-brain technical and operating systems factors have received by far the greatest attention in quality research, but what our research has revealed is how important the softer right-brain organizational, cultural and human factors are in improvement efforts – issues such as identity, aesthetics, politics, leadership, value systems, organizational 'slack', and learning, none of which have received anything like the same amount of attention. We argue that future research, policy and practice need to address the sociology of improvement in equal measure to the science and technique of improvement, or at least expand the discipline of improvement to include these critical organizational and human processes. Practitioners especially should refer to the wonderful example set by Luther Midelfort hospital (*see* Chapter 6) in achieving the perfect balance between the socio and the technical, and also by San Diego Children's Hospital (*see* Chapter 2). Modern 'Lean production' practitioners should also take note, as did Luther, that Lean without the socio may improve system performance and efficiency but not necessarily service quality or the patient experience.

Study methods and approach

An orientation to our journey

We could have gone out seeking answers to the many challenges posed by this research armed with hypotheses to test, and there is an abundance of these in the TQM and CQI literatures, but we decided instead to start with something else: the practice rather than the research. We wanted to find out what people are doing (and not doing) in the QI arena, and the reasons they give for doing or nor doing it; that is to say, the rationales that are driving their policies and practices.

This book is based, therefore, on inductive, grounded (i.e. ground-up; cf. Glaser and Strauss[60]) research, where theory and empirical development unfold together and feed each other, ending with some clear hypotheses about how you implement, spread and sustain quality rather than beginning with them. The broad goal of this kind of research is a *richness* of understanding, which in terms of preparation calls for a 'head full of theories'[61] and what Paul Schulman (cited by Weick[61]) calls 'conceptual slack': a diverse set of theories, models and causal assumptions that serve as a hedge against premature closure, while at the same time allowing the mind to remain open to all kinds of explanatory possibilities (what designers call 'fluidity'). The word 'open' is important because what we are talking about here is going into organizations with an open – as opposed to an empty – mind.

In our case we wanted to try to understand at a deep level the kind of processes that enable healthcare organizations to achieve QI; what was it that had taken them to the heights of excellence (as perceived by their patients and peers and supported by clinical and performance data), and had then enabled them to remain there for what, in most of our cases, had been a considerable period of time?

But where to look for these? As Stephen Barley noted some years ago,[62] one does not always go to the academics to find the new and emerging theories, but to the practitioners. Contrary to popular belief, academic theory often follows rather than leads practice theory. Accordingly, the task we set ourselves was to go and find out what the lead practice theories were, particularly among the frontline innovators in the quality arena where they would most likely be found. That was our quest. So where did we go and what did we end up actually doing?

Fieldwork

In-depth fieldwork was carried out initially in nine healthcare organizations: five in the US and four in Europe (*see* Table 1.1). These organizations were selected on the basis of

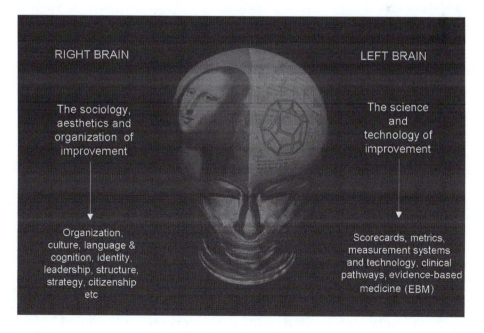

FIGURE 1.1 A human as well as a technical challenge

peer recommendations from international experts working in the improvement field in the UK and US, and from surveys of various kinds of awards and recognitions that these organizations had received for outstanding performance in the quality arena. Following site selection, high-performing micro-systems were chosen on the basis of soundings taken from a variety of internal staff at different levels of each organization. We were thereby able to obtain the view downwards from the top team and upwards from a micro-system, which enabled us to explore the interrelationships and dynamic interplay between them and to distinguish the roles each level was playing in the overall improvement effort.

The fieldwork[63,64] took place intensively over an 18-month period, involving approximately 15 people days' work in each organization and carried out by two or three researchers. We used intensive qualitative methods, including face-to-face interviews and informal discussions (all tape-recorded and transcribed), observation of staff meetings and day-to-day clinical practice, and collection of organizational documents as well as any published external reports for all the selected macro- and micro-systems.

Table 1.1 Case study sites: selected macro- and micro-systems with meta-narratives

MACRO-SYSTEM	MICRO-SYSTEM	META-NARRATIVE/KEY THEME
United Kingdom		
Royal Devon and Exeter	Orthopedics center	Organizational identity
Peterborough	Radiology department	Empowerment
King's College	Breast cancer clinic	Organizational citizenship
United States		
Children's Hospital of San Diego, California	Allergy and immunology clinic	Mindfulness and sensemaking
Cedars-Sinai, California	Emergency department	Organizational learning
Luther-Midelfort Mayo, Wisconsin	Critical care unit	Socio-technical systems
Albany Medical Center, New York	AIDS treatment center	Social movements and mobilization
SSM Health Care, Missouri	Intensive care unit, St Joseph's Hospital	Spiritual capital
The Netherlands		
Reinier de Graff, Delft	Varicose surgery	Collective leadership

We also show in the third column of Table 1.1 how it was possible in each case to identify a dominant theme – what we call here and elsewhere[65] the meta-narrative – something that stood out from other factors, that gave each organization's approach to QI its uniqueness and distinctiveness, and to which other factors (many of them overlapping between the cases) seemed to connect, root and branch (related approaches to analyzing complex sets of qualitative data in this way include meta-ethnography[66–68]). On the other hand, in talking about meta-narratives it is important to emphasize from the outset that we are referring to a higher level of abstraction, or superordinate theme in the narrative, and in no way seeking to undermine or contradict the multi-factorial nature of improvement systems and processes described earlier. As we have said, the meta-theme is what stood out from other processes in each of the stories, but this is not to say that all of these other themes and issues did not exist.

As always, the writer Rudyard Kipling acted as our guide and mentor for the research journey, providing in his poem a high-level checklist of the different kinds of research questions that needed to be covered (*see* Box 1.1):

BOX 1.1 Research questions

'I have six honest serving men,
They taught me all I knew,
Their names are WHAT and WHY
And WHEN
And HOW and WHERE and WHO.'

The WHAT in this case being 'thick description', observation and collection of 'quality' stories (*see* the 'richness' issue, described above);

The WHY being the interpretive, sensemaking element (*see* explanatory emphasis also discussed above);

The WHEN being the task of reconstructing the chronology of issues and events with the players themselves;

The HOW being the interactions, dynamics and processes involved in the evolution and development of the quality journey;

The WHERE being the contextual element, near (organizational) and distant (the healthcare sector);

The WHO being the actors and how they viewed things from the position of participant.

Drawing on the data collected through all of these methods, we then prepared draft case study narratives,[69] piecing together the various accounts of each individual organization's journey to quality. These original full-length drafts were then fed back to key informants in the participating organizations, where possible accompanied by presentations of the key findings to a wider audience for additional feedback, discussion and comment. In-depth case studies of quality programs of this nature are rare enough in healthcare research,[70] but feeding them back (not only for validation purposes but also in an 'action' context for stimulating further reflection and discussion) is, we believe, relatively unheard of in quality research. In the end, for reasons of length and not being able to do full justice to all the material we had gathered, we were compelled to exclude two of the cases from this book (King's and SSM Healthcare). Readers can be assured that many of the themes and issues revealed in these two cases will surface here in various forms and guises. Again for reasons of length, the original full-length versions of the remaining seven case studies have also had to be shortened considerably for this book.

The metaphorical journey-based narrative approach[71] used in this research provides a unique perspective on what leading healthcare organizations on both sides of the Atlantic were able to achieve and the various processes associated with their successful QI efforts, but also a temporal perspective on how sustained improvement was accomplished and how failures and 'bumps in the road' led to alternative directions and solutions. As already stated, although research has provided an abundance of data on key success factors in QI efforts, very little was previously known about how these combine and interact with each other in the improvement process over time.

Analysis

Before diving headlong into the first of the seven case studies we would like to give the reader both a preview and an overview of the places to be visited and the kind of issues and key themes encountered (i.e. the meta-narratives of each case).

'Mindfulness', a concept that figures prominently in the work of organization theorist and social psychologist Karl Weick, holds that quality or excellence is essentially a human accomplishment – an individual or group mindset characterized by a constant and intense awareness or alertness to the prevailing situation – and draws attention to the importance of the social, social-psychological and organizational dimensions of QI efforts. This notion of quality as a social construction draws attention to the meanings, values and beliefs that people bring to the organization care setting, summed up in Weick's concept of sensemaking. The story in Chapter 2 of one organization, San Diego Children's Hospital in California, focuses on a micro-system (the Allergy and Immunology Clinic) to illustrate the practice of mindfulness and sensemaking within the context of the methodology laid down from the top for the practice of quality: clinical care pathways.

The central thesis of Chapter 3 is that QI efforts need to address the issue of identity because it is a source of (a) standards and excellence (b) pride and commitment, and (c) sustained quality of care. The stories and tales we were told by those we met and interviewed at the Royal Devon and Exeter NHS Foundation Trust led us to speculate throughout this chapter about the importance of 'identity' in relation to sustained quality of healthcare: in particular, the influence of corporate identity, professional identity and personal identity, and how these may impact on quality and service improvement efforts. The micro-system under study in Exeter is the Princess Elizabeth Orthopaedics Centre.

The story of QI at Cedars-Sinai Medical Center in Los Angeles (Chapter 4) stretches over two decades, representing a journey of accumulated organizational learning, change, and customization of quality approaches, methods and tools. This chapter recounts the journey at both the executive level of the medical center as a whole (macro-system) and within a clinical unit (micro-system) with notable achievements in QI, the emergency department. More important than the particular QI approaches and tools that Cedars-Sinai has learned, however, are the processes by which this accumulated 'bricolage' of quality has been constructed and the glue or mortar the institution has used to bind these elements into a coherent path of sustained improvement. Three elements crucial to the organization's journey in this regard include: (a) a *learning culture* rooted in the particular history and identity of the institution, (b) a *learning infrastructure* for sharing knowledge and bringing focus to improvement activities, and (c) *communities of learning* that engage the energy and commitment of individuals toward a quality agenda.

Following the trend in leadership writing over the past 10 years or so, but one that with certain exceptions has remained stubbornly absent from healthcare research until now, Chapter 5 proposes a view of leadership that is more depersonalized, de-individualized, more collective and systems-based than the one that is normally associated with the organization and quality literatures. Veinal surgery within the Reinier de Graaf Groep in the Netherlands is the micro-system which forms the setting for this chapter.

The goal of Chapter 6 is to understand how the Luther Midelfort Mayo Health System in Eau Claire, Wisconsin – a healthcare organization serving a relatively small, rural community – has become a nationally recognized leader in sustained QI. The case analysis points to the character of Luther Midelfort as a smartly designed sociotechnical system. The institution as a whole exhibits a great deal of attention and insight into both the social aspects of the organization (its culture, the commitments and motivations of staff, the informal patterns of relationships among groups) and the technical aspects of work systems (the transformation of effort and resources into products and services, the transfer of information, and the use of technologies). The chapter explores the ways in which senior management at the macro-level and the leadership of the critical care unit at the micro-level of the organization manage the interaction between these systems to achieve a synergy that furthers the organization's goals, particularly in relation to quality of care.

Chapter 7 and the recent literature on 'empowerment' provide strong evidence for the need to adopt a wider conception of the term than has been the case up until now, one that embraces not only the usual power and control issues, but also issues of organizational style, relationships, motivation and culture. We use the broader, deeper sense of the term here, one that resonates with an organic view of empowerment and that moves away from the tired literature and management-speak on this concept. Here we examine the impact empowerment as a process and a relationship has for employees, and its consequences for organizational creativity, flexibility, learning and effectiveness. The radiology department at Peterborough forms the micro-system for this chapter.

Unlike most of our chapters, which give fairly equal weight to analysis of the macro-system and the micro-system, our focus in Chapter 8 (our final case study) is primarily on the micro-system: the AIDS Treatment Center (ATC) of the Albany Medical Center (the macro-system). This is because the factors that have led to its high performance are attributable as much to the internal characteristics of the micro-system and the unique features of AIDS care in the US as to the influences of the larger medical center of which it is a part. Given ATC's principal identity as a clinic serving HIV/AIDS patients, it is not surprising that the organization has been strongly influenced by the AIDS movement, one of the most successful movements in American health during the past three decades and closely associated with wider movements for gay rights and patient rights. For example, staff exhibit the hope, caring and idealism that is associated with commitment-based movements, whose goals or cause focus on improving society. This chapter therefore examines sustained QI from a social movement and mobilization perspective.

Looking back over the journey

Journey completed, the final thing that needed to be done was for us to find a suitable high point on the landscape from which to look down and back on the places we had visited, and allow us to gain an overall sense of what we had seen and experienced. Siggelkow describes this as 'cutting through' and 'rising above' the idiosyncratic case and 'unearthing similarities across cases', and argues that this is essential if case studies are to be more than interesting vignettes and be capable of making a bigger and wider contribution to theory and practice[49] (see also Eisenhardt and Graebner[72]).

At ground level our eyes had naturally been drawn to the variety and detail in the organizational landscape, but from higher ground we could at last let our eyes run over and between all of the sites, and ponder whether there were commonalities we may have missed. The more we compared the stories and the more we tried to look above and beyond the details, the more common contours and features we began to see. Another way to represent this idea would be to say that just as the skyline of every city is never the same, so it was the case here with our different organizations, although this is not to say that there are not common issues and challenges that any city – or QI process – will face as it seeks to put the foundations in place, begin construction, and then start to grow and thrive.

We shall leave the details of this notion – what is known in social science as the 'universal but variable thesis' – to a later chapter (Chapter 9). However, we believe it may be worth alerting readers in advance to the core challenges we found, so that they can begin to look out for them as they read the case studies, and be able to appreciate the varied and infinite ways in which people in the different organizations sought to address and manage them.

Drawing generalizations from case study research is always an issue, but this notion of 'common challenges, diverse solutions' has hopefully enabled us to do this without losing the uniqueness and individuality of each organization's approach to quality excellence. Here, though, the rationale for doing this is more of a practical than a conceptual one: we firmly believe that the reason why these organizations have been able to achieve, and then sustain, high levels of care is that they have recognized and been extremely successful in addressing the challenges in question, on an ongoing basis and in ways that have been appropriate to the local contexts in which they have found themselves. In short, the challenges we have identified, or rather, the way that the organizations have taken up these challenges, provide important insights into why these particular healthcare organizations have been successful in the quality arena.

Here are the six common challenges we identified from across the nine in-depth case studies:

- structural (organizing, planning and co-ordinating quality efforts)
- political (addressing and dealing with the politics of change surrounding any QI effort)
- cultural (giving 'quality' a shared, collective meaning, value and significance within the organization)
- educational (creating a learning process that supports improvement)
- emotional (engaging and mobilizing people by linking QI efforts to inner sentiments and deeper commitments and beliefs)
- physical and technological (the designing of physical systems and technological infrastructure that supports and sustains quality efforts).

Building on this framework in Chapter 9, and at this point with our sights set firmly on practice and the needs of the practitioner, we draw on the stories from the seven case study organizations included here to illustrate the array of approaches and means of addressing them as they were described to us. This takes the form of a checklist, map or guide that readers can use to identify where the organizational gaps in their local improvement efforts may lie and what they may need to do to address them.

In chapter 10, which takes the form of an advanced guide for theorists and the more venturesome and intrepid practitioners, we introduce a novel methodology that utilizes formal network analysis techniques for examining and visualizing the particular constituent processes and the ways they are inter-related. These 'process mappings' provide a way to make useful comparisons across organizational contexts in order to generate insights into organizing for quality in healthcare.

Finally, one of our hopes for future improvement journeys is that practitioners and researchers, currently, and all too often, strangers to each other – will come much closer together and share their knowledge, learning and experience, in so doing avoiding some of the mistakes we so obviously made. To this end Chapter 11 looks at some of the implications of our work for both of them and the roles they will need to play if it is to be a fruitful joint endeavour.

2

The art, the science, and the sociology of improvement: San Diego Children's Hospital

ORIGINAL CASE STUDY RESEARCHED BY PAUL BATE AND PETER MENDEL; NARRATIVE
PREPARED BY PAUL BATE

One can begin the story of an organization's 'journey to quality' almost anywhere. This particular story begins with the appointment of Blair L Sadler to the post of president and chief executive at San Diego Children's Hospital (*see* Box 2.1) in 1980 and ends in 2002 when the hospital received the prestigious Ernest A Codman Award in recognition of its achievements in healthcare quality outcomes. This national Joint Commission award recognizes 'exemplary performance', and the hospital (which we shall refer to as 'Children's') was the first children's hospital in the US ever to receive it. Sadler himself has described the first half of this period as 'a decade of surviving', and the second as a 'decade of thriving'.

The main focus of this case study is on the second decade, because it offers a good fit with our inclusion criterion of 'sustained quality,' showing both empirically and through the words and perceptions of those involved that the improvement path wound consistently upward during this period, marking what may go down in the organization's history as its golden age of quality.

Organization stories like these rarely have fairy-tale endings, however. From 2002 the hospital entered a more turbulent period in its life, and what Sadler originally predicted would be a 'decade of soaring' became more a case of stalling. The hospital had to take a breath. As a result of financial problems, staff and budgets for further improvement work were cut, and attention switched from concerns about quality (improvement) to those of quantity (revenue).

This case study will not go into these recent troubles in any detail, nor for that matter the deeply impressive turnaround and recovery from them under Sadler's stewardship in the two years leading up to his retirement in 2006. This is simply because we have little interview or factual data about the period or issues in question beyond hearsay and anecdote. However, we return to this at the end of the case study to speculate on how fragile quality efforts can be within this kind of challenging context, and what future stories are likely to get told about Children's.

BOX 2.1 Case profile: Children's Hospital and Health Center of San Diego

CASE PROFILE

Type of Organization:	A non-profit, integrated pediatric health care system comprising the main campus hospital in Kearny Mesa and a number of neighborhood centers offering primary care and specialized services.
Focal Micro-System:	Allergy and immunology (Asthma) clinic
Size:	The San Diego region's only designated pediatric trauma center, including 225 beds. It provides 75% of all inpatient pediatric care in San Diego County and treats 78% of all hospitalized poor Californian children under the age of 5.
Location:	San Diego, California, the second largest city on the US west coast, with substantial levels of uninsurance, immigration, and ethnic diversity (e.g. over 50 languages spoken in San Diego schools).
Country:	United States
Awards and Recognitions:	First pediatric hospital to win the Joint Commission's (JCAHO) Ernest A Codman Award for quality achievement (2002); ranked 7th in *Child Magazine*'s US Top Ten Children's Hospital survey (2001); voted 1 of 15 hospitals with a 'heart' by *Modern Maturity Magazine* – the only pediatric hospital selected.

KEY CONCEPTS

Mindfulness: a heightened state of involvement and wakefulness or being in the present. A mindset associated with organizational cultures having a preoccupation with failure, reluctance to simplify issues, sensitivity to operations, commitment to resilience, and deference to expertise. Characteristic of 'high reliability organizations'.

Entrainment: the adjustment of behaviors at one level of organization to be in timing or tune with events at another. A key process linking macro- and micro-systems and the *meso*-level interactions between them that support the improvement effort.

The science of improvement: 'standardizing to excellence'

The 'science of improvement' at Children's is synonymous with the Center for Child Health Outcomes and Clinical Innovation and with nephrologist Dr Paul Kurtin, its director since its establishment in 1996. Under his leadership, the Center has developed a strongly evidence- and measures-based approach to quality improvement.

Interestingly, the story behind the birth of the Center is not only about quality for its own sake, but also about quality and quality measurement being good *business* sense. Sadler describes the 'business case for quality' that he put to his board in the mid-1990s and which ultimately secured the funding for the new Center:

> Our cornerstone belief was that hospitals that commit to providing *optimal experiences* for their patients, families and staff through relentless and measurable quality improvement will significantly differentiate themselves from their competitors ... [The defining moment] was when I became convinced, and we were able to convince the board, that we were at financial risk and market risk if we were unable to *prove* our qualities and our outcomes.

Thus, *measurable* quality improvement was expected to give Children's a strong competitive edge and a unique niche in the market, enabling it to deliver its plans for growth and expansion and increased market share (as indeed it did – market share went from 48% to 75%). This had particular appeal to the board, who at the time were being seriously courted for a merger by a bigger hospital.

The Center replaced a quality department that formerly collected, analyzed and reported data needed to meet Children's external regulatory responsibilities. The new Center consisted of a group of change and improvement professionals, together with some internal clinical staff, whose task was not only to measure quality and outcomes but also to facilitate and enable improvement efforts across the whole organization. This 'Faculty of Improvement' sought to bring about a change of emphasis from quality assurance to quality improvement, and to move 'quality' out of the organizational margins and into a core organizational strategy and discipline.

Having Kurtin as head of the Center was crucial, because he both brought a good deal of knowledge about service improvement and was a highly respected clinician in his own right who, as described later, could engage physicians on their own terms. Kurtin himself takes up the story:

> I came to San Diego with the *science of improvement and measurement*. We documented variation in care throughout the organization; for example we documented variation between providers in caring for children with asthma, we documented variation in individual providers over time. [We found] that we don't treat asthma the same way two days in a row. And we asked: Is that the way it should be? And so we not only documented variation, we also documented not following national guidelines and explained how everybody has problems with national guidelines. And then I tried to bring in the idea of systems thinking and how complex medicine is and how a doctor trying to do it alone isn't going to work. So, after documenting variations, we worked with the medical staff to determine what [an ideal] treatment plan or 'pathway' would be, and the first one was asthma.

Thus began Kurtin's integrated care pathways (ICPs), by now a well-trodden path in healthcare but not so much the case then. The aim of the 'clinical care pathway' (as it is commonly called at Children's) is to stamp out the tremendous variation that exists in practice, much as car factories wipe out variation on the production line, standardizing treatment according to the state-of-the-art 'gold standards' of care. In its definition of care pathways, Children's put the emphasis on it being 'a *process* of care, designed to increase the likelihood of positive outcomes, based upon the effective and efficient use of resources'. It was framed in terms of a *'promise'* that the clinical pathway would ensure 'every child will receive optimal care: . . . effective, efficient, safe, timely, equitable, and patient-centered,' thereby aligning with the wider organizational vision. The stated overarching *aims* of the pathway program were to 'decrease unnecessary variation in care, improve resource efficiency, decrease the gap between knowledge and practice, establish a collaborative, systems approach to care delivery, and assure patient safety'.

Having chosen the arena of engagement (asthma) and the weapons (integrated care pathways), the next stage involved what Kurtin describes as 'putting on the flak jacket' and going into battle. Asthma had been chosen for a number of reasons, not least because there were one or two influential opinion leaders within the clinical department who were prepared to give it a try and would champion the cause. This notion of finding and using clinical champions – the innovators on the front edge of the Rogers innovation curve,[1] and the peer-to-peer leaders according to the principle of 'homophily'[2] – was to become an important part of Children's overall change methodology (as with so many of the cases in this study). Back to Sadler:

> We basically said find physician champions, and that was the key thing . . . someone who was more of a risk-taker . . . who was intellectually curious about and open to change, had credibility, and had a connection with a relatively large number of patients at a relatively high amount of resource utilization. So, if successful, it was going to create a ripple effect.

Even with such 'champions' there was a great sense of reluctance and resistance from clinicians early on, with many of them couching their apprehensions in substantive criticisms of care pathways as being 'cookbook medicine' and back-door clinical de-skilling. Kurtin replays the kind of heated conversations that took place during this time:

> 'I've been practising pediatrics for 25 years and I don't need a pathway to manage asthma.' I would say, 'I'm sure you're right, and I am sure you are very good at it, but tell me how your kids do, what are your outcomes?' No doctor knows their outcomes. So I would say, 'Let me show you ours, the 400 kids on the pathway and how they are doing. These are kids on the pathway and these are kids off the pathway.' And we have quality, length of stay, cost, readmission rates, transfers to higher level of care, any outcome anybody could think of. 'Why don't we compare your results to these?' 'Oh yes, but my patients are sicker.' 'Oh well, we took that into account, we've severity adjusted everything.' I tried to have every question answered before they asked it, and the data was overwhelming.

Kurtin was able to use the data as 'ammunition' that allowed him to say, 'This is sub-standard care; 50% of patients receiving the appropriate care isn't good enough. There's a shortfall in quality here and I can prove it.' Nevertheless, it was only by dint of his being a clinician that he was able to stand up in front of his peers and be able to say such things and get away with it. As one of his senior managers, a non-clinician in the Center, put it:

> How Dr Kurtin approached it is one very effective way to engage, it's very much on a peer-to-peer basis. I don't think that I could walk into a room of general surgeons and get them to agree on how to all do an appendectomy the same way like Dr Kurtin or another peer could.

Kurtin emphasizes that the data were never intended to be confrontational but motivational:

> I mean, the nurses for the first time had proof that they were taking good care of kids . . . There is a lot of pride in feeling good about saying here is the national average, here's us. Give me some names, oh, Boston Children's, here's their data, here's us. Cincinnati Children's, here's their data, here's us. We beat everybody.

Patients on the asthma pathway were found to have improved quality of care on all sorts of measures. Length of stay was reduced from 4.4 days to 2.2 days in the first year and later to 1.7 days, with similar year-on-year improvements on numerous other key indicators (e.g. oxygen use, steroid use, readmission rates) that were demonstrably sustained over the first seven years.

The pathways made good clinical sense but proved good financial sense, too, giving Sadler a lever for gaining the support of wider sponsors and stakeholders. The data showed that pathways dramatically reduced variation in the cost of care per child, and enabled a far larger proportion to be cared for at lower cost. For example, the direct cost per child treated dropped from $2,518 before the asthma pathway program to $449 afterwards – a saving of over 82%.

The early successes in asthma made it much easier when the time came to spread pathways to other parts of the hospital: 'We moved from forcing or pushing people to do pathways to their calling us' (Center member). Push became pull; the pathways program gathered pace, spread and momentum, resulting by 2003 in more than 60 pathways covering most of pediatrics, such as urology, medicine, neonatology, intensive care, and hematology/oncology, thus including an estimated 40% of all patients.

A 'watershed decision' that changed the procedure whereby the clinician had to positively opt to put a patient on a pathway to one where pathways became the default method of care unless the clinician specifically ruled that they should not, proved another crucial factor in accelerating the spread of the pathways program organization-wide. This was about two years into the program and all the more significant because it was a clinician – the chairman of the pediatrics department – who proposed it. As Sadler states:

> And then overnight we went from 15%, 20% compliance to 80%. And then after that, it just steadily moved on. And they've kept learning from the technology that took nine months to a pathway and now takes 30 days, and how to make it easier for the physician to learn and try and do and not be threatened.

The graph in Figure 2.1, described by Sadler as a 'tipping point', shows just how powerful this intervention was, moving the organization from an initial 20% adherence to pathways before they became the 'default' method of care, to 92% adherence by 2002.

The sociology of improvement

It would be easy to credit all this success, as indeed many in Children's hierarchy do, to the 'appliance of science': targets, data, measurement and the pathways methodology

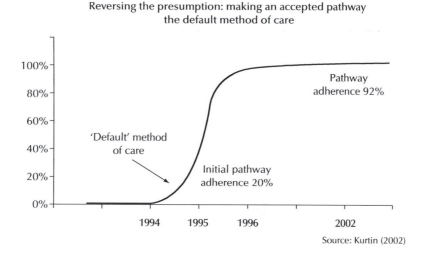

FIGURE 2.1 Reaching the tipping point: a transformational moment

itself (the left brain issues described in Chapter 1). While it is undeniably the case that the science of improvement, and pathways in particular, has made an enormous contribution, it does not explain the variation in the effect of pathways that has been observed between this and other organizations: why have the results been so dramatic at Children's while experience elsewhere with pathways has been more mixed?

For a more complete picture of causation, we need to shift our attention from *what* was done to *how* it was done, to the process of implementation and development itself, and the ways in which the 'people', process and change management issues were addressed. Our contention is that what really made Children's special was the maturity, professionalism, knowledge and skill with which the change leaders and key staff managed the whole 'sociology of implementation' within the organization. This takes us back to an earlier assertion that the implementation of pathways is a *human* accomplishment. In other words, the skills, science and technology around pathways may be one thing, but getting the understandings, agreement, buy-in and commitment to them (as opposed to simple compliance) is quite another.

Pathways at Children's represented a new and largely unfamiliar approach to quality, and had to be defined and made sense of from scratch, and then translated into a whole set of new practices. Thus, the methodology of pathways was only one part – albeit an important part – of a much bigger cultural change around the 'mindset' and definition of quality.

Although leaders at many levels of Children's have contributed to this sensemaking and change-making process,[3,4] a key group in this regard has been the improvement leaders who make up the core of the Center and who have been working at the coalface of the change endeavour since pathways began more than 10 years ago (managers, researchers and redesign facilitators, educators, and so on). It is they who must take a lot of the credit for the impact and success of the quality program at the hospital. Especially in light of the criticism of clinical pathways as the 'McDonaldization' of healthcare and 'Julia Child cookbook medicine' from some of the most influential gurus in healthcare improvement,[5] it is all the more significant that the pathways facilitators at Children's were able to end up with a strong consensus behind their program.

So how did they do it? Interviews with members of the Center revealed an acute awareness of the sociological, human dimension of change, and the kind of change model and philosophy that would be needed to address it: a model that engendered trust, openness, participation and inclusion, ownership, personal responsibility, peer-to-peer leadership and mutual learning.

The quotes from the interviews that follow reveal their impressive grasp of organization development (OD), total quality management (TQM) and continuous quality improvement (CQI) theory, procedures and skills, as well as a clarity about the kind of 'change rules' needed to get people on board: 'the whole business of building buy-in' as one of their number described it. By integrating the pathways philosophy (the what) with wider TQM and CQI philosophies (the how), the Center members were able to create a model for improvement that was stronger than any of these elements alone. A senior Center member summed it up when she said that the pathway is not about 'one way' but rather a continuous improvement process that involves everything from measures and targets to human and organizational change processes:

> Care pathways and TQM, they're not separate. They're absolutely integrated. How we do the pathway, it's all basically PDSA [plan-do-study-act]. You know, continuous cycles, PDSA. And the people on the teams know that, too. *I think we have created a new way*

of doing the pathways that makes it different from other hospitals. I think absolutely that's why we had the buy in and didn't do the conventional cookbook care pathway.

Using the Center members' own words we can begin to disentangle the various strands of their model of change, as follows.

Getting people's attention, and then their intention

We raised the organizational noise factor around improvement with pathways . . . there was a lot of chatter and discussion . . . just getting a dialogue helped. (Center member 1)

Actually we don't sit down, we go up and stand on the unit and just talk because these people are busy . . . maybe we'll walk up to someone who's got a new patient who's just come in and we'll say, 'Did you know we can do the pathways?' and hand them data and literature and stuff. (Center member 2)

Correct 'framing' of pathways and quality improvement

You find . . . what's in it for them. Is it going to make their day easier, is it going to be easy to do, is it the right thing to do, and can I prove that? . . . It's whatever you can find to be the hook. It's bargaining. It's salesmanship. I guess I should sell cars, huh? (Center member 2)

If you improve quality you reduce cost. But when we go into pathways work, we don't say that we're going to reduce the cost to this diagnosis by 15 or 80 or whatever percent. It's, 'We're going to create a pathway that's based on quality.' I think if we had gone at it from a cost standpoint overtly from the beginning physicians really would not have been buying into that, because [they] want to provide quality care. (Center member 3)

Using physician and nursing leaders: pathways champions

In addition to Kurtin, as mentioned earlier, and senior colleagues in the Center, there was also a wider network of clinical leaders at the next level down (some formal, others informal) who ended up playing a key role in championing pathways within their own departments:

If I need to get something done and I need a reasonable surgeon to go talk to, I pick up the phone and I call [Surgeon B] because he understands quality improvement and the value of it and he also has informal influence over all the surgeons and can speak to them in a way they understand . . . the dialogue gets started. (Center member 2)

Inclusive and team-based

In the first part of the pathways, the plan phase . . . we invite everyone who has any stake in the diagnosis, so the first meeting's going to be pretty big. We invite any physician who has admitted more than just a kid or two for that diagnosis, community and hospital, nursing – every department that touches the child. (Center member 4)

It's definitely a team process. And I think it's probably more my job than anyone else on the team to see how people are interacting and how things are going, and making sure that people feel good about doing this. And also that they get credit for it. (Center member 4)

Authorship equals ownership

One pathway we did early on wasn't very successful and the reason . . . was because we didn't take the time to get our doctors on board, to make them really understand all the ins and outs of it. The pathway is the end result, but the real change happens – culture change happens – in the process, because . . . if you're in a pathway group then you take this back to your area and you share it and you talk about it and you bring back your ideas. So you're building 'buy in'. There's a story, I think Dr Kurtin tells it, about a tree house, build your own versus someone builds it for you. Dad built the kid a tree house and the kid wouldn't go in. (Center member 2)

Collaborative not coercive

We say, 'It's okay, if you don't want to do the pathway that's fine, come back here and give us your opinion.' We're very careful not only to approach people that are opinion leaders and want to do the pathway, but maybe some of those who don't. So they can see what the process involves, it's based on the literature, it's based on our data, it's based on their expert opinion. *So it's not really a cookbook, it's their book. So they actually are creating it* . . . the whole idea is this is a learning process and they have to think about it . . . it's educational development. (Center member 1)

Neutral and non-partisan

You need to be completely dispassionate about it . . . I'll have someone call me that night or the next morning [after a meeting] and say, 'I didn't agree with this, this and this, and you can't put that in the pathway.' So then at the next meeting I'll have to take a few minutes to say – and I've only had to do this a few times – 'Dr So and So called me after the meeting and had some discomfort with this, and I think we should discuss it,' and I leave it very open. There's no advocacy on my part and I don't take sides. (Center member 1)

Conducive to learning

What we like to do is fully embed our staff in the learning experience rather than medicine experience . . . so that physicians get excited and want to show you their pathways graphs. (Center member 3)

There is a lot of teaching that goes on here. It's got that kind of atmosphere of learning, so we use pathways not as a tool but a way of building intensive learning. Also on a clinical level we use it for intelligent decision making, not as the cookbook. (Center member 1)

Easy to do and user-friendly

Anything we can do to make it easier for the nurses, the physicians, and anybody up there, is going to make it more successful. I think everybody wants to do the right thing, but when it becomes difficult to do so they may not always do it. (Center member 2)

We made it easy to do the right thing. Our standardized order sets mean that at three in the morning you're not relying on the house staff to remember the right thing to do; it's there. (Center member 4)

Tied together into a single change philosophy, these attributes provided a powerful way of dealing with the sociological dimension of improvement within Children's, yet always aligned and integral to the pathways methodology and the science of improvement itself. Listening to these accounts, it is hard to see how the science could have progressed as far as it did without the 'effective' sociology.

For the last element of the macro-system story at Children's, we move to the right brain side of the improvement equation – the 'art,' aesthetics and environmental dimension. Of the three areas, this is probably the one where Children's has the greatest claim to uniqueness.

The art of improvement: 'so how does it 'feel'?'

No story about San Diego Children's 'journey to quality' would be complete without reference to the vital role played by the arts and the environment in its service improvement philosophy and practices. Ironically, according to Sadler, this was yet another largely unanticipated and unplanned development:

> I think how a lot of this came together was serendipity in that we started out very much on a left brain cognitive path and then, independently of this path, the real transformational experience was when we treated this as a 'sick building', when the architect said, 'We want to ask you each to give 30 seconds thought to this one question: *What do you want this new facility to feel like?*' Well, we hadn't thought about that, we'd thought about the functions, how many beds, how many treatment rooms, not what it was supposed to feel like. So, we all filled in this stuff, and came out with things like how playful, how comforting, and inspiring the San Diego architectural environment should be.

The aesthetic dimension of 'quality' was to open up many different branches of the arts to Children's improvement efforts: art itself, architecture and building design, music, sound, and many more, all of the things that have a direct impact on the patient's *experience* of the care they receive.

Trying to answer the 'How should it feel?' question brought with it the dawning realization that by following the route of science one could come up with the world's most perfect pathway – no delays, no errors, best practice, and so on – and yet the patient's *felt experience* of going down that pathway might still be little better than it had been before.[6] Unlike manufacturing, where the pathways technology was first invented, patients are not cars. They pay heed and are sensitive to the world around them, taking it in through all five senses, defining the experience of the journey in affective as well as cognitive and cold clinical terms. Because of this, 'quality care' can never just be about the typical outcomes described by models like the US Institute of Medicine's (IOM) influential 'wheel of quality'[7,8] – laudable and necessary though they are (*see* Figure 2.2).

What was needed, sitting alongside, was another wheel that included all the subjective, sensory and environmental issues that the IOM model missed out. And because there wasn't one, Children's had to invent it (*see* Figure 2.3).

Just as Kurtin was always the scientific leader at Children's, there was never any doubt who the environmental or aesthetic leader[9] would be, and that was Sadler himself. Looking back, he identifies a number of 'transformational experiences' in his personal and professional life that brought him to this professional philosophy. There was the moment of 'awakening' in 1993 when the architect asked his question, 'What do you want this hospital to feel like?' – not so much the question, but Sadler's realization that he had never thought about it quite that way before. Another was seeing the aesthetic design principles finally bearing fruit on the opening day of the new hospital. Sadler and his colleagues had no idea how people would react, and confidence was not helped by some adverse publicity just before the opening. They need not have worried: it was judged a huge success. Sadler still gets emotional when he talks about the weekend in question:

> What actually happened that weekend – which was the one time we opened for the public – we ran out of all the maps and all the brochures because people had heard by

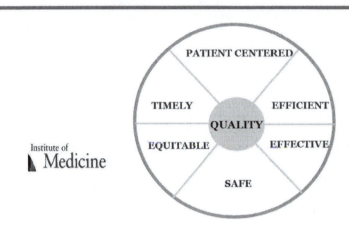

FIGURE 2.2 The components of quality: Institute of Medicine

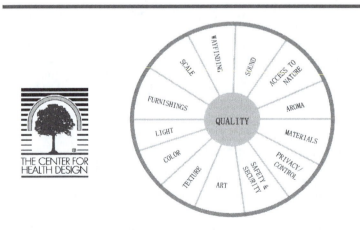

FIGURE 2.3 The components of quality: Children's Hospital and Health Center of San Diego

word of mouth. I will never forget a couple who had just finished a tour on a Sunday afternoon and they said, this is wonderful, why can't any other hospital in San Diego feel like this? And then we moved in, and there was this extraordinary reaction and people loved it. So that was 1993 and from 1993 to about 1998, we systematically went though creating the same 'feeling' in all the other parts.

For Sadler, one of the transformational experiences representing the essence of what the hospital stood for – and for him still stands for – is the story of Carley, a little girl who died from a rare form of cancer after having spent three of her four short years of life at the hospital. After her passing, her parents decided they wanted to create a legacy to Carley and raised the funds to transform three grey drab courtyards into 'magical places' (*see* Figure 2.4).

Opened in November 1999, and paid for entirely out of $450,000 in private donations, Carley's Magical Gardens were designed to provide a soothing, calming, healing space for patients, families and staff (it was awarded the Architectural Design Showcase Citation of Merit by *Healthcare Design* in November 2001). This is just one of a number of soothing spaces that have been fashioned from reclaimed courtyards and parking lots at Children's, creating a unique and special ambience for all who visit. 'Customer' surveys confirm this:

> I loved the architecture and interior designing; it made for a very relaxed and comfortable environment for kids of all ages.

> This is definitely a great hospital; the best bit was the star lights above the nurses' station at night and the mobiles and playthings in the walls of the hospital.

> The children's activity room was wonderful, as was the healing garden.

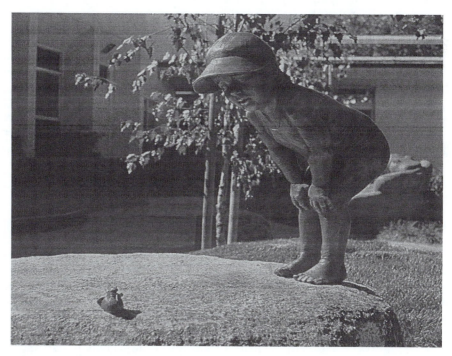

FIGURE 2.4 Statue of Carley Copley

> This is an excellent facility. It is too bad more hospitals have not followed your example.

> The best hospital we have ever seen or been in. Everyone we know says the same. Our five year old cried when we took him home.

Although art, architecture and design are integral to Sadler's 'quality' vision of optimal care and the perfect place, he has never concealed his view that they are also integral to the business side of the hospital. The view is that creating an optimal healing environment 'pays' in terms of competitive advantage and increased market share, improved recruitment and retention, increased philanthropy, higher patient satisfaction, and reduced medical errors, patient falls, infections and drugs use. Stress, anxiety, depression and fatigue levels have also been shown to decrease, thereby improving recovery speed and reducing average lengths of stay.

He is not alone in this view: it was the field of private-sector, profit-oriented service marketing that first put the business case for 'whole experience' service onto the agenda. One such book is a favorite of Sadler's: *The Experience Economy: work is theatre and every business a stage*, by Pine and Gilmore.[10] It describes how companies can gain competitive advantage by providing a 'whole-life' *experience* for the customer. The conclusion from the evidence is simply that aesthetics pay: they attract customers and allow an organization to command additional premiums for its services.

It can be seen that the 'quality' bar is set much higher in the experience-based – as opposed to the solely service-based – organization, and this applies particularly to a hospital or healthcare system. Services put the emphasis on getting the job done, but experiences must do this *and also* provide that something extra that will remain in the memories of the patients and their families for long afterwards. This brings us to the importance of the part played by the micro-system.

The Allergy and Immunology Clinic: the micro-system perspective on quality

Having already heard a good deal about the early breakthrough successes with care pathways in asthma, and the strong support given to them by clinical and nursing staff in that area, we were not at all surprised when that same micro-system, formally known as the Allergy and Immunology Clinic, was recommended to us for the next level of our study. However, rather than being simply the Center 'writ small', it was clear quite early in the fieldwork that department members viewed and thought about quality and service improvement in very different – although not necessarily conflicting or contradictory – ways from their senior managers and improvement professional colleagues in the wider system.

Voltage drops in meaning

The situation we found was one where the messages and meanings emanating from the 'top' of the organization appeared to diminish in strength and intensity with each level of the organization they passed through. To avoid any possible misconception about a clash between center and frontline, we have chosen the term 'voltage drop' to describe this. Take the Center's 'vision for quality'. Sadler is big on vision, and talked with passion about 'perfect care' as something that 'we never reach, but like the North Star . . . serves as a beacon to guide us'. But as far as the local impact of this North Star, Fitzgerald's wry observation springs to mind: 'Visionary light, like any other, diminishes in proportion to the square of the distance.'[11] Not that staff were in any way dissenting from that vision; just that, in their world of trying to achieve that 'perfect care', doing things was more important than having visions.

An even sharper voltage drop was found in relation to the 'healing environment'. Leaving the main hospital to walk across the expanse of a mainly empty car park to the outpatient asthma clinic, we were reminded of Alice leaving Wonderland for the everyday world. Offices, waiting areas and treatment rooms were colorful but cramped and austere, and the reception desk and windows (staff pointed out) were set at child-unfriendly heights. Some nice touches had been added to make it more personal and child-friendly, but despite these local efforts things fell a long way short of the Wonderful World of Disney on the other side of the car park. However, more noteworthy was the fact that while staff said they would welcome more pleasant and spacious working conditions, they did not seem to attach anything like the same importance to physical environment as was articulated higher up in the organization.

Care pathways? What care pathways?

Further surprises were to follow. After all we had been told about the Clinic being the champion of care pathways, we had expected them to feature prominently in the story of its own 'journey to excellence'. Not so, as we discovered on the very first day of our visit. Following our request to view the various pathways' algorithms in more detail, two of the senior staff, looking a little embarrassed, said they had not seen them for some time. They were 'probably in a drawer somewhere', and not to worry, they would find them for us before we left that day (which they did).

The issue turned out to be more than just administrative. Pathways, staff later explained, were important, but were only one of many items in the baggage they had packed for their quality journey. They were described as 'only a tool' – to aid clinical decision-making, reduce variation (especially among community physicians practising in the hospital), and test consensus around a particular clinical process, but a tool that was only as good as the craftsperson using it. And it was more the 'home-grown human process of going through the pathways method' than 'what came out at the other end' that was important: 'The pathways simply gave us another reason to come together and talk about the care we give' – a form of quality dialogue.

There was no inconsistency here, they told us, for contrary to management folk-lore, they had always been ambivalent about pathways, and had remained so. And for very good reason. Their belief was that such ambivalence (as opposed to nega-tivity) was necessary if pathways were not to end up being used inappropriately or dangerously.

Mindful as opposed to mindless use of clinical care pathways: 'missing the zebra'

Staff in this particular micro-system had not rejected or resisted pathways, but had chosen to deploy them in a particular way to establish what they called the 'bedrock' of their service. They were the beginning, not the end of, the quality journey. They believed the success of pathways depended on how they were *used*, in particular that pathways were never accepted at face value by members of the department but were constantly challenged as part of an ongoing, intelligent, critical process:

> People keep up with the literature. They also *challenge* the pathway. They put the references down at the bottom and so you can go back to the literature, and say maybe that's what it says in your pathway but I don't believe it, or you know, this paper is flawed and I don't know whether I am going to do it this way, or this is a great paper and I hadn't

seen it and this is the way I'm gonna practice. So I hope that is why pathways work here, because people *think* about it. (Clinician)

Staff in the asthma clinic constantly stressed that care pathways should never become a substitute for active vigilance and attention. We seemed to have arrived at the nub of the quality issue: those actually 'doing' it felt that 'quality' was less a technique or methodology than a frame or habit of mind, something in the head, an attitude.

Without this level of awareness and critical evaluation, there is a risk often described metaphorically in healthcare as 'missing the zebra', where, because of the conditioning of routine clinical decision-making, everything is seen in terms of the standard illness or the standard patient (everyone a black horse), while unique and often consequential features of individual illness episodes (the zebra – the exceptions to the rule) do not get noticed and picked up. Also described as 'schematic myopia' or inattentional blindness,[12–14] this is clearly what critics are referring to when describing pathways as 'cookbook medicine'.

Staff in the clinic were able to give a clear explanation of how, by developing a psychology of what Weick and others[3,15,16] have called 'mindfulness', they could safeguard against the danger of missing the zebra:

> Medicine is cookbook up to a point, and then every single person is different. The kids sometimes come up from the emergency room with a certain diagnosis, and as the person sits on the floor and evolves you realize that it is not actually what the patient has. They may have pneumonia but also they have this other underlying problem which is why they have pneumonia. You can't just fill out the pneumonia pathway and say ok, I'm going to give this patient ceftriaxin and they're going to get better. (Clinician)

They did not necessarily reject pathways, or even cookbook medicine – after all, one could not go around challenging everything all of the time. Clinical routines, protocols and recipes were a necessary aid in clinical decision-making, not least at three o'clock in the morning! But the stress was on 'aid' as opposed to 'substitute' for thinking. *Using* the pathways was fine, but *relying* on them, they said, was a serious mistake:

> They are great at three in the morning when you are half asleep. I think pathways are good in the right context. *I think they are useful if you already know what you are doing, you've already thought about differential diagnosis, you already know your treatment options.* Then it's a good thing; you're not going to forget to do something; so nobody's gonna stay in the hospital longer than they need to be there because oxygen wasn't weaned at ten a.m. because you didn't read that order. It's good for that part of it.
>
> But I think the danger of pathways is *you just don't think about it.* You calculate the drug doses, you check your boxes, you sign your name, and it's done. You haven't necessarily thought about other things the child could have, other tests that might be useful. Could this be done as an outpatient where it's less costly than keeping them in hospital? Do I really need this particular test on every single person that gets admitted? This is the danger. But they are very helpful at three in the morning when you are tired and you may forget something. (Senior clinician; our italics added here and below for emphasis)

Staff told us that this 'attitude of mindfulness' – of *questioning* not *accepting* – infused all aspects of their practice. It was their local philosophy of quality, part of their culture. This, for example, was what lay behind new interns being barred from using pathways during their first three months in the clinic.

Developing 'community' within the micro-system

Throughout the interviews and observations it was apparent that the culture of the micro-system was sustained, as in so many of the cases in this study, by a tight-knit core team, or, more accurately (given the multiple teams in a micro-system) a 'community'. But tightly knit in what sense?

First, virtually all staff in the micro-system were quick to wax lyrical about the 'quality' of their local clinical leaders, defining this in a similar way to staff in Batalden *et al.*'s[17] micro-system as mentor and teacher, the person who acted as your guide through the whole learning cycle, from acquiring and building knowledge, through taking intelligent action, to reviewing and reflecting on that action. For example (our italics):

> Dr X is one of the best teachers I have ever worked with. If we could all learn to think like him we'd be real smart . . . A lot of the 'art' part of it in medicine just comes from watching people like him and seeing how they think about it. I mean with a really good Doctor *it's fun just to watch them think*, and see what they come up with, and hope one day you'll be able to think in the same way. I mean he teaches even when he's not teaching! It comes from loving what you do. (Clinical fellow)

When interviewed, the leader in question also underscored the importance of being a mentor and role model, but claimed it was as much about style as content; for example, acting in an inclusive, democratic, informal and above all 'collegial' manner:

> I think probably you should kind of, first of all, lead by example. Try to do things like be on time, show concern, compassion, and that type of thing. And it's a little bit more . . . it's not hierarchical, *it's more a kind of egalitarian thing*. Everybody kind of contributes and everybody's voice is heard, I think. And it's fairly informal, so it's more of a democratic type of team. (Clinical leader)

But at the harder end it was also about protecting your staff and the clinic from the icy winds that blew down from the mountain top from time to time, recent examples being the downsizing, cost-cutting and re-engineering at Children's.

Staff also frequently referred to close, family-like ties and the unspoken understandings that come from these types of bonds as a primary glue for the micro-system community:

> We all have lunch together every day, we just like working with each other. (Nurse)

> It is everybody, not just our leader, that sets the climate. (Occupational therapist)

> The people here are special. *They know how each other thinks*. I'm sure any one of them can tell you what Dr B is thinking and what prescription he is going to favor over another. (Pharmacist)

Helping to foster these ties, team members saw their jobs as different but still of equal status and importance within the clinic:

> It's not really a hierarchy. It's very much a team effort, and I think that's a big part of it. People feel like they are equivalent and have different things to add to a child's care. (Clinician)

> The team work here is great; you feel a little bit more important than elsewhere. In this part you are involved with the whole treatment. (Nurse)

It is interesting that 'collegiality' and 'equality' were likewise identified as key factors in Godfrey and colleagues' study of 20 high-performing micro-systems.[18] The clinic also displayed a great deal of flexibility, interchangeability, and blurring of roles, similar to what Godfrey and colleagues described as 'cross-cover' for one another:[18]

> It really is a team. I can do the nurse's job or the pharmacist can do part of my job, so we all do what we can at the moment. (Nurse)

> There are many people who do not have very discrete or defined roles . . . It's about them having flexibility and being able to do things you might not classically do, so they'll, I guess, *feel free to do*. (Unit clinical leader)

Much of the flexibility described above hinged on the ability to trust each other's judgement and expertise, mirroring what Weick describes as 'respectful interaction' in which 'trust, trustworthiness, and self-respect develop equally and allow people to build a stable rendition of what they face':[19]

> Trust and commitment to each other: that really is the lifeblood of it. You know what, for me as a nurse it's really important to know I'm working with F or I'm working with R, and I've worked with that nurse before and I trust her, so if something's going on with my patient, I know I can say, help, and that person's going to be able to come and we're going to work as a team and bail me out. I can trust her judgement skills and her assessment skills . . . her level of quality of care. (Nurse)

These features of the micro-system as a whole reveal unmistakable similarity to the organization studies concept of a 'community of practice'.[20,21] The basis of this concept of 'community' – also reflected in Judge *et al.*'s 'goal-directed community',[22] Borei's 'community of purpose'[23] and Peck's concept of community as individuals who have learned to communicate honestly with each other[24] – is binding commitment between the members, a commitment from which patients will be the beneficiaries because it is this commitment that leads the group to work to a high level day after day.

A community is a place where you would do anything not to let your colleagues down, where you feel a strong sense of loyalty and shared identity to them and the task, and an unerring commitment to the high standards and values of the group, such as keeping a 'mindful' eye on practice and quality. High quality standards are not maintained in a community because of targets, measures, programs or improvement methodologies: these may be important, but as mere tools they do not achieve quality care on their own. This comes because the ethos of the group frames the giving of high-quality care as a social imperative.

Putting it all together

This story of Children's 'journey to quality' has detailed the contributions of many people at many different levels and in many different parts of the organization, and it is the collective, multi-level nature of this achievement that must feature prominently in any explanation of its success in getting further than most on this journey.

For example, following the pathways story from its source, we had been brought by the staff themselves to the realization that it was not so much about method as human agency. At each level we had found a different kind of human accomplishment: at the top the framing and articulation of a vision and strategy for quality; in the Outcomes Center in the middle the day-to-day implementation of that strategy by the organizational development professionals; and finally at the front-end the translation and application of all this to day-to-day care – a chain of human agency that had finally given some meaning to the term 'organizing for quality'.

This multi-level perspective suggests that various strata of the organization can play different but equally important roles in relation to the quality endeavour. Top teams cannot actually 'do' the care, but they can provide the right receptive context[25-27] or cultural soil for quality processes to flourish, grow and spread their roots within the organization. If the role of the macro-system is about providing the necessary supply lines, staging posts and base camps to allow frontline teams to mount their (daily!) assault on Everest,[28] the role of the actual team is to ensure the members have all the necessary skills, and are sufficiently prepared, both mentally and physically, for the climb itself – preparation, as always, being more important than planning because conditions will change and it is impossible to know precisely what to expect.

A number of organizational theorists have emphasized the need to understand and address change at many levels across the organization simultaneously, given the complexity of organizations,[29] the key role of links across levels,[30] and the likelihood that changing only a few system elements at a time will not come anywhere near to achieving all the benefits that are available through a fully co-ordinated approach, and may even have negative pay-offs.[31-35]

Applying these insights to the experience at Children's suggests several propositions about the multi-level nature of quality efforts.

- ❏ The nature, direction and impact of quality improvement efforts are never unilaterally determined at any one level or single part of the organization.
- ❏ 'Quality' is accomplished by different individuals and groups taking different actions in different parts of the organization.
- ❏ Underpinning and driving these actions are various meaning or interpretive systems, each with its own distinctive logics and each fulfilling different functions in relation to the overall quality process.
- ❏ It is the pattern of relationships between these different roles and behaviors that determines the nature and outcome of a quality improvement process, but particularly the extent to which they provide 'interlocking functions'.
- ❏ 'Successful' quality improvement is about achieving synergy and complementarities between these different functions and levels.

And what of the future?

We described at the outset how, in the past several years, Children's had entered a more difficult period in its life, involving downsizing, loss of senior figures from the top team, and cut-backs to departments like Kurtin's Outcomes Center for work on quality. Sadler himself refers to this as 'The Perfect Storm', including simultaneous increases in service demands and consumer expectations; rises in costs related to pharmaceuticals, medical technologies, and capital and information technology investments; and substantial declines in reimbursement rates, philanthropic giving, and certainty of earnings from endowment investments, among other challenges.

So what are the future prospects for Children's quality journey? Faced with these pressures, will it be able to retain its reputation as one of the leading organizations in healthcare 'quality work' in the US? We can speculate on two very different scenarios. On the one hand, it might be argued that because the 'quality ethos' is so deeply woven into the cultural fabric of the organization it will take more than a few local difficulties to do it any permanent damage. In sharp contrast to the book and Hollywood film by the same name, the boat will weather the storm and sail off into the sunset.

On the other hand, the very fact that 'quality' is so deeply embedded in the culture may be what makes it vulnerable. When an organization has espoused a cause in a way and to an extent that employees have come to believe it gives their work real purpose and meaning as part of a larger effort, an 'ideological contract'[34] can be said to have formed that binds employees to the organization, becoming an inducement to elicit employee contributions and commitments. The question here – and it is highly relevant to Children's because there is no doubt that 'quality' has attained the status of a cause over the years – is what happens if staff feel their organization has 'violated' or abandoned this cause?

According to Thompson and Bunderson,[36] it is almost as though a 'hot button' has been pressed, creating a deep sense of disappointment, betrayal, even moral outrage among employees. Pasmore[37] comments on the similar effect of such violations of the 'trust contract' between employee and organization during the aftermath of downsizing, weakening an organization's ability to respond to further change. Not that everything comes to a halt, or even that there are any measurable short-term effects on targets and productivity or quality of service. Nonetheless, the damage to the socio-cultural fabric, and to trust and good faith in the organization, can be deep and lasting.

By way of conclusion, we have to say that there is no way of knowing whether or in what way any of this might apply more narrowly to quality and service improvement efforts within organizations. However, we can see no reason why it should be any different, especially where quality is a core cultural concern. More importantly, neither do we know whether there has been any serious breach of the ideological or trust contracts in the context of San Diego Children's Hospital. This is a question that only the people at Children's themselves can answer, but it is one, at least, that needs to be asked.

Journey highlights

Stories rarely tell it exactly 'how it is', and this one is no exception. Our aim in telling it has been to highlight those aspects of the hospital's journey that make it interesting or unique and might offer scholars and practitioners some new insights into issues of healthcare quality. Following is our selection.

The art and science of improvement

The story underlines the importance of attending to, and skillfully bringing together, both the science and the art of improvement – not forgetting the sociology – in the quality improvement arena, seeking to demonstrate through the Children's case just how powerful their combined 'intelligence' can be (*see* left brain / right brain, Figure 1.1). Through the case we have also endeavoured to draw attention to a lacuna in the wider field concerning the aesthetic and sociological dimensions of improvement, which is, we believe, a consequence of a preoccupation with the 'science' of improvement and with more technical concerns. We discuss this further in Chapter 11.

Macro-system and micro-system connections

The link between the macro-system and micro-system levels of the organization is of vital importance. The precise word for this is 'entrainment', which refers to the adjustment of behaviors at one level to be in timing or in tune with events at another.[38] In recent years quality studies in healthcare have become increasingly concentrated on the micro-system, frontline level,[18,39–41] and the present case study provides strong justification for this: it reveals that many of the keys to quality are indeed to be found at the 'front end' of care, especially in the psychological, group and cultural dimensions of micro-system working.

However, the danger for any researchers looking solely at this level is that they run the risk of missing the influential role played by the organizational macro-system in the working and effectiveness of the micro-system. There is also the danger of failing to recognize the wider strategic management challenge of any improvement effort, which must seek to achieve synchronization or complementarities between these levels – 'two horses pulling the same chariot'. To focus too narrowly on the micro-system is to underestimate the importance of, and the need for fit with, the wider organizational context.

Table 2.1 Different but interlocking and complementary roles

MACRO: STANDARDIZING	MICRO: INDIVIDUALIZING
framing and gaming!	the 'doing' of quality
protecting	challenging and redefining
visioning	socializing
resourcing	mobilizing
devolving	bonding and team building
structuring/embedding	'retrospecting' and learning
knowledge harvesting and diffusing	redesigning, improvising and customizing
measuring and evaluating	
protocolizing	

Table 2.1 sums up this idea by showing the different but interlocking and complementary roles being played by the macro- and micro-systems at Children's, the former focused on standardizing processes (achieving consistent high-volume care), the latter on individualizing processes (delivering high-quality personal care).

The meso paradigm for quality

The question of levels of analysis takes us beyond the immediate realms of this particular case study to a consideration of the whole way in which healthcare researchers approach 'quality', change and improvement. Drawing on the work of Robert House and colleagues[30] in organization theory, we invite readers to consider a new model for looking at quality, one which goes by the somewhat unattractive name of the 'meso paradigm for quality', and which argues that it is not only the processes and variables at each level that are crucial to quality but the nature of the interaction between them. Children's provides a clear case for why quality research requires the simultaneous study of the micro and macro, and the interactions between them, and why researchers and practitioners need to incorporate such 'meso paradigm' thinking, which for the most part has been lacking in the field.

Mindfulness and mindful organizing

If one issue stands out as being of special importance in this particular quality journey it would be 'mindfulness'.[42–47] For some time the concept of 'mindfulness' has featured strongly in the organizational literature on high-reliability organizations, and is said to account for much of the difference between a high-quality safe organization and a low-quality unsafe one, even when all the scientific monitors and controls are in place in both.[15,48] An examination of mindfulness and the process of 'mindful organizing' in the quality context, which may be done culturally in terms of a culture of mindfulness or personally in terms of an attitude of mindfulness, reveals that healthcare researchers have either been looking in the wrong place or even perhaps been using the wrong conceptual lenses to identify the keys to quality and service improvement. The literature has always accorded priority to material issues and technical and behavioral 'variables' such as the nature and degree of information technology support, measurement, leadership, method and structure, but what the mindfulness theme offers is a strong reminder that quality is not only about method and technique, but also outlook and frame of mind – the immaterial (and therefore easily missable) subjective dimension of life.

3

Organizational and professional identity: crisis, tradition and quality at the Royal Devon and Exeter NHS Foundation Trust

ORIGINAL CASE STUDY RESEARCHED AND NARRATIVE PREPARED BY GLENN ROBERT AND PAUL BATE

The story of high-quality care at the Royal Devon and Exeter (RD&E) NHS Foundation Trust and its Princess Elizabeth Orthopaedics Centre (PEOC), one large clinical department within the organization, demonstrates the distinct importance of organizational 'identity'. By identity, we mean the collective self-definitions of an organization and the groups within it of 'who we are', the collective role 'we' play, the distinctive characteristics 'we' possess, and the image 'we' wish to project,[1–3] another immaterial and therefore invisible phenomenon like 'mindfulness' in the previous chapter. In particular, this case study highlights the influence of organizational identity, sub-unit identity, and professional identity and how these can sustain the contribution of additional discretionary effort from individuals to tasks that benefit co-workers and the organization as a whole,[4] such as achieving and maintaining high levels of quality and continual QI.

In addition, the macro journey of the Trust and the micro journey of the PEOC are, in a number of ways, stories in contrast, differing in timeframes and in the nature of the insights they give on the role of identity in sustaining quality. The former represents a redemptive tale of overcoming recent crisis and, in so doing, redefining the culture and ultimately the self-image of the organization. The latter chronicles a longstanding reputation for innovation and clinical excellence and the lasting impact this has had on the pride and esteem underpinning the routine performance of members within a high-functioning clinical unit. These two stories together also provide an enlightening perspective on how various forms of identity at multiple levels of an organization may interact – indeed, be managed, guided or nurtured – to productively reinforce each other towards the goals of service improvement and quality.

At the level of the Trust, the quality journey begins, according to many at the RD&E, in the mid-1990s after the appointment of the current chief executive, the fourth person to have held the position in the previous five years. Her appointment was quickly followed by a crisis – in part a crisis of identity – for the organization, the response to which is still viewed by staff as a turning point. Members of the senior team at RD&E characterized the transformation over the last 10 years as that of a defensive, inward-looking organization seeing itself become much more open, informal, collegial and outward-looking. During this period the RD&E also provided specific mechanisms and resources to support and enable high-quality clinical care. An important element of this new identity – the outward-looking, opportunistic organization – led to much greater involvement with formal QI initiatives.

BOX 3.1 Case profile: Royal Devon and Exeter NHS Foundation Trust

CASE PROFILE

Type of Organization:	A regional National Health Service (NHS) trust comprising a comprehensive system of healthcare services and medical education programs.
Focal Micro-System:	Orthopedics center
Size:	The predominant provider of acute health services for 470 000 neighbouring residents, and of specialist services to a wider population of 750 000. The system includes 850 inpatient and 62 day case beds. It is the largest employer in the local area, with over 5000 full- or part-time staff.
Location:	Exeter, south-west England, a rural, although relatively affluent region. The area population is older than the average served by other trusts in its 'coast and country' group and contains a very low proportion of ethnic minorities (less than 1%).
Country:	United Kingdom
Awards and Recognitions:	Top-ranked '3 star' rating in NHS performance tables 3 years running; one of the first 10 trusts in the UK to be granted Foundation Trust status, which permits greater independence in managing local budgets and services; one of only 4 UK sites in 2001 selected for the Pursuing Perfection initiative sponsored by the Institute for Healthcare Improvement and Robert Wood Johnson Foundation.

KEY CONCEPTS

Organizational Identity: a shared sense of 'who we are' and 'what we stand for' that conveys the distinctive character of an organization and the groups within it. Related to cultural notions of image and reputation. As markers of the enduring and central traits of groups, identities represent a reservoir of commitment and motivation within organizations that can help sustain service quality and improvement.

Discretionary Effort: additional effort expended by employees of an organization beyond what is contractually required. Such 'extra role' effort includes the creativity and energy typically necessary to generate innovation, high standards of performance, and continual improvements in service.

The journey to quality for PEOC was described as dating from much earlier, in fact beginning in 1927 with the initial founding of the orthopedic hospital, as it was then. The long history of the PEOC is characterized by commitment to the local community, innovation, professional pride, clinical research and continuous audit. The department developed a deep-seated sense of identity and self-esteem through the continuing influence of strong role models and international recognition for the quality of the care provided. However, this was not without some of the disadvantages that often accompany such achievements, including a certain aloofness and detachment acknowledged by staff both within and outside the department. Until 1997 the PEOC had remained to some extent separate from the hospital – culturally, operationally, and physically. However, a transfer from the PEOC's original site to new facilities attached to the main hospital has been accompanied by a re-connection to the corporate body and identity of the RD&E.

We propose that this is where the two stories come together in the present day: the corporate identity of the RD&E (enacted by the senior executive team through the development of a new 'style of working'), largely forged through crisis, has been shaped and implemented in ways that reinforce, rather than clash or attempt to tamper with, PEOC's own long-established local commitment and professional identity, traditionally fuelling the department's pre-existing focus on high-quality clinical care. This case study traces these stories through the words and accounts of the senior leaders of the RD&E and staff within the PEOC. Relating these accounts also calls attention to the key role played by those individuals who, to the benefit of both the wider Trust and the PEOC, have worked collaboratively to (re)build the bridges between the macro- and micro-system under study.

Managing 'who we are' at the RD&E Trust

The 'then'

At the RD&E the chief executive uses the story of how the organization traveled from 'then' to 'now', framing this journey in terms of how the organization's 'style' and identity had changed quite dramatically over its course.

'Then' the organization, as she described it, had a negative reputation, the result in part of high turnover in senior management and the influence of particular senior clinicians who were widely viewed within the region as 'a difficult bunch of consultants'. Accordingly, the organization was considered to have an arrogant and inward-looking 'style':

> If you had asked the question five maybe seven years ago, our style as an organization was to be quite conservative, to keep our head down, only raise it above the parapet if there was proven experience or expertise that said this was the right way to go. (Director of operations)

This attitude, also described as a 'we will do what we want because we are Exeter' mentality, resulted in a number of service developments taking place elsewhere in the region but not at the RD&E. The reluctance to work with and learn from others outside the organization, coupled with a refusal to recognize that such behavior is detrimental to the organization itself, prompted the new chief executive to set formal objectives for her senior colleagues aimed at improving outside participation as well as the external recognition and image of the RD&E:

> It was about trying to bring the management out and saying, 'Yes, you've done a good job internally but unless people out there know what you are doing...' The objective for each of the execs was, 'You will get yourself actively involved in one project regionally and if you get yourself on something nationally, then that is what you do – your agenda is partly outside as well as inside.' (Chief executive)

However, in order to induce fundamental change, it is often the case that an organization must be destabilized – virtually shocked or jolted – calling into question customary actions or performance and convincing members of the necessity for a different way of seeing and doing.[5,6] Such 'precipitating' or 'triggering' events present some of the most extreme challenges for organizations, as well as some of the most substantial contexts for change and adaptation.[4,7] Events would soon conspire to put the RD&E into a predicament of this kind beyond what anyone within the organization could have predicted.

Crisis as a turning point

In the late 1990s an event, or rather series of events, at the RD&E came to light that would be variously described by members of the senior management team as 'extremely traumatic', 'awful', 'hair-raising stuff' and 'catastrophic'. The alert was sparked after NHS medical staff raised concerns over the mammography films of 12 women who had been screened and cleared by one of the local breast cancer services, but each of whom eventually developed cancer before their next routine examination. Staff expressed concern over the interpretation of tiny calcium deposits shown on the original mammogram film, and asked the NHS National Breast Screening Program to review the 12 scans. Problems were identified with the interpretation of the films of nine of the women, which led to almost 4000 screenings being reviewed. About 2000 women called help lines set up by the hospital. The errors took place between January 1991 and June 1997, during which, as best could be determined, 82 victims were wrongly given the all-clear, with 11 of them dying.

Two radiologists left the hospital after the errors were uncovered (*see* Figure 3.1). They were both found guilty of serious professional misconduct by the General Medical Council's Professional Misconduct Committee (although not ultimately struck off the national register). The chief executive's response was candid:

> We had failed and there's no point in covering up something as catastrophic as that. There is no excusing it – you can come up with all sorts of reasons as to why it happened but for those individual patients, we failed them. We tried to get the message over to staff that it's not about criticizing them but about saying *we have failed as an organization* and the very least we can do is say, 'We're sorry, we failed and we are liable.' (Chief executive)

It is not uncommon following such an explicit admission of failure for members within an organization to engage in various defensive reputation repair behaviors, such as simple denials of the problem, finger-pointing, or scapegoating of others.[8] In the case of the RD&E, however, the crisis, was used to bring people – particularly the clinical and managerial teams – together:

> And we have been thrust into the limelight to a certain extent by some events we would not have wanted to have happened – such as the breast screening incident that took place just when [the chief executive] arrived here. There is something about managing those types of circumstances out in the public arena really well. People feel we are the type of organization that can cope with adversity. The way the clinical and managerial teams worked together over that time has been well received. (Director of operations)

This result was no accident. In addition to publicly and forthrightly addressing the failures of the organization, the chief executive also viewed this 'shock to the system' as an opportunity to inculcate a belief of constant self-questioning[9] (*see* also Chapter 2) and institutionalize an organization-wide ethos of learning.[10]

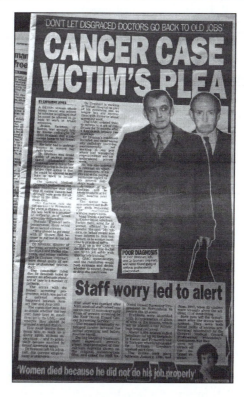

FIGURE 3.1 Local media coverage of the breast cancer screening scandal

> It makes you much more systematic in how you review these things. The question it opened up was, 'I found this one – what else is there lurking around in this organization that I don't know about?' What I am going to be sure about is that I have systems to allow people to raise concerns, systems where we can begin to ask the right questions. With the breast service incident the indicators were there but they weren't picked up on until it was too late – a classic in governance terms: when you look back you can usually see. How do we get a system in place that gives the organization intelligence? We have more work to do to get people to question more. (Chief executive)

Note the emphasis in the quotation above on the need to 'give the organization intelligence' and to 'get people to question more'. In this way the breast cancer screening incident afforded leaders of the RD&E space to strategically appropriate collective experiences into a 'sustainable corporate story' and response,[11] or, as the chief executive described it, as a 'vehicle to get the message across' that quality is important and that the organization has to take quality and governance much more seriously.

The crisis played another role: it demonstrated that the then newly appointed chief executive could 'stand up to' clinicians for the so-called 'good of the organization' as a whole:

> ...a huge dilemma was when she had to confront the clinicians – breast radiologists – and that was a testing time for her, but she demonstrated that she could stand up to them for the greater cause of the organization. Historically, that is what had her accepted. It is hard coming in from an outside culture – they don't have many people coming in at

this level from outside Devon even. My gut feeling is that since she has been completely consistent with them; that has stayed. (Director of nursing and service improvement)

The crisis also served as a character-building and, in a deep sense, an identity-defining moment[12] in the life of the RD&E. Many of those interviewed echoed the observation of the medical director that coping with such 'adversity' in what has been perceived as a constructive and successful way has led to increased self-confidence for the organization as a whole:

> I think the individuals who work here are proud to work in the Trust because it does well. They like the fact that members appear on television to talk about their problems, so I think people do have a pride in the organization. (Medical director)

Thus, the breast cancer screening crisis at RD&E combined with other factors – a new chief executive and greater public scrutiny of healthcare providers – to put 'service improvement' at the top of the organization's agenda, the challenge being defined by the specific failure as one of providing safer, better and more reliable services for patients going forward.

'Walking the talk'

'Walking the talk', a phrase used by the chief executive, in essence refers to concretizing a new identity and intent into the strategies and structures of the organization; in other words, putting the espoused identity and the values associated with it into institutional practice.

Similar to other NHS trusts, clinical governance is defined by the RD&E as 'the continuous improvement of the quality of services provided to patients' and relies on a clinical governance committee at the level of the board and executive to oversee organization-wide activities on these issues.[13] Its agenda includes clinical governance, controls assurance, risk management, health and safety, clinical audit, patient advice and liaison services, and patient complaints[13] (*see* Figure 3.2).

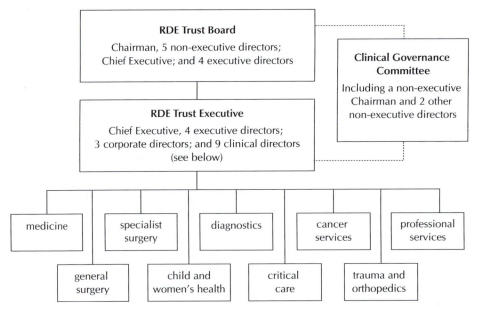

FIGURE 3.2 Clinical governance structure at the RD&E

The Trust's clinical governance committee meets quarterly with senior management and representatives of clinical specialties throughout the RD&E. It also holds formal quarterly performance reviews with each directorate, which must submit a written report covering areas such as finance, operations, waiting lists, risk management, adverse clinical incidents, and clinical audit. This quarterly review process is considered one of the lynchpins of the Trust's approach to performance and quality monitoring and has been recognized by district audit as one of the actions taken by the Trust to ensure that it is in a position to respond efficiently and effectively to the requirements of clinical governance.[14]

Although predating the arrival of the new chief executive, these performance reviews were restructured and refocused directly as a result of the breast cancer screening crisis:

> . . . we had a quarterly review process already in place – mainly financial – but we streamlined that and made it much more focused . . . things will come up in the quarterly review: 'We've got a problem with whatever' and they'll say 'I'm talking to the modernization team about some help with some process mapping or running a day with us.' Or if they haven't we'll say, 'Well can you talk to so-and-so as they are doing some similar work in another project and some of the learning may help you.' (Chief executive)

In addition, the RD&E has instituted monthly meetings between the executive team (the chief executive, medical director, director of operations, and director of nursing and service improvement) and each of the nine clinical directorates (represented by the clinical director, directorate manager and senior nurse). These monthly meetings are important because, despite the relatively large size of the Trust, they allow 'active engagement of the executive team with directorate affairs'. For the director of nursing and service improvement, the meetings are a particularly useful and, within the NHS, relatively unique mechanism introduced by the RD&E:

> It's the one extra that I haven't seen anywhere else and this is on top of quarterly reviews. There is a small agenda but it gives open discussion. It's not like the quarterly review where you are looking at performance. In this way you keep a handle on what's happening but there is mutual respect: you are not someone sat over here who only goes to them with a problem; rather there's an ongoing interest. For me that's what makes the difference. (Director of nursing and service improvement)

As mentioned in one of the quotations above, the RD&E also employs a small, central modernization team to support service improvement work throughout the RD&E. This team includes a head post created in the summer of 2002, 'services development manager', filled by a senior administrative member who can take an organization-wide perspective on quality, 'join up separate pools of activity', and 'scale up' the impact of efforts within the organization as a whole.

Within this remit there is a clear commitment to the training and ongoing development of project managers in order to form a core group of frontline clinical staff with QI expertise:

> I've inherited a number of project managers who are different in lots of ways. My role is to develop their skills and . . . to really put that project management expertise out into the directorates at the right level . . . What I am developing much more with them is their role in going out there, showing, demonstrating, coaching, supporting and then leaving the skills out there. (Services development manager)

Reflecting this objective, the chief executive emphasized that the modernization team is not the 'quality' team, *per se*, but rather a resource providing core QI competencies and expertise for the wider organization, 'time-limited in terms of the particular projects they are working through but where you need . . . some focused attention and facilitation'. In other words, a 'change management' team.

As befits such an emphasis on ensuring that quality is delegated down to the departmental level (to the PEOC, for example), the Trust does not have a formal quality strategy as such:

> We don't have a quality strategy. I believe in quality and I believe in having a framework and a sense of direction, but I am also very opportunistic and the organization has to keep on its toes. The environment we work in changes rapidly. I couldn't produce for you our quality strategy and I have almost deliberately not put a quality strategy together.
>
> But there are a number of initiatives in terms of how we measure what we do for patients, how we measure what we do with the staff, what's the learning that comes out of complaints and the governance work and how do we put that all together . . . So we don't have a quality strategy and equally we don't have a quality department – it has to be bedded into the work of every directorate and we monitor their performance against a range of indicators that demonstrate quality outcome. (Chief executive)

The dominant change management approach was described as 'focusing attention and facilitation', with the emphasis on 'the softer, emotional networking stuff' and a belief that the 'less formal spin-offs are much more productive'. As a result, there is no top-down, standardized approach to QI imposed upon departments within the RD&E. Instead, Trust leaders have encouraged frontline staff to own and express the quality agenda in locally meaningful terms:

> It's about having a style that's sufficiently flexible to say they will work in different ways, they will learn in different ways, what's important to them they will express in different ways. It's all about delivering quality patient care, but they will express it and the bits that are important will be different – that's fine, if I can get them started on something they want to do then we can move it to the other bits . . . 'Have you thought about applying it to . . .?' (Chief executive)

Likewise, the Trust has embraced a more organic – as opposed to a strict command-and-control – approach towards quality improvement, as related by the director of operations when referring to the Pursuing Perfection initiative described later in this case study:

> I've got this thing about excitable atoms – that's how I feel about quality improvement. I never thought I would say anything like that! I feel like an excited atom, and then there are a few more excited atoms and it's sort of all going through everything we do. Pursuing Perfection isn't about this big tent that sits on top of us – it's about an octopus and tentacles that goes out through the organization, scooping people up and gathering them in as it goes on. It's from within the very body of the organization. (Director of operations)

This decentralized, organic approach to QI is further enabled by a relatively flat organizational structure and an accessible senior management team:

> The first thing I always say when asked is that 'it's this relationship thing'. I have heard of trusts where people dare not go see somebody higher up without an appointment. There is a very open structure here. It's not particularly flat, but it is pretty flat, and that

> I think would mean the open relationships, the respect for each other's area of work, and the mutual support. I think those things make us stand out and . . . allow us to do the things we do. (Medical director)

The decentralization and local ownership of the quality agenda fostered at the RD&E mean that clinical and non-clinical departments can retain a strong sense of identity for themselves and their staff while belonging and contributing to the wider Trust. This dynamic is mutually beneficial to both levels and the result of a deliberate strategy from senior management. It relies on harnessing the power of various group and professional affiliations (and the commitment they invoke) within an inclusive corporate identity, rather than on uniformity or standardization, as the core driver of quality throughout the organization as a whole.

The 'now'

To take present stock of the Trust's journey as it was related to us is to portray a move from a rather closed and narrow organization (the 'then') to one that is much more open:

> We also have – I believe we have – an open style. There is a lot of one-to-one coaching that takes place, fairly informally. I will see – not in a structured way – regularly the directorate managers who will pop in . . . You can go through very formal briefing mechanisms – we have formal briefing mechanisms – but . . . [it] is the openness and frankness, the engaging people in the process that means you have more chance of getting through something. Do ask questions but do it from a position of respect rather than ill-informed judgements behind closed doors. (Chief executive)

> Now clinicians continually come up here, they don't have to make appointments, they open my door, they go and talk to [the chief executive] about whatever is on their mind so she will know what the issues are. We've always said we don't need processes to find out the problems, we know from the noise on the street. When each of us hears something, it's very quickly communicated to the others. (Medical director)

This informal, cross-professional dialogue is what creates and reinforces the prevailing corporate character and identity. This culture (or 'style') of openness is the context in which identity is formed and enacted.

The shift to a more open style has also naturally led to a more informal and collegial organization, as exemplified by the notion of 'pre-meeting work' and keeping the 'human bit':

> There's a lot of pre-meeting work that takes place within the Trust to try and understand where people are coming from and how they see things . . . People are quite willing to go off and have an informal chat about something to try and work their way to a reasonable solution rather than just waiting for the formal meeting to be called. (Director of operations)

> With a big organization still trying to keep the human bit. I deliberately from time to time use the park-and-ride scheme – it's important that you are seen to be chatting to people using it. Those fairly intangible things. We had a major bed crisis on Monday night and the director of nursing and I were moving patients, wheeling trolleys down the corridor. (Chief executive)

At the same time, this shift within the organization has supported a less defensive, more receptive attitude towards external influences and opportunities. The most vivid and ambitious example of this is the RD&E's participation in Pursuing Perfection, an international initiative sponsored by the US-based Institute for Healthcare Improvement (IHI), which seeks to radically transform patient care. The Trust's Pursuing Perfection program involves partnering with 10 other healthcare organizations in the local community on a range of health system improvements. Senior managers described this initiative as recognition of the change that has occurred in the 'character' of the organization and its agenda, which is now truly 'outside as well as inside'.

In summary, the 'now' for the Trust is a relatively happy organization, more at ease with itself, one that is increasingly receptive to opportunities for learning, with an open, informal style and a very different external image from that of a decade prior:

> The perception from outside – as we have been involved in a lot of organization pilot sites – so we've had the exposure, our name splashed all over the various different publications, so it's almost like that's fulfilling the prophesy and . . . it's great for us because, you know, it's this thing about motivation. (Services development manager)

The macro-system in this case study has played a clear role over the last 10 years in nurturing this change in organizational identity in order to advance the quality of healthcare. It has done this partly through challenging the old corporate identity in response to a crisis, partly through providing a redemptive organizational narrative that individuals can relate to, and partly by implementing policies and procedures that reflect and reinforce the new shared self-image of the Trust and values that underpin the organization.

Next, we take up the story of the Princess Elizabeth Orthopaedic Centre (PEOC), a micro-system within the Trust with its own long-standing identity and particular set of implications for understanding how organizational identities can serve to underpin high-quality care.

Tradition, reputation, and the delivery of high-quality care at the PEOC

'The journey starts in 1927'

When the current clinical director of the PEOC was invited to relate the story of the department and its journey to quality, he began by saying, 'The journey starts in 1927', when the hospital (as it then was) opened:

> That is when the orthopedic hospital was started as a hospital school, by local people, at the instigation of Sir Harold Blatter, who was one of the people responsible for services around the country, mainly because of TB, polio, osteomyelitis and, in particular, crippled children who were being hidden away. (Clinical director)

The historical origins of the PEOC clearly resonate with staff from among the different professions in the unit, expressed as a sense of both history and pride:

> I think it's a sense of pride and a sense of history. And I know that sounds crazy – I don't live in the past, I'm not that kind of person, but actually it does make a difference if there is a history to a place or a team of people. It's . . . not the building that makes the place, it's the people that are in it, and I truly believe that . . . I think those people are the people that care about what they do very much and they have a sense of pride in what they do. (Senior nurse)

This sense of history also encompasses a commitment to quality that can be traced back to the opening of the original hospital, as evidenced by that fact that clinical audit has been 'standard practice for years ... from 1927 there is a record of every orthopedic operation that was done since the hospital opened'. This heritage is still referenced – literally, as illustrated by the following orthopedic consultant – and continues with the ongoing, routine monitoring of performance and patient outcomes at the PEOC.

> ... and there are all these pictures of the Queen and pictures of the old TB hospital and I am quite a traditionalist. I reviewed a lot of old x-rays and old notes and people in the TB unit and hip and things like that in the 1900s and I was reading these notes and seeing all these famous names ... (Orthopedic consultant)

From 1932 until 1964 the orthopedics hospital was run by one clinician, Norman Capener, an orthopedic surgeon who would later become president of the British Orthopaedics Association and vice-president of the Royal College of Surgeons. The medical director related how when Capener wanted to appoint a new member of staff he just did it and then informed the management committee and his colleagues afterwards. This practice allowed the orthopedics hospital to maintain a select team of clinicians, but resulted in 'a sense of isolation and a perception ... that all orthopedic surgeons were difficult and that their chosen method of negotiation was to put their heads down and butt you as hard as they could'.

The 1960s was another key period in further defining the PEOC's own self-identity and clinical reputation. During this time surgeon Robin Ling led the development of the world-renowned Exeter hip system, one of the first successful 'metal on plastic' hip replacement prosthetics and designed on biomechanical principles with input from the engineering faculty at the University of Exeter. This work was seen by staff as 'having put the Centre on the map'.

Much of this pride in the longevity and achievements of the department is magnified by the affection held for that 'old hospital across the road', where the department was physically housed between 1927 and 1997. This period was referred to as the time when 'we were a little family on our own over there'. The 'old hospital' seems to represent the physical embodiment of the commonly held view, by both staff and 'outsiders', of the department being somehow 'different'.

Relationships between the PEOC and the RD&E were not further helped by various negotiations and discussions relating to the introduction of the first NHS trusts in the early 1990s, which 'created some very deep wounds' and left 'feelings of betrayal and even despair'. In October 1997 the PEOC moved from its original site to the far end of the RD&E hospital, retaining their 'name, front door and flagpoles', a move seen by staff as having begun to redress some of the misperceptions of the PEOC:

> Historically, I think it's [the department] been perceived as a bit aloof, a bit too separate not quite team players for the Trust and I think that's less since we've been over here. When we were across the road, it was much stronger. (Physiotherapist)

Despite some of these antagonisms between the PEOC and the RD&E from the earlier phases of the Trust's development and the historical view of the orthopedics department as being 'difficult' (a view echoed by the current directorate manager prior to his existing appointment), the quality of care and surgical reputation of the Centre have been consistently very high, a fact that was often lost on those in other parts of the Trust. When the directorate manager did take up his post he:

> ... found that everybody always talked about the bad things, the confrontation, the

> fact that they couldn't get on with anybody, their waiting lists were long. [But] nobody within the organization outside of orthopedics ever picked up on the good things, which were the fact that they literally like to stay on the cutting edge, that their standard of surgery was really high, the training for the junior medical staff was great, that almost anywhere you went in this country, somebody would say, 'Its great, I've heard about it.' (Directorate manager)

This continual delivery of high-quality care has been particularly rooted, in the case of the PEOC, in the strong sense of tradition and good reputation enjoyed by the department – frequently remarked upon by various members – which, as sources of commitment and self-esteem, contribute to maintaining a cohesive micro-system with high internalized standards of care and behavior among staff.

Commitment and tradition: 'two very big things'

The sense of history and a tradition of excellence in the PEOC translates in a number of ways into a commitment among staff to the department and to uphold its legacy of achievement. The directorate manager succinctly puts the two together: 'commitment and tradition . . . those are two very big things here'. Others in the department elaborate:

> It's history, it's having leaders to follow. I look at the current consultants here and I think x is one of the best hip surgeons in the world and what he says you believe it because I know him as a person and he's not self-promoting. I look at the spinal surgeon and I think if I had a back problem I would have it fixed by him . . . each person gives the best care they can . . . I know if somebody comes into this unit, they are going to get some good service. (Orthopedic consultant)

> I do think if somebody has set very high standards – and certainly in my trade the standards that Robin Ling had set himself and his predecessors were what I accepted as being the norm . . . all the people that have trained have come across those high clinical standards, and not only the clinical standards but the priorities that one has, whether your duty is to your community or to your bank balance to put it crudely . . . (Clinical director)

This tradition and commitment are reinforced from one generation to the next through the training of registrars,* the department being described by one consultant as able to 'attract the cream of the registrar world', often explicitly to partake of the department's heritage:

> . . . when you are in surgical training, you always look for the figureheads and people you admire as surgeons, and I think here – 90% of the surgeons here who have trained me – and I look at them and I think you are some of the top surgeons in the UK and in some respects, some of the top surgeons in the world in terms of hips and things like that. And I think with that tradition behind it, I feel to see my name at the end of that list is great. (Orthopedic consultant)

Much of the sense of continuity felt throughout the micro-system comes from the tendency of registrars to return there after they have qualified and become consultants.

> We've got surgeon consultants that have been here a long time and then we've got those who come through within their training programs, registrars who come and then come

---

* Registrars in the UK are the equivalent of medical resident trainees in the United States.

> back as consultants . . . we've all started here many years ago and most people have gone
> away and come back once, twice, more times than that sometimes. People come back:
> they want to work here . . . it's a nice hospital, they know people, people always remember
> you and that's important. (Theater nurse)

Having trained in the department, newly appointed consultants know many of the
non-surgical staff:

> It's got a good feel about it . . . the operating staff are very much 'we are orthopedic
> theatre staff'. I've come back after being away for two and half years . . . but I still know
> most of the porters and all the nursing assistants and most of the theatre staff, and all
> the secretaries are still the same. (Orthopedic consultant)

They have also experienced the particular culture within it:

> History I think has a large part to play in it . . . At least four of the current consultants
> were registrars, so they've had that cultural thing sort of drilled into them as well.
> (Physiotherapist)

Others within the PEOC echo the importance of familiarity and strong personal
relationships that facilitate social interchange, such as putting 'a face to the people you're
dealing with, which makes relationships easier, even when things are tense and when
things aren't quite right', as described by a theater nurse. This level of social interaction
and quality of relationships help maintain the cohesion within the department and
provide members with a feeling of group purpose and distinctiveness:

> I've worked in other good hospitals but you just didn't feel you were part of a unit really.
> You just felt you did your little bit and if you didn't do your little bit nobody would
> notice and you'd go home. Maybe you get a bit carried away and you think what you do
> is more important than what it really is, but I think there is genuinely the feeling that you
> are doing something that is recognized hopefully for what it really is. (Physiotherapist)

The shared sense of tradition and 'mentality' of group cohesion and commitment
within the unit has endured over time into a resilient and lasting identity. To some
in the PEOC the strength and durability of the department's distinct identity is
remarkable and, at the same time, a great collective asset:

> I can't explain it as I was actually watching and waiting, when people who have been here
> a long time leave, for that sense of pride and the mentality to go, but it hasn't actually.
> I think in these days of great conglomerates and corporations there is still a sense of
> identity and I think that's what does it. (Senior nurse)

Reputation and self-esteem

Highly cohesive groups provide the sort of security that heightens participants' self-
esteem and increases co-operation within the group.[9,15] This dynamic is especially
operative in the case of the PEOC, in which the unit's long-established reputation for
clinical excellence and innovation generates a great amount of pride, sense of efficacy,
and intrinsic motivation for individual members to perform at the levels of their
current and historical peers.

Staff in the department often talk about past and present surgeons in terms, for
example, of 'x has a very big reputation world-wide', 'the hip research unit has become
world renowned', 'y has been the major speaker at symposiums and meetings in 22
different countries and literally all five continents of the world', and 'z is very much
an international name'. One effect of such reputations[5] or 'living history'[16] is that it is

'much easier to work hard in a unit where you have well-known people and you have foreign visitors coming' from outside to learn and observe:

> Just historically it has a good reputation for being at the forefront, so the innovation that goes alongside the research . . . The calibre of surgery is high: you go to other units and you think, 'Oh my God, I wouldn't send my mum there.' (Physiotherapist)

> . . . there is a kudos about it and I sort of can't believe that I'm good enough to be an x consultant, but I'm here and I'm enjoying it. (Orthopedic consultant)

> [The consultants] are proud as well of being here: it shows with them. (Ward nurse)

The PEOC's celebrated clinical reputation is similarly motivating not only to surgeons but to staff throughout the department:

> I think we're all very proud of where we work and I think that shows that people have high standards – we've all got high standards and I think that's quite important actually because it means leading by example . . . I mean the medical staff are world renowned and it's up to us as senior nurses to make sure that the nursing staff keep up to that level too. It makes people motivated as they really enjoy the challenge. (Senior nurse)

These sentiments have fuelled a propensity for continuing innovation in practices that extend beyond clinical treatment to various processes of care within the PEOC. For example, a senior nurse who had recently joined the department from another district hospital was struck by the amount of thought and effort spent on designing the unit's discharge process and its efficiency in handling a workload that otherwise she expected would have the department 'grind to a halt every day'. Similarly, a physiotherapist recounted how Robin Ling, famous for developing the Exeter hip prosthetic, also pioneered expanding the role of non-medics in orthopedic treatment.

These practice innovations have gained similar notoriety for the department as its clinical advances and, as described by the physiotherapist, highlight the special multi-disciplinary systems and cohesive relationships that staff find rewarding and empowering:

> . . . now it's more or less widespread practice really. We got involved with other medics coming here to see how it works, business managers coming to see how it worked. For me it led onto quite a lot of things.

The services development manager further points out the ownership and efficacy underlying this continual improvement, it being both commonplace within the PEOC for years and done without the pomp of formal pronouncements or initiatives typical in much service improvement work.

> They do a lot of quite innovative stuff but they've been doing it for years and they don't necessarily use the 'packaged' techniques . . . [T]hey've got a lot of ownership . . . when they really think there's a need from a patient perspective or from the staff, they'll make those changes and they just do it without any flag waving . . . (Services development manager)

Shared stories: 'crossing the road'

As we have seen, shared stories represent 'institutionalized repositories' of organizational history[17] that organizations and their members can use to draw inspiration from and to encapsulate, preserve and transmit central aspects of culture and group identity.[16,18] One particular story frequently referred to by interviewees as a key milestone in the

PEOC's recent history was the department's move from the 'old hospital' to the main site in 1997. Despite the transfer to the main hospital site, the department has retained its own entrance and reception area in its new purpose-built facilities. The frequent telling of this narrative suggests its use as a morality tale of sorts to convey how the department has retained its separate identity while at the same time becoming more incorporated into the Trust:

> . . . the identity, that is still separate, and I think it works fantastically well because it is at the end of the building . . . [w]e have our own entrance and we've got our own theatres and our own wards, and I still think that's very good. (Orthopedic consultant)

> . . . I think it managed to keep its separateness. And people thought a lot about that sort of thing to have the entrance, to have their own reception area and all that sort of stuff and people fought quite hard for that. (Physiotherapist)

On balance, staff in the PEOC tended to view the move as positive, especially considering a number of tangible benefits for patient care in terms of better access to specialties and support services in other departments, such as testing, x-ray, and intensive care that are now available 'on our doorstep', as a senior nurse put it. Another nurse sums up the general sentiment:

> I think there's always good and bad when you move from a hospital to a Centre, from an old site to a new site, from being on the ground floor – which was like a bungalow looking out onto wonderful grounds – to then being on the level three of another unit. But then it's like anything; what you gain somewhere you lose somewhere else. We've now got access to so many more facilities, from a staff point of view but also from a patient point of view, clinical point of view, all the services are here on site whereas we were isolated before. It opened our eyes to the big wide world of what is available in the general hospital. (Theater nurse)

This exposure to the 'big wide world' of the main hospital was also reflected in increased opportunities for staff to network with their peers in other parts of the Trust:

> You see colleagues that you would never see other than at meetings and usually it's at those meetings that you're trying to sort out problems. It's that informal social interaction that takes place in the corridors that you weren't part of before that I think is hugely important. (Senior manager)

The PEOC's move to the main hospital site was similarly perceived by staff and the chief executive as having impacted positively on the wider organization as well:

> I think there was a tendency in the past to blame somebody across the road for not playing ball, because it's easier when you don't know the people very well and there isn't that personal relationship . . . No matter how hard you try, it feels different if you've got a second site. What surprised me was, whilst there was pride in the orthopedics center, the bulk of that pride was over the road. There was what I call adolescent pride here [in the main hospital], almost a sibling rivalry. What we've been able to do in getting a single site is actually exploit and get rid of those sibling rivalries, by . . . focusing people to work together in a different way. (Chief executive)

Interactions and interpretations: bridging the macro- and micro-systems

Having separately explored the macro- and micro-systems, we now turn our attention to identifying how the interactions between the two levels – and the interpretations used to frame these relationships – lead to sustained quality in frontline healthcare. In particular, this section addresses how the two levels work together to manage and sustain the unique identity of the orthopedics department while ensuring it contributes to the performance and goals of the wider organization. We focus first on a key role that bridges the macro- and micro-systems (leaders as 'issue sellers'), and second on a critical enabling attribute of the relationship between the two systems at the RD&E – the high levels of trust.

Leaders as 'issue sellers'

Micro-systems are often more relevant to an individual 'than a more abstract, complex, secondary organization' (such as a macro-system).[19,20] Therefore, a key role for leaders at the macro-system level is finding ways to secure employees' attention to and understanding of events, developments and trends that may have implications for wider organizational performance,[21,22] a process also termed 'issue selling'.[23]

From this perspective it is not necessary for the macro- and micro-systems to be strictly aligned in all respects of their culture and operations, merely jointly articulated and compatible. On the one hand, as we have seen, an important role of macro-system leaders is to cultivate a corporate sense of identity and commitment; on the other, leaders in the micro-system under study here attempt to cultivate and harness the same on a departmental and professional level. In the absence of any mediation, the two systems could easily become disconnected or dysfunctional (working in different directions) due to the inherent tensions between corporacy and professional autonomy that exist in most healthcare organizations.[24]

The classic task for those at the interface of these levels is to manage the tensions involved.[25] For example, if leaders and other key individuals located in such positions fail in this regard, there is a clear danger that the micro-system in particular may become parochial, xenophobic and excessively inward-looking. Therefore, these roles are lubricants, acting as translators between the macro-system (the 'organization') and the micro-system. The ability to interpret between the managerial and clinical languages of both levels is especially important when the different identities of each are so strong, as in this case study:

> They're the jam in the sandwich. If you think about the role that [the directorate manager] undertakes, and all the directors undertake, they have [a] top team and the clinical teams and they have to create some kind of mutual language, so that when we talk targets, there's an interpretation that takes place about what that individual patient needs. I think that's the critical factor and if their translator isn't working then nobody's translator is working. (Director of operations)

'Selling' QI initiatives – notably those originating from central government imperatives, such as the NHS's targets for booked admissions for patients – is not necessarily an easy task in micro-systems with an ingrained sense of their own professional identity, where frontline staff often perceive there to be greater and more immediate priorities:

> Booking is actually really important for a lot of people . . . But on the other hand, in the grand scheme of things and with some of their [PEOC's] other priorities, I can understand where they're coming from. That's about me working with them at the right level to recognize where it fits in with their priorities, and how we ensure that it fits in with something else. (Services development manager)

Similarly, the chief executive felt that as long as such QI activities were framed in terms of improving patient care and finding a close fit between the external NHS context and the service priorities of those at the micro-system level, then the organization could still deliver and staff would not feel disenfranchised:

> We are part of the NHS and we are taking the King's shillings and therefore we have to do some of these things, whatever we might feel about them. You will still see the same level of commitment, lots of people getting involved and doing it, because . . . in the end it always goes back to making a real difference in patient care. Where it's making a difference in patient care, people will engage with it, whatever their reservations are about the process. (Chief executive)

This 'interpretive' work is of special importance in healthcare organizations in which managers typically are unable to use traditional rewards or punishments to influence the behavior of busy clinical professionals who often have multiple and competing loyalties – to patients, to their practice, and to hospitals.[26,27] Thus, such efforts often require overcoming not only a great deal of ambivalence among clinicians, but in many cases cynicism as well. Speaking about one of the orthopedic consultants, one interviewee remarked, 'He takes cynicism to new heights. If it was an Olympic sport, he'd be the marksman for cynicism.'

In some respects actions speak louder than words, and dissipating such cynicism depends on the direct experiences that staff have with Trust-wide quality initiatives that demonstrate the benefits to the work and care provided to patients. For example, members of the PEOC viewed participating in the work of the Trust's modernization team and quality improvement programs such as the Pursuing Perfection initiative (mentioned earlier) as contributing both to the PEOC and to the wider hospital:

> We've been involved in modernization work and all sorts of bits and pieces really: looking at getting patients in for hip replacements the same day, so they come in in the morning and go for surgery thereby reducing the length of stay. This ward is one of the pilot sites for Pursuing Perfection and we've managed to reduce our discharge time, which helps the rest of the Trust because it means we have a quicker flow-through of patients. (Senior nurse)

Once the framing of the quality agenda in terms meaningful to clinicians is achieved, and direct experiences prove it of mutual value to both the macro- and micro-systems on the ground, clinical staff can become one of the driving forces behind the success of quality and service improvement initiatives:

> . . . the doctors know if they work with us they get more. So long as there are winners on both sides it keeps things moving along. (Senior manager)

> Once they take ownership, they're amazing!! You know you can put it in there and it will go. But it's getting them to take ownership, because once they [do] they make it a success. (Services development manager)

Trust and respect

The shock to the organization's identity caused by the breast cancer screening crisis had led us, via 'walking the talk' and issue selling, to the 'now' of the organization: open, informal and collegial. One particular attribute of the relationship between the macro- and micro-systems in the current organization stood out from our fieldwork: the high level of trust between the leaders and staff at both levels of the RD&E.

This began with widespread respect for the chief executive, who set the tone for relationships between the administrative and clinical staff throughout the Trust:

> The reason this Trust is so enjoyable to work in is the relationship between managers and medical staff. We get on well together, we communicate well, there's a mutual respect and it stems from [the chief executive]. (Medical director)

> She [the chief executive] is so accessible. You walk into the dining room and she'll come and tap you on the shoulder – not just me but an A grade or anybody – and I think that's what makes the difference. It's the same with any of the directors: you know them all and see them in the corridor, they will talk to you. You're not just there as a worker; you're also a person and that's what makes a difference and I think that's what comes down. (Senior nurse)

Trust (or mistrust) is based on expectations of others' behavior, typically as the result of past experiences and interactions with those individuals or groups.[28] The objective of members of the macro-system in interacting with frontline departments and staff was that they perceive the Trust as being honest and 'playing it straight'.

> There might be times when negotiations have to take place and they might not necessarily always be what they wanted but . . . [b]ack to honesty – that there would be an honest exchange. I would like them to think that they were always dealt with honestly and that there wasn't any kind of underhand manipulation that took place that they were uncomfortable with. (Chief executive)

The members of the macro-system also have striven for frontline departments and staff to truly believe that the RD&E leadership sincerely 'have the best interests of the organization and patient care at heart . . . to care about what happens . . . and are prepared to put themselves out'. Similarly, they have sought to develop a spirit of comradeship such that staff at the micro-system level know that the executive team, and the chief executive in particular, 'will be there batting with them', that 'they are not fighting alone', and that the Trust would be 'fighting their corner'.

The high level of trust between members of the macro- and micro-systems was partly attributed to the clear recognition of interdependencies between them, and in particular the respective roles and responsibilities of managers and clinicians. While recognizing the role they had to play in 'protecting' and 'defending' the micro-systems, members of the macro-system were also clear about the most important contributor to quality of service and image of the organization: the quality of the clinical practitioners:

> My philosophy is 'let's be clear about why patients come to this organization'. They come here because GPs believe we have clinicians who are good: they don't come because I am here, or because the Trust board is here. They come because we have clinicians delivering a good service. You have to value that – you may have to deal with deviate behavior from time to time, but if people believe that you are valuing the majority, the message that goes around the organization when 'she' has dealt with somebody is generally 'for it to have got to that point it must have been serious because that is not the way they normally behave': the body of the kirk says, 'on balance she's usually right'. (Chief executive)

At the same time, leaders within the PEOC showed respect and appreciation for the role of the macro-system and the collaborative and mutually beneficial manner in which the executive of the Trust pursues the mandate for the organization as a whole.

> I don't think the quality of patient care is any better or any worse now than it was when we were on another site. What has helped has been since we've come here, we've had this target-driven NHS that we're all working for. I think we now deliver the same quality of

service but in a much happier management environment we have to hit these targets, it's in our shared interests. (Directorate manager)

A consequence of this understanding – and valuing – of each others' roles and, in essence, the distinct identities of the macro- and micro-systems, is a deepened trust upon which both levels can pursue improvement of the organization.

The implications of identity for sustained quality

Clearly, the journey to quality at the RD&E has not been solely about identity. There is certainly much in the macro-system story of the Trust that concerns general cultural change towards openness, informality and collegiality, leading to structural and operational changes, such as a particular governance and 'quality' infrastructure and decentralization of the quality agenda in response to the breast cancer screening crisis. Yet it is difficult to ignore the extent to which these cultural and institutional changes have become ingrained in the Trust's identity, or deeper cultural sense of 'who we are' and 'what we stand for'.[1] This sense or identity is considered to represent the central, enduring and distinctive character of an organization[3] that encapsulates and helps preserve the core values, beliefs and shared attachments of individuals and groups within the organization.

It is also hard to disregard how, as relayed to us by those we interviewed and met more informally during our fieldwork, the particular governance and decentralized approach of the Trust has allowed clinical micro-systems such as the PEOC to retain a strong sense of their separate identity, so essential to their own ability to maintain consistently high levels of performance and quality of care.

Identity, performance and quality

The extent to which individual employees identify with their organization has long been recognized as affecting both the satisfaction of individual members and the effectiveness of the organization.[19,20,29] For example, research in the US has showed that physicians who perceived the identity and external image of the healthcare systems to which they were affiliated to be relatively more attractive tended to identify more closely with their respective organizations, which in turn was related to co-operative behaviors.[8] Similarly, attachment to one's organization has been positively correlated with greater amounts of 'extra role' behavior,[30] such as spending time helping newcomers, working on long-term projects, pushing others to perform to higher standards, or providing ideas for improving the organization.[4]

As we found in both the RD&E and the PEOC, the feeling of solidarity that emerges among individuals through group affiliation can serve as a powerful catalyst for collective action; they become 'linked together in a number of ways that generate a sense of common identity, shared fate and general commitment to defend the group',[31] which also resonates with recent work exploring the concept of communities of practice in the healthcare setting[32] (see also the San Diego case in Chapter 2 and Cedars-Sinai case in Chapter 4).

It was clear that the very sincere attachments within the PEOC to the department's tradition and reputation played a significant part in engaging staff, particularly clinicians, to apply the creativity and energy – what might be termed 'discretionary effort' – necessary to generate innovation, high standards of care, and continual improvements in service that are so difficult to mandate or contractually coerce.

Of course, affiliation with an organization may also confer negative attributions towards its members. If individuals find themselves at odds with the espoused identity of their organization or perceive its external image as unfavorable, they may de- or dis-identify with the organization,[33] reducing co-operation, withdrawing effort, or even leaving the organization entirely. The leadership of the RD&E was able to avert this danger during the breast cancer screening crisis by using the sharply critical public treatment of the Trust as a rallying point to bond members and redeem the institution, as opposed to letting the crisis devolve into a situation in which members would feel compelled to detach themselves from the organization (either figuratively or literally). As a result, the RD&E was able to transform the crisis into a motivator for change, maintaining (or even increasing) the devotion of its staff while redefining the identity of the organization in the process.

Furthermore, the very distinct identity of the PEOC and the method of its incorporation into the overall Trust lend an interesting slant and insight into the dynamics between the macro- and micro-systems within healthcare organizations and their joint ability to achieve and sustain high-quality care.

Multiple identities within the RD&E and PEOC

Typically, 'organizations have multiple identities in multiple contexts with multiple audiences'.[3] The healthcare setting is a good illustration because of the multiple and competing identities typically found therein (i.e. specialty based, professionally based and organizationally based).[34–36] In the context of UK healthcare, these 'fabricated, pro-jected pictures have to be aimed at various constituencies': the Department of Health, strategic health authorities, regulatory bodies, local healthcare community partners, as well as internally to a healthcare organization's own staff. Given this complexity, the senior executive team – and particularly the chief executive – have a key role to play in shaping organizational identity and as image makers for the organization.[5]

As discussed above, the PEOC has retained its unique identity while becoming more closely incorporated within the Trust and aligned with the performance and goals of the wider organization. This accommodation was not by accident, nor only specific to the PEOC. The chief executive explains that it was, in fact, a deliberate strategy of the macro-system to deal with seeming paradoxes of identity arising in a large healthcare organization:

> Orthopedics isn't the only one that has its own front door, [although] it has the best front door coming in. We've done that deliberately, because we've rationalized from five sites down onto this site, and most of the departments that came from separate hospitals have their own entrance, and that's critically important in terms of identity and not being swallowed up. That's very important . . . I think if we hadn't put their own front doors in, they may feel they have to establish their own identity and the barriers become more fixed. (Chief executive)

As a consequence, the identities at the macro- and micro-levels are allowed to co-exist (and perhaps reinforce each other, to merge and overlap to some extent) rather than being expected or forced to become synthesized or uniform. Hence, this case study of the RD&E shows how it is possible for organizations, especially in healthcare, to accommodate and leverage the distinct professional and group identities within sub-units without appearing hopelessly fragmented or ludicrously schizophrenic.[37]

Organizational identity: an untapped resource?

Identity and identification are 'powerful lenses for explaining change, action and inaction by individuals and collectivities'.[38] As demonstrated in this case study of the RD&E, they help to explain why individuals act on behalf of the group or the organization, and the direction and persistence of collective behaviors such as efforts that contribute to high-quality care and continual improvement.

In addition, identity – whether corporate, departmental or professional – represents an internal, implicit and consequently deeply embedded 'check' on the quality of care. Strong positive identities can provide managers and employees with a sense of meaning, purpose and excitement, which can arouse commitment and even passion.

Another valuable finding from this case study is how multiple identities in an organization can accommodate each other in constructive ways. The interactions between the macro- and micro-systems at the RD&E came to mutually reinforce (as opposed to, at best, have no effect on) the quality of care provided. This reinforcement is revealed in the protective behaviors, both downwards ('keeping issues from outside away from' the micro-systems) and upwards (as evidenced by micro-system staff concerns for the chief executive if the Trust was unable to meet targets). It is also revealed in their mutual actions: the recognition that both are 'fighting for each other', and if they work together both will benefit. Such accommodation of identities and respect for each others' roles has not only served to build trust between the different levels of the institution, but also allowed the RD&E to tap into the multiple professional and departmental identities common within healthcare settings to engage staff in the quality agenda across the organization.

At the RD&E the catalyst for this process was a crisis within a particular service, indicating the potential and importance for leaders to manage and shape organizational identities. Such identities can then act as invaluable organizational supports for specific initiatives and infrastructure to improve quality.

As the enduring and central traits of an organization and the groups within it, organizational identities constitute a relatively stable cultural 'bedrock' on which to support and anchor a quality agenda. Understanding this property offers the potential to address the key imperative of sustainability that continues to plague quality research and practice in healthcare; i.e. the persistent tendency of quality efforts to flounder amidst the ebbs and flows of forces acting upon and within healthcare organizations. Thus, organizational identities represent a steady – yet all-too-frequently unacknowledged – reservoir of commitment and motivation, and an often untapped resource in healthcare that can sustain quality performance and improvement over the long haul.

4

Organizational learning and sustained improvement: the quality journey at Cedars-Sinai Medical Center, Los Angeles

ORIGINAL CASE STUDY RESEARCHED BY PETER MENDEL AND PAUL BATE; NARRATIVE PREPARED BY PETER MENDEL

The story of quality improvement (QI) at Cedars-Sinai Medical Center stretches over two decades, representing a journey of accumulated organizational learning, change and customization of quality approaches, methods and tools (*see* Box 4.1). During this time the US healthcare field in general has gone through a similar period of experimentation with various innovations and approaches to quality, but, interestingly, with less impressive results. As a system, we are still left with the challenge of how to spread and sustain QI throughout healthcare and make continuous improvement a normal and common feature of the typical organization providing health services,[1] and in this regard we may have much to learn from the Cedars story.

This challenge can to some extent be understood as developing the ability of the organization itself to learn (including learning how to improve). Learning can be considered 'organizational' in the sense that lessons from an institution's experiences are incorporated into the formal and informal routines that comprise the operating life of an organization, independently of any of the particular individuals who perform them.[2] There may also be different depths to which organizations learn: from first-order change that results in new procedures or the use of new technologies, to second-order change in mindsets and patterns of decision-making that augment the capacity of the organization to absorb and act on new knowledge. This latter 'double-loop' learning,[3,4] in essence learning how to learn, is arguably at the heart of current notions of continuous quality improvement (CQI) and is, as the Cedars-Sinai case demonstrates, crucial to sustaining an improvement trajectory within an organization.

For organizational learning to occur requires engaging in two related processes: exploration and exploitation.[5] Exploration involves a search for new knowledge and technologies, and learning about new ways of thinking and working. Exploitation involves taking advantage of what the organization and its members already know and profiting from investments in intellectual and social capital accrued through prior exploration. A main focus in this line of research has been the degree to which organizations must balance the risks and costs of exploration and the stagnation of over-exploitation.[6,7] Achieving effective organizational learning, however, depends not only on the relative balance of resources devoted to each activity, but also on understanding how either process can be accomplished successfully. In the case of healthcare organizations especially, this understanding is not entirely clear.

BOX 4.1 Case profile: Cedars-Sinai Medical Center, Los Angeles

---

CASE PROFILE

Type of Organization:	Acute care hospital center, founded by the Jewish community. Includes integrated health, mental health, and research programs and services.
Focal Micro-System:	Emergency department
Size:	One of the largest non-profit hospitals in the western US. 875 acute care beds, over 6600 employees and 1700 affiliated physicians.
Location:	Los Angeles, California. Primary service area covers 2 million urban residents from gritty parts of West Hollywood to posh Beverly Hills.
Country:	United States
Awards and Recognitions:	Most Preferred Hospital in Southern California, Consumer Choice Award (NRC, several years running); No. 2 Ranking of National Metropolitan Hospitals (AARP 2002); California Council for Excellence Award (2000); Magnet Excellence in Nursing (ANCC 2000); Top 100 Most Wired Hospitals (Hospital and Health Networks); reputation as Hollywood's 'hospital to the stars'.

KEY CONCEPTS

Organizational Learning: the encoding of organizational experiences and lessons into an institution's formal and informal routines that will outlast the tenure of any specific individuals. Includes 'second order' changes in organizational mindsets and information processing that augment the capacity of the organization to absorb and act upon new knowledge.

Bricolage: literally meaning 'brick laying', this term refers to the disassembling of diverse sets of organizational forms, models and paradigms, and the recombination of selected components into distinctly new and coherent organizational structures and practices. A key process in the ability to customize quality approaches to the context of a particular organization.

This case study recounts the journey of organizational learning at Cedars-Sinai Medical Center at both the executive level of the medical center as a whole (macro-system), and within a clinical unit (micro-system) with notable achievements in QI, the emergency department (ED). The study examines not only what Cedars-Sinai as an organization has been able to develop and incorporate in terms of quality approaches and practices, but also the process of this accumulated learning and how it has been maintained over the past two decades.

At first blush this might not seem so surprising. Cedars-Sinai, one of the largest non-profit voluntary hospital centers on the west coast of the United States, is a relatively well-endowed institution with a national reputation for clinical innovation and the expertise of its medical staff. Such clinical excellence, however, does not always equate to service excellence, let alone to continuous improvement in organizational systems. In fact, an organization's prior success may serve as a barrier to learning new practices and willingness to change and adapt to new circumstances.[8,9]

In particular, it should not be underestimated how difficult it is for any organization to learn adaptively. Many organizations fail to explore to any significant extent, succumbing to internal inertia and becoming calcified, closed systems.[10] It is also easy for organizations to derive the 'wrong' (i.e. maladaptive) lessons, given rapidly changing external conditions, and the problems of selective attention, limits to human cognition, and reliance on available information that is more often than not imperfect or ambiguous.[11,12] Indeed, the environments facing organizations are chock-full of solutions and recipes for improvement, a veritable (and noisy) 'market of reform'.[13]

Organizations must therefore selectively search, filter and make sense of this information,[14] and generic descriptions of new practices must be translated and modified when they are imported into local settings[15,16] and actively rendered salient, familiar and compelling in order to take hold.[17] Organizations also show a tendency to adopt new reforms as fads or fashions; i.e. in name or gesture only, as 'talk' and not action.[18,19] Such symbolic adoption may help legitimate a medical institution as a modern organization but not necessarily be associated with changes in its core operations and performance.[20,21] As a result, when a hospital adopts a particular quality approach, such as TQM, there is a question as to whether this represents mere conformity to prevailing management trends or customization in terms of deeper organizational learning and change.[22]

In the case of Cedars-Sinai, both the medical center and the ED managed this customization or translation of new quality paradigms and techniques by constantly sifting, weeding, taking apart, and retaining, absorbing and refashioning the useful aspects of externally sourced or internally generated approaches. Students of culture and organizations have termed this type of process *bricolage*, the piecing together and layering of components from seemingly distinct models into new, identifiable and coherently functioning sets of practices.[23,24] For example, this case study describes how 'key aspects of care', distilled from the institution's experimentation with clinical pathways, were melded with the Joint Commission's later requirement to monitor 'core measures', and how in the ED the unit's academically oriented health services research has provided a basis for more hands-on continuous improvement activities.

Probably more important than the specific QI approaches that Cedars-Sinai has learned, however, are the processes by which this accumulated bricolage of quality has been constructed, and the glue or mortar the institution has used to bind these elements into a coherent path of sustained improvement. There are three elements crucial to the organization's journey in this regard:

- ❏ a *learning culture* rooted in the particular history and identity of the institution and actively oriented towards supporting organizational improvement
- ❏ a *learning infrastructure* comprising boundary-spanning roles within the organization, a series of interlinked committees and governance boards, and other resources for sharing knowledge and bringing focus to improvement activities
- ❏ *communities of learning* that help to engage the energy and commitment of individuals toward a quality agenda at both the micro- and macro-levels of the institution.

History, culture, and the journey towards improvement at Cedars-Sinai

The current Cedars-Sinai Medical Center is the product of the merger in 1961 of two hospitals, both founded at the turn of the twentieth century by the local immigrant Jewish community in Los Angeles: Cedars of Lebanon Hospital established in 1902, and Mount Sinai Hospital established in 1918. The merged institution moved into its present campus location in 1976.[25]

Although retaining homage to particular religious traditions, such as a Jewish chaplain and kosher food service, the Judaic heritage of the institution is most strongly reflected in what the medical center's own literature describes as devotion to both the 'art' and 'science' of medicine; i.e. medicine as a healing profession as well as medical research and education.[26] To one senior vice president, a veteran of the institution of over 20 years, Cedars-Sinai is a rare 'hybrid between an academic and community hospital'. Staff strongly 'hold to a mission' of serving the community and humanistic treatment towards patients and staff. They also display the 'depth of intellectual capacity' and affinity for 'constant learning' that are characteristic of an academic institution.

Another senior vice president describes the implications of this academic orientation in terms of a general sense of collegiality ('never personalizing issues', 'opinion is okay, but show me the facts'), and an emphasis on consensus-based decision-making ('carrying a consensus' from one level to another, particularly among the executive ranks). Another top executive with over 20 years' tenure sees the lasting cultural imprint[27,28] of the institution's immigrant roots in its continuing 'ethic of striving for excellence' and 'passion for excellence in everything that we do'.

A senior leader of the medical staff describes how this striving for excellence is manifested through expectations regarding the expertise and reputation of the hospital's clinicians:

> I think what makes [Cedars-Sinai] outstanding is our physicians . . . We're not a medical school, but we function in many respects like one. We have a huge resource of attending physicians who, in their private practices have become leaders in their own fields . . . We have on purpose tried to set the bar a little bit higher here than other institutions in terms of the medical staff, and in terms of quality issues and so on . . . (Senior medical staff leader)

In addition to the influence from Cedars' community constituents, the expectations of particularly high-end clientele, although only a small proportion of the patient population, can create self-reinforcing pressures to maintain the reputation of the institution. As a top management executive explained:

> . . . there is a feedback loop that goes on as well. Were we a great institution that ended up taking care of high demanding people, or did we just happen to be a good institution that was around high demanding people that made us great or strive for greatness? . . . The irony is . . . we have this reputation as the 'hospital to the stars', but the [high end] clientele is really a very small percentage of the people we see. Still, the image of the 'hospital to the stars' drives a lot of the culture. (Senior executive)

Physician leaders in the ED similarly describe the self-reinforcing pressures of the hospital's reputation applied through the expectations of patients:

> One of the downsides of Cedars is the expectations of people. For whatever reason, they expect more here. Even the ED. If somebody comes to the Cedars ED, they expect to be seen right away, taken back right away, put in a room right away, get all the tests right

> away . . . go upstairs right away. None of which happens unless you're lucky or it's not
> very crowded. And sometimes when somebody is nasty, they'll use it against you. They'll
> say, 'Is this Cedars-Sinai?' (Co-chair of ED)

The image of the 'hospital to the stars' and the remark 'Is this Cedars-Sinai?' indicate that the striving for excellence represents not merely an ethic or element of the working culture at Cedars-Sinai, but has also become ingrained into the identity of the organization and its participants' sense of 'who we are'[29,30] (see, in particular, the Royal Devon and Exeter case study in Chapter 3). This identity is further reinforced by a host of external recognitions and national awards,[31,32] which lend a sense of external validation to the image held by the various constituents, both within and outside the organization (see Box 4.1 above).

Despite its national reputation, Cedars-Sinai experiences many of the same short-comings and challenges to providing quality care as other healthcare organizations. The account of one senior physician leader suggests this can be a humbling experience, prompting questioning and self-examination:

> The Quality Council meets every two weeks or so. The first half hour is a presentation
> of significant adverse events that the chief of staff chairs. We have the same [types of
> issues] . . . as everybody else, and at that meeting . . . we all hear the [events] and try to
> analyze what happened . . . and it kind of makes everyone humble, because even in what
> is perceived to be an outstanding institution in the States, mistakes and errors happen
> . . . (Senior medical staff leader)

Cedars-Sinai not only shares many of the same challenges to quality of care as other healthcare institutions, but it also faces similar fiscal pressures endemic throughout the healthcare field in the US. Since the advent of 'managed care' insurance and competitive changes in the 1980s and 1990s, Cedars-Sinai, along with other hospital and health systems, has experienced cyclic swings in financial margins. As described below, these profound changes in the wider healthcare environment would provide one of the initial impetuses to the institution's 'quality journey'.

The journey towards improvement

In the early 1980s the conception of quality at Cedars-Sinai, as in most healthcare organizations, rested on the traditional definitions of the medical profession; that is, almost solely in terms of individual clinician training and judgement. Assessment of clinical quality was the province of professional peer review panels, which focused on *post-hoc* examination of clinician behavior and procedure, but less on systematic appraisal of the organizational context and process of care. To the extent that the latter were addressed, this occurred through the accreditation process, which, as described by a senior medical administrator who practised in the hospital at the time, was considered a 'paper obligation' handled by 'more clerical' people and 'generally irrelevant' to the medical staff.

The first turning point in the hospital's shift towards QI took place in the mid-1980s with the formation of a Health Services Research section within the department of general medicine (see Box 4.2).

Although an admittedly academic approach, it focused attention on the relationship between the process of care and outcomes, and on the use of that information for improvement within the organization:

> We began taking information analyzed internally and presenting it to medical staff
> committees and administrative areas, because we felt that if people actually had

information, they would be able to use it and make rational decisions, and if we can do that compared against the literature, that means we would have some real opportunities for improvement, and that was one of the major turning points. (Senior medical administrator)

BOX 4.2 Milestones in Cedars-Sinai's quality journey

1986:	Health Services Research section formed
1991:	QI 91 – Xerox quality training
1992:	Medical staff task forces, training in service data and analysis
	Hiring of MD/MPH with strong QI background and connection to IHI
	IHI training and collaboratives began
1994/95:	From Clinical Pathways to Key Aspects/Core Measures
	Quality Council, chaired by CEO
1998:	PICOS lean manufacturing – GM consultants, via IHI
2000, 2001:	Institute of Medicine reports
2000:	Physician Leadership Development Program
2001/02:	Physician–Administration Compact, Code of Conduct

As one of the hospital's top executives describes, this reflected an academic medical center 'changing with the times' as it adapted its core mission and research expertise to new ends:

> And there you have the evolution of the core historical mission of the institution as an academic medical center changing with the times of the environment around it; health services research became a legitimate discipline. (Senior executive)

Soon after, profound changes in insurance, market and governance conditions culminated in what would be known by the early 1990s as the 'managed care' revolution in American healthcare, resulting in a new and intense set of competitive and cost pressures on hospitals and medical providers of all stripes.[33] In the case of Cedars-Sinai, such external trends again were translated in a manner commensurate with its historical values and mission, yielding another major turning point in the journey towards QI:

> The next major turning point was about 1990 . . . We were once again facing economic pressures . . . cost pressure on all hospitals and looking at ways to reduce length of stay, reduce cost per case in a safe evidence-based way . . . So our position was rather than just cutting X, Y, Z off the budget, we would work with our medical staff to identify opportunities based upon institutional comparisons and literature searches and things of that nature. (Senior medical administrator)

As part of this response, the hospital engaged a consulting firm to begin organizing a series of task forces and training in service data and analysis for the medical staff. These committees would later form the basis of the Performance Improvement Program, the backbone of Cedars-Sinai's infrastructure for improvement described later. In the meantime, the hospital introduced a more short-lived quality training initiative in the administrative ranks, called QI 91, based on a program developed at the Xerox Corporation. Although exclusively focused on non-clinical, back-end business processes, the program represented an important 'baby step' towards 'structured quality'.

By 1992 the medical staff task forces had evolved into standing 'performance improvement committees', or PICs, addressing a wide range of QI issues throughout the hospital:

> I think that was a major change by the beginning of the 90s, when we started having the PICs. We had pretty much monthly committee meetings in place for years, but the structure has evolved from a medical advisory group, which had a different direction, to actual performance improvement. (Senior medical staff leader)

During this same time, a physician had recently completed an internship at Cedars-Sinai towards his master of public health (MPH) degree. Such hybrid physicians–management professionals – medical doctors who also acquire managerial training and thus more easily bridge the clinical and administrative worlds – had become increasingly common as the result of managed care trends.[34] In this spirit, the hospital decided to hire this physician to lend clinical background and credibility to the quality effort. He would also prove to be a 'boundary spanner'[35,36] in another sense, acting as a pivotal conduit of ideas and contacts from wider networks of QI in healthcare emerging at the national level:

> So he ... and [a previously hired non-clinical consultant] ... became a team and began to bring to the institution a whole discipline around analyzing process, flow diagrams, cradle diagrams ... and we began to infuse the organization with that approach. We linked up then with the national demonstration project, later becoming the Institute for Healthcare Improvement. [He] became faculty in the IHI and kept us connected with a network of people who had a growing similar interest around these kinds of things. (Senior medical administrator)

At this early point in the medical center's quality journey, the challenge of changing traditional mindsets about quality from an academic or strictly clinical perspective to an 'improvement' orientation loomed especially large. This change included both how to systematically conceptualize organizational processes, as well as how to implement improvement:

> ... I mean in 1991 when you start with a flow diagram on the wall, people looked at it like, 'What is this?' But that was part of the learning curve to getting people to think about processes ... now the lingo is you're sitting in a meeting and somebody is talking about running a 'test of change', and that's a giant leap forward ... [I]n those days ... we'd pilot on one floor and ... if it works here – as is – we'll go house wide, instead of testing it in one place, seeing what's wrong with it, redesigning it, then adding another floor. But that was the healthcare model, that wasn't unique to Cedars. (QI director)

One of the first quality initiatives from this period illustrates the gradual organizational 'learning curve' in implementing QI and how the initial process of introducing change was conditioned by the culture of the institution, particularly among the medical staff. This early effort was directed at restricting the prescription of Demerol based on the extensive literature that had emerged contraindicating many uses for the drug:

> The culture and the rules of engagement still tilt in favor of respecting the individual physician's prerogatives. For example, we had an issue with the use of Demerol for pain. We went through education, we went through cajoling, we went through a year and a half and watched the graph get better, get worse. Get better, get worse. And finally, after paying respect to the individual physician prerogative ... the MEC [Medical Executive

> Committee] finally . . . put the auto-substitution in place . . . [N]ow maybe in theory, that ends up with more lasting acceptance. I'm not sure. But, speaking to you as someone that's actively involved and my own frustration about not moving fast enough, part of it is that ethic within the medical staff to give their colleagues a lot more latitude. (Senior executive)

Despite the time and difficulty of the Demerol project, the experience was encapsulated as a story which has been invoked to speed along later efforts:

> It makes it easier, because you can always tell the story. So, in the middle of the beta-blocker discussion somebody says, 'We're really not going to spend the two-year Demerol project on this, are we?' There is an institutional recollection . . . (QI director)

Such organizational 'stories' represent a major repository of culture[37] and an important mechanism of organizational learning by encoding the lessons of collective experiences into readily understood institutional shorthand. Moreover, culturally relevant stories and metaphors can be imported from outside the institution – another role of boundary spanners in organizational learning:

> In the current thinking of most physicians, the VA [Department of Veterans Affairs Health Administration] is a pit . . . but today the VA is one of the safest places in the world. So when you start telling stories about what's happened in the VA, that is helpful as well, in the sense that if the VA can change then we can change. (QI director)

In addition to importing ideas and concepts, boundary spanners can facilitate the connections of others within the organization to external networks and experiences. As mentioned above, the physician brought on board to guide quality efforts at the medical center also served as one of the initial faculty for the IHI, whose 'collaboratives' and other programs bring together groups of organizations interested in learning and working on specific QI issues. Cedars-Sinai participated in a number of these collaboratives from the early 1990s onward, which have provided staff with quality concepts and skills, as well as inspiration and experiences that have helped deepen the culture and commitment towards QI in various areas within the hospital.

> Well, for example, IHI had a collaborative on C-sections. So we sent a team . . . [It was] this concept of taking some people who were believers and non-believers and making them the team . . . they develop a relationship with one another and then come back and become the champions in the OB group to do that. So, where you didn't have a 'knee-deep' situation, that certainly works. (QI director)

In the mid-1990s Cedars-Sinai experimented with clinical pathways, an approach to standardize typical processes of care that had begun to gain increased prominence in health services. Although Cedars' experience with pathways was not as promising as that of other healthcare organizations (*see*, for example, the San Diego Children's Hospital case study, Chapter 2), the approach was not wholly abandoned, but distilled into what the hospital termed 'key aspects of care'.

> In mid-1994, 1995, we were doing a lot of pathways work and it started to get complicated . . . especially when a patient had two or more other co-morbidities . . . We finally came to a point in realizing it doesn't work for us. We said there were things that worked out of it though . . . For the care for the total hip patient . . . as I recall, there were three: getting the patient out of bed in 24 hours, the pre-op antibiotics, and DVT prophylaxis. If you did those three things, your outcomes in hips are better. So we moved to what we call 'key aspects of care', which were those key details. (QI director)

Not long after, the key aspects of care merged relatively easily into the Joint Commission's (JCAHO) accreditation requirements to track performance on a set of 'core measures':

> We started the 'key aspects of care' and then the Joint Commission came along with the core measures, and in essence the core measures are really the Commission's key aspects of care – we would like to think. So, for those things where there are core measures, they are transparent key aspects of care. (QI director)

The road from clinical pathways to 'key aspects of care' and the core measures is a central and striking example at Cedars-Sinai of how components of quality paradigms from various sources have been extracted and layered into new and unique programs and practices. This process of bricolage, as described by a senior clinical leader, is motivated by an underlying pragmatism to exploit new approaches in ways best suited to driving improvement within the organization:

> . . . we realized that [clinical pathways] was adding a lot to paperwork but it wasn't actually having significant input to change, whereas the core measures are really narrowed down, they're measurable and they seem to have a much bigger impact. (Senior medical staff leader)

As Cedars-Sinai's experience suggests, arriving at a new approach through this process can qualitatively affect the application in practice and its implications for the organization. For example, the core measures have been integrated into a set of aggregate trend indicators, or 'dashboards', with much more of an emphasis on analyzing processes and identifying areas for improvement than might be expected if the approach had been adopted solely for compliance reasons:

> The concept of measurement has snowballed. So, as opposed to the early years, people now say, 'Where is the data?' . . . [And] I think more and more . . . one of the advantages of having the dashboards is there is an obligation to measure the foundation and look at the data when [they] come out, and by putting a cover memo on a dashboard, we're pinpointing what the issues are and the observations. (QI director)

By this point in the mid-1990s a myriad of activities and structures supporting QI had clearly begun to flourish within the medical center. In 1995 the Quality Council, an important capstone to this quality movement, was established. Chaired by Cedars' chief executive, and comprising other top executives including the vice president of finance and senior leaders of the medical staff, the Council consolidates oversight and vision for quality across the hospital and elevates QI efforts and goals into the strategic process of the organization.

Despite all of this quality activity, in the next several years Cedars-Sinai continued to explore new quality approaches and techniques, taking considerable care in deciding which to adopt and how they were to be utilized. For example, PICOS, a 'lean manufacturing' program developed at General Motors and introduced to the medical center in 1998 through its connection with IHI, appeared applicable mainly to non-clinical and ancillary areas of the hospital. Six Sigma, a popular quality methodology developed by Motorola, was still under scrutiny as to whether 'it's right for clinical care'.

As with the core measures, the implementation of new external requirements continued to be modified to better suit the purposes of the hospital. For instance, JCAHO's mandated sentinel event process to identify and examine instances of medical errors was reworked into a 'significant adverse event' process that also includes 'near miss' events. How such new processes are imported into the organization may be as important as what is adopted:

> ... if I brought something in from the Joint Commission and said, they dropped it here on our doorstep and we have to do it, then there would be resistance. But if you take that and say there is something good here that we can work with, I think that's helpful. (QI director)

Around the same time as the sentinel event process, the Institute of Medicine issued its two landmark reports on healthcare quality, *To Err is Human*[38] and *Crossing the Quality Chasm*.[39] The national attention generated by these reports provided a degree of external validation to Cedars-Sinai's past efforts. Senior advocates of the quality agenda were also able to successfully capitalise on the attention, using the reports as a vehicle for further mobilizing various constituencies within the hospital around patient safety and QI.

> The IOM report was powerful. There was great public credibility about that and suddenly people were talking about safety and harm and that was different ... We went around with a PowerPoint presentation on it, and we didn't get stuck in the details ... Thousands of people a year were dying and there might be something we could do about it. (QI director)

Throughout this period the transformations taking place in healthcare were unsettling not only to the medical center but to physicians as well, serving to leave many of the hospital's affiliated doctors disaffected. Motivated by these changes, the medical staff instituted another milestone in Cedars-Sinai's quality journey, an innovative clinician-led physician leadership development program. The objective of the program was to create a collegial community to reinvigorate and prepare physician leaders for the new healthcare environment facing the medical staff and the institution in general, as described in more detail below.

It was not long before the leadership program resulted in a physician–administration compact, outlining mutual obligations between the medical staff and hospital administration:

> ... by the end of the second year [of the physician leadership program] ... one of the doctors said, 'Wait a minute, where's the administration?' ... So we had a mini-retreat with the administration and basically said, what are your expectations and what are our expectations? ... [W]e developed a compact ... [which] never would have existed if it weren't for the leadership development program. (Senior physician leader)

This spirit of forming and bridging communities committed to improvement across many areas within the institution was further extended through a code of conduct detailing expectations for physician treatment of nursing and other staff, and by the implementation of the 'MD/RN collaboratives', a series of interdisciplinary meetings and joint grand rounds for physicians, nurses and other clinical professionals within each department.

Customization, bricolage and organizational learning

As we have seen, Cedars-Sinai's quality journey demonstrates a long-term accumulation of innovations and organizational experience into an infrastructure, culture and set of communities supporting QI. Crucial to this organizational learning has been the process of customizing new paradigms and techniques through the pragmatic layering of disparate – perhaps even seemingly discordant – elements. This can be seen in the progression from academic health services research to training in service data and analysis, and eventually medical staff committees addressing quality issues in different areas, as well as in the transition from clinical pathways to key aspects of care and core measures.

The experience of the ED has mirrored, and in some cases foreshadowed, this journey. Like the hospital, the ED's own program in services research has served as a basis for QI in a number of areas:

> Initially, a lot of this [quality] stuff came out of research methodology, kind of old fashion and not rapid cycle, test of change methodology. For instance, some of my first quality work was really a research project. Stuff that I presented in papers at meetings, but they obviously had value as a quality tool. For instance, we had an earthquake in 1994, so we studied that from an operational side to present at the meeting. In fact, it had applications in both fields. (ED physician leader)

Also like the wider hospital, the ED has explored a variety of specific approaches to QI. Since the 1990s these have included several benchmarking and throughput analyses conducted with outside consultants, such as the VHA (Voluntary Hospital Association) and the Advisory Board, which the department engaged on its own accord. The ED was also one of Cedars-Sinai's earliest departments to participate in the IHI QI collaboratives.

The first of these collaboratives in 1993/94, which addressed emergency room waits and delays, introduced staff in the department to various QI techniques and rapid-cycle change processes, such as plan-do-study-act (PDSA) methodology, and, just as importantly, the 'language' used to frame quality concepts. Several initial projects reflect the application of these improvement methodologies and the accumulation of learning and expertise over time from one effort to another.

For example, the ED early on addressed an emerging standard for timely antibiotic treatment of pneumonia even before it became part of the JCAHO core measures. This initiative became a 'prototype project' for similar time-to-treat processes for cardiac interventions. These initiatives provided experience collaborating with the hospital's cardiology division and managing a multi-disciplinary implementation effort, which then permitted a relatively easy transition to implementing new standards for cardiac care as they came on line. Similarly, the ED's participation in a later IHI medication safety collaborative resulted in a 'natural flow' into further quality applications within the department and, as described by one of the ED nurse administrators, exemplified a rather easy coexistence of QI techniques taught in the collaborative with more traditional 'quality assurance' methods, such as audits and compliance.

As a consequence, the ED, as with the hospital in general, has pursued a quality journey incorporating a variety of QI paradigms and methods. At times these local efforts have presaged those from the wider medical center. They also indicate how bricolage in practice allows for a mixing of traditional and conventional approaches to quality particular to the local setting. Thus, the micro-system perspective illustrates the porousness of organizational change and learning, and that the exploration and importation of new ideas and the blending of new practices can occur at many levels, not simply from the top down.

Organizational fads or learning?

Some critics warn that an emphasis on constant experimentation with new approaches may signal or lead to a preoccupation with managerial fads and fashions, distracting from real change and improvement in performance.[13,40] However, different movements for organizational reform can offer vital opportunities for learning if organizations are properly oriented and proficient at doing so.[41,42] As an experienced member of the hospital's central QI staff commented, walling the organization off from these trends may not be the most effective strategy, nor entirely possible:

> I think that is the part of the healthy wealth and experience that a hospital needs to go through. Learning about all these different things only makes us better by going through these different fads and fashions. I don't know if you can get away from that [anyway], and part of it is regulatory driven. (Senior QI staff member)

The emphasis on customizing new approaches allows one to take advantage of these opportunities for organizational learning while helping avoid succumbing to mere conformity or blind adoption. The process of bricolage, or pragmatic layering of various elements from different approaches, also permits the effective blending of methods that to some may appear contradictory to conventional QI, whether these are more academically oriented health services research or more traditional quality assurance techniques. These processes, evident at both the macro- and micro-levels within Cedars-Sinai, are what make adaptive organizational learning so beneficial and challenging, a view articulated by a senior leader within the hospital's medical staff:

> And I'm convinced – and this is what makes this so difficult – is that each hospital has its own microenvironment, its own uniqueness . . . (Senior physician leader)

An infrastructure for learning and improvement

Thus far, the story of quality at Cedars-Sinai has chronicled a myriad of structures and activities supporting QI. Figure 4.1 presents an organization chart of the main infrastructure that has emerged from this journey. As one might expect from the process of customization and layering that produced it, this 'performance improvement program' exhibits a distinctively organic character, interlaced within the mainstream structures of hospital governance: as much a 'wiring diagram' (in the words of many we interviewed) as an organization chart.

The primary backbone of this infrastructure are the performance improvement committees, or PICs, in the lower right of the figure, which as we have seen grew out of the medical task force committees established in the early 1990s. The PICs are multidisciplinary committees, chaired by physicians, which focus on QI within specific departments or clinically based populations. They are complemented by the QI committees, or QICs, in the lower left of the figure, a set of cross-functional, 'process-based' committees bringing together members from various departments and 'filtering up' information and effort on quality issues that cut across the medical center. Although there are no direct reporting relationships between the QICs and PICs, there is a good deal of staff rotation and cross-pollination between the two sets of committees.

The Medical Executive Committee, or MEC, the main locus of medical staff influence and decision-making, has oversight over all clinical issues, including the QICs and PICs:

> MEC plays an important role in this too, because all these different performance improvement committees report on up to MEC. This is where MEC gets all the actions

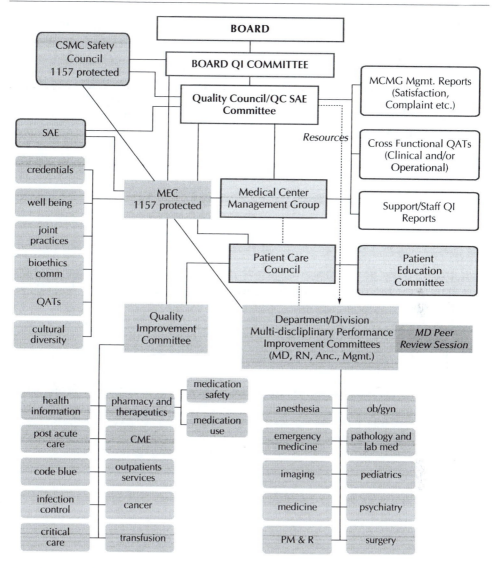

FIGURE 4.1 Performance Improvement Program organization chart

identified at these committees for approval, but they also have each one of these areas give a quality report on a quarterly basis. So, they are the kind of analytical force, but they are [also] asking each one of these different areas to focus on an important quality initiative and give updates at the MEC level. (Senior QI staff member)

The Quality Council, as mentioned earlier, provides a 'capstone' to the quality efforts of the medical center. The Council, chaired by the chief executive, includes the senior executive team, as well as the major players from around the institution involved in quality. It is also the place where QI efforts from the clinical and non-clinical areas of the hospital meet. The Quality Council reports to the Board of Directors Quality Committee, further reflecting the strategic importance of the quality agenda to the organization.

Other key components of the improvement infrastructure not shown in Figure 4.1 include a central quality and performance improvement staff, and what QI leaders at Cedars refer to as 'sub-PIC' processes. The Performance Improvement Group consists of approximately eight full-time staff who co-ordinate the collection and tracking of data, facilitate QI meetings and projects, and conduct the annual data and quality plan reviews. The role of this central staff is not to manage QI *per se*, but to provide expertise and logistical support for the quality functions and activities of the PICs, QICs, and Quality Committee. 'Sub-PIC' processes refer to the plethora of QI projects, studies and change efforts at the department and frontline levels. These are the 'tests of change' and improvement cycles which comprise the bulk of the quality work in the institution. In this way, the PICs act as an open funnel and forum for these diverse efforts within a department.

> [The PIC] is where the sub-PICs report, and then there are other people in this direction who are on the larger PIC. So, it's a way of disseminating the information in a collaborative way. (Senior medical staff leader)

Functions of the improvement infrastructure

One of the most important functions of such an extensive and multi-tiered infrastructure is to provide strategic direction to the medical center's quality agenda. Part of this function, as mentioned above, is to incorporate quality into the strategic process of the institution. Not only is the Plan for the Performance Improvement Program reviewed annually and approved by the Quality Council and Board QI Committee, but quality in turn has become an integral element in the medical center's overall strategic plan.

> . . . going into next year, we have five strategic goals in this organization and one of them is about quality and safety. That's going to be on everybody's plate next year and that's a long way from a decade ago when we were looking at finances as number one. So, it's setting the institutional priorities for quality and safety, and then asking what's going to happen in any particular neighbourhood in the institution. (QI director)

Another part of this function is to bring coherence and direction to the quality agenda itself:

> . . . and what impressed me when I came to Cedars was the whole structure here really . . . looking at quality in the entire medical center as opposed to individual initiatives. (Senior medical staff leader)

Without such a strategic framework to guide QI, it 'will happen in little pockets, and certainly in the early 90s we had lots of little projects going on – but it doesn't happen as an institutional strategy' (QI director). It also serves to direct activity and emphasize specific quality goals and initiatives as needed:

> I think what [the PI structure] does is target the goals to be very specific. It kind of isolates projects; for example, post acute care [PIC] was very much involved with the Demerol initiative. Our department committee has been very much involved with initiatives in patient safety . . . So, it's actually helped direct activity . . . (Senior medical staff leader)

Even more importantly, Cedar-Sinai's improvement infrastructure serves as a knowledge management system,[43] not so much for reporting and control, as to share information within the organization – both vertically and horizontally – and to signify top-level support, visibility and recognition for QI activities. This mechanism for internal diffusion of ideas and practices keeps people abreast of the latest goings-on in quality across the medical center, 'funneling' organizational experiences and learning up and down the infrastructure, as well as through cross-cutting flows for 'disseminating information in a collaborative way'. Indeed, it is these informational processes and flows that tend to generate the particular structural mechanisms that develop:

> Very often some of those successful projects have really been collaborative efforts between physicians and pharmacy and physicians and nurses and so on and that's evolved a whole bunch of different parallel mechanisms. That's why I used the example of the biological organism as an example. (Senior medical staff leader)

The visibility the infrastructure lends to local QI activities provides both accountability and recognition. The latter is especially important in fostering a sense that the discrete initiatives throughout the medical center have greater collective significance, and that QI represents a legitimate priority that matters to the organization:

> . . . what gets to the upper echelon of the organization is, in my opinion, complete work that carries our recommendation, and frankly, work that oftentimes has already been completed and they are actually asking for a blessing or a sanction. (Senior vice president)

The nature and limitations of the improvement infrastructure

Any organizational structure has both benefits and limitations. One of the oft-noted drawbacks and frustrations of the QI infrastructure has been the slow movement of information and 'certain inertia built into a system like this in terms of reaction time', given the extent of committees, sheer numbers of issues the PICs and other committees must address, and consensus-oriented decision-making. Although the spread of information and consensus may require time and some structural redundancy, especially in such a large organization, these may simply represent the costs of sustaining QI in the long term:

> I wouldn't call it a downside as much as I would call it a challenge. Sometimes [in] drawing consensus . . . you need to be able to pull the right people together and you need to build in the time to do it. (Senior vice president)

In this sense, the infrastructure is a 'double-edged sword', suggesting a strategy that focuses on managing the tensions inherent in such a system:

> We kind of believe in the medical center, although we get frustrated at times with the bureaucracy, and the bureaucracy is a big issue. It's the same bureaucracy that's often effective in the things it does, so it [is] a double-edged sword. (Senior medical staff leader)

In the end, the performance improvement system is not simply structure for structure's sake, not an empty infrastructure, but a living, 'organic' system, animated and supported by the swelter of department-level and frontline quality activities and embodying a specific culture and philosophy of improvement and learning:

> When I look back at other hospitals I worked at . . . that were to some degree really proactive in their quality programs . . . their priorities were different. They say they have their structures, they have the corporate quality person and also have to ensure that everything is in place, but they weren't building the culture. They were building the structure for it, but it wasn't really embodiment or belief in that philosophy. (Senior QI staff member)

Communities of learning and engagement

Animating and guiding Cedars-Sinai's infrastructure for quality, as described above, has been a specific culture supportive of learning and improvement. This cultural dimension of the institution's distinct focus on QI is pronounced, even in the everyday attitudes of staff around the medical center.

> I think the culture here is different from most hospitals. I mean, if you talk to people on the nursing staff, people are more attuned to safety issues and quality issues than most hospitals I've worked in. I really think it's that cultural . . . (Senior director)

Some of the foundations of this culture have been touched on, such as the institution's strong academic inclination, research tradition, and culture of striving and questioning. However, aspects of these traditions are not always compatible with an improvement orientation, as demonstrated in the effort required to shift from a 'pilot test' to a 'test of change' mentality. The experience at Cedars-Sinai and its ED suggests that developing such an ethos of learning and improvement is a long-term process, which involves a number of facets, most notably engaging staff (particularly clinicians) and forging a sense of community and shared commitment at both the micro- and macro-levels of the institution.

Clinical ownership and leadership

Although the prominence of physician–administrators in key executive and service improvement positions at Cedars has lent credibility to the quality agenda, this is only a precondition. According to these and other leaders within the medical center, truly engaging physicians in QI has required fostering a sense of ownership of the process among the medical staff itself:

> Until the doctors believe that this is their issue, their problem, it isn't going to get better . . . [There's an] expression, 'No one in the history of the world has ever washed a rental car,' which I love because that is exactly true. (Senior physician leader)

Central to this objective has been the clinical staff taking up leadership of the quality agenda. Such physician leadership can take the form of many roles throughout the institution. Certainly, the initiative by top levels of the medical staff helps set the tone for the whole organization:

> There is an elected physician who rotates every year, and [in this chief of staff position] were some people who really had great vision. In many respects, if I say 'I want to go here' and the political leader says no, I'm not going to go anywhere. But if you find a political leader who really has vision around this, we can move mountains. (Senior medical administrator)

Physician leadership and ownership of QI are, of course, equally important throughout the organization. As in other healthcare organizations, the advocates of the quality agenda at Cedars have emphasized enlisting and developing 'physician champions' – leaders in the trenches of the medical staff, so to speak, whose clinical knowledge and credibility can determine the support for and success of quality efforts in specific areas of the hospital. The experience at Cedars-Sinai also suggests that, given the variable supply of such physician champions and the challenges of maintaining QI across the hospital, this local physician leadership works best when complemented – or even supplemented – by other forms of leadership within the institution.

> Finding physician champions is always desirable, but there is a sort of dance between

finding physician champions and executive leadership. In the case of the hip project, the CEO made that a priority, physician champion, you're going to get resistance, but you keep driving ahead. And it doesn't have to be the CEO, it could be the chairman of the department, whatever. (QI director)

Fostering this sense of ownership and leadership for QI among physicians is no simple task, especially among a medical staff comprising over 1700 practitioners with widely varying degrees of affiliation, backgrounds and interests. The underlying motivations of 'such a large, disparate medical staff' are similarly diverse, implying a varied set of methods for engaging physicians:

> ... for some it's money, for some it's power, for some it's the right thing to do. So I don't think that any one way works. (Senior physician leader)

Among the primary ingredients at Cedars in this regard has been:
- one-on-one peer-to-peer influence and persuasion among physicians, depicted as an often protracted and 'painstaking' process
- persistence in maintaining a dialogue (also described as 'not backing off . . . until they were tired of listening') in order to reach resolutions around quality issues
- preserving a sense of collegiality, partnership and atmosphere of mutual respect among professionals (e.g. implementation that is open to concerns and not too heavy-handed), which is particularly crucial – and difficult – in mobilizing collective change within a culture that so strongly reifies the autonomy of individual clinicians.

Despite the progress that Cedars-Sinai has made in engaging physicians over the course of its quality journey, there is a delicate balance between ownership of QI and the perceived professional interests of the medical staff:

> You can't have somebody who is administration telling the doctors what to do, because we just don't like people telling us what to do, even if it's the right thing. So the doctors have to think about it, and they have to drive the change, but then if we do it too well, then we become one of 'them' and then we're suspect. (Senior physician leader)

Consequently, even in an institution as clinically driven as Cedars-Sinai, partnership and ownership of QI between both sides of hospital governance appear essential to sustaining a quality agenda:

> The quality work . . . seemed to be initiated and energized from the clinical side, and on one hand it's a good thing because you've got the medical staff generally connected, and that's . . . the sore point in most . . . organizations. On the other hand, it's not sustainable without an equal measure of support on the management side. (Senior medical administrator)

Learning environments and community at the micro-level

An organization with a learning environment engages members through continual enhancement of knowledge and skills and encouragement of learning from each other, from mistakes and errors, as well as from innovations and successes. A very visible component of the learning environment in the ED has been an emphasis on staff development and training, a particular cause célèbre of the nursing leadership over the past several years. In addition to raising the certification requirements and developing an extensive internal training program for the nursing staff, the department established a system of three career 'tracks' to allow nurses to advance according to different sets of competencies and interest: a management track for those who want to learn QI and management skills, an education track for those who like to teach classes and assess educational needs, and a clinical track for those who prefer to focus on taking care of patients and sharing their skill through one-on-one training. This has since been adopted in other areas of the hospital.

Another key aspect of a learning environment is creating a safe space in which organizational participants can learn from errors and 'near misses', as well as from positive experiences and achievements. This open learning and sharing of mistakes can be modelled by example from the top:

> I believe very strongly in sharing my screw-ups with the staff . . . absolutely in public and apologizing . . . They know it, because my job is to teach them to do my job. (ED nurse administrator)

The department also made great strides in developing a 'non-retaliatory' atmosphere for bringing errors to light through its work with the IHI medication safety collaborative. This effort established reporting and education mechanisms with safeguards that encourage the free flow of information. These systems highlight the role of trust and respect among peers, such as with the dedicated nurse educator, and maintaining a proven record of integrity.

> Our educator started safety briefings where he would meet with the staff and . . . he [also] created a safety hotline. And these are things that they learned at the IHI. Even though he is in the assistant manager group . . . he has got a fantastic personality . . . and is perceived solely as an educator. They will tell him things they will never tell another CN4 or me, because he's not perceived as management . . . And we respected it. So no matter what he heard, he would turn it into an education, and he would come to me and say, 'Listen, we need to do this, this and this.' But I would never know to this day who the individual was, what the mistake was . . . So that track record of his proved it and encouraged it – by word of mouth, he's safe, a safe haven. (ED nurse administrator)

The department reinforces this open learning environment further by providing mechanisms through which staff can learn from their own and others' behavior. For example, the physician leadership regularly gives feedback to the department's medical staff on their working 'attitude' and handling of patients, as well as celebrating local 'heroes' who embody the department's desired ethos and behavior:

> I personally handle all the complaints that come through the department. I communicate back with patients. But also I'll provide . . . feedback with the physicians . . . I think it's important for people to understand how they're being perceived. Some of them they don't, and I think once people do, then they have a chance to modify themselves. We have a . . . physician here named [Dr. BBB]. He's a sweet guy, he also just has a kind face. Whatever he's got he could put it in a bottle and sell it and become a billionaire because he really gets so many compliments. And the other physicians recognize it. We have a term for it. If a patient needs a little bit of [bedside manner] . . . just go in and BBB-ize them. (ED co-chair)

Selecting staff who already possess some of these qualities has helped strengthen and encourage this environment. One of the physician co-chairs of the department relates an early conversation that raised the importance of this lesson and also represents an example at the micro-system level of the 'exploration' of new ideas from outside the organization:

> I had never been in a Nordstrom's [department store] in my life. Every girl I went out with talked about Nordstrom's and how good it was. I actually tracked down one of the vice presidents for HR at Nordstrom's . . . and I said, 'I'm a physician at this hospital,' and I think I was associate administrator at the time, 'and I want to know how you train your people to be so good?' She said, 'We don't train them.' I said, 'What do you mean you don't train them?' She said, 'We hire them.' (ED co-chair)

Even so, the department on occasion has identified individuals who habitually violate the ethos of the department and do not appear willing or able to change. In these rare instances, maintaining this environment has required making the eventual decision to let go of the individual, despite the person's clinical expertise:

> We actually had a physician who . . . was pretty well trained, but I kept getting complaints . . . I knew she had a bad attitude . . . [T]hen there finally was [a patient letter] that came about the end. I read his letter and I said, '[How can I let this person] take care of patients . . . in the middle of the night when I'm not here because that person is representing me?' We called her in and I'll never forget it . . . She was in the office . . . It wasn't the first time we'd talked . . . but the talking was done because I didn't feel like you could change [this person]. (ED co-chair)

Shared commitments and community

As the discussion of the learning environment alludes to, trust and openness are essential enabling conditions for organizational learning and improvement.[44] At times it can be difficult to ensure these conditions, such as under the constantly rising service volumes experienced by the ED, which have tended to exacerbate tensions between nurses and physicians, particularly over the management of patient flows. The ability of the department to work through tensions and conflicts, maintain communication and broaden dialogue among the staff has rested in many respects on an underlying sense of shared commitment and purpose, that 'in the end . . . everyone realizes we're . . . in this together'.

This sense is partly aided by the greater inherent cohesion afforded by the ED's structure as a relatively closed contract department in which all staff, including physicians, are employed by the ED. Leaders in the ED also point to a number of defining moments in the department's history that have contributed to such an underlying community sentiment. These moments represent peak periods of performance that could only have been achieved by working collectively, or points in time when the collective mission of the group has been publicly validated:

> When we had the earthquake here in 1994, it was tremendous how the department came together and saw at that time, and I'm not sure we've ever beaten it, three hundred patients that day. When we had the riots and all those kind of things make people realize how important we are. The big thing with the riot was one of the firemen was shot in the neck and they took him past seven or eight hospitals to bring them to us on their rig. We have his picture out there. He was actually at the dedication of the new ED. We need those every once in a while . . . (Co-chair of ED)

More than merely a dedication to the department, this sentiment reflects commitments that individuals display to each other (*see also* the San Diego Children's Hospital, Chapter 2, and Albany AIDS Treatment Center cases, Chapter 8, in particular), manifested by looking out for each other, concern for each other's emotional wellbeing, and an authentic camaraderie and shared social bonds:

> Staff work hard to make sure that each other takes their breaks. When I came here . . .
> I discovered that it's such a sacred cow that no way was I going to touch it. They need
> to physically get away, and they need to mentally get away. And they watch out for
> each other . . . So the camaraderie exists when they have to need each other. Often the
> camaraderie exists for the social thing afterwards. And when it's quiet around here,
> which is not often, you can see it. (ED nurse administrator)

For its part, the leadership in the ED attempts to encourage this natural camaraderie.
For example, the department participates in the hospital's critical incidents debriefing
team, which provides support for staff emotionally affected by events at work, reinforcing a shared concern and commitment for the wellbeing of individual staff. Similarly,
the department provides various acknowledgements and rewards that recognize
the contribution of staff throughout the department, helping to create a sense of
inclusion.

What gives this community sentiment greater meaning is not only a feeling of
inclusion in a larger collective whole, but one that, at heart, is committed to a common
purpose. In the ED this centers on serving the patient, so that even in scheduling shifts
'we do what's best for the patient in the end'. As the physician leadership make clear
to potential candidates during the hiring process for new physicians, 'This is our core
value. You have to understand that the patient is the one who counts. You've got to see
it from their perspective' (Co-chair of ED).

It is this belief and knowledge that others in the department are equally committed
to the fundamental mission – 'what's best for the patient' – despite obvious other
interests and disagreements (often deep) on how to realize this common purpose,
which sustains dialogue, learning and improvement, even through the friction and
strain that inevitably arise in organizational life.

Learning communities across the organization

Overlaid on these local learning environments, similar communities supportive of
learning and improvement have been formed across the organization. To some extent,
the performance improvement committee structure and quality infrastructure as a
whole – with its knowledge management function of sharing information, experiences
and lessons across the organization – serves as just such a community of individuals
from throughout the medical center, whereby people learn from each other, gain skills
and expertise, and are committed to improvement.

One of the most explicit examples of this kind of macro-level community at
Cedars-Sinai is the Physician Leadership Development program. In many ways this
program constitutes what has been termed a 'community of practice'.[45,46] This concept
has been used to define groups of individuals with like interests, typically of a technical
or professional nature, who share knowledge and skills in a free-flowing manner to
transfer innovation, skills and best practice.[47,48] Over time these communities also
tend to acquire a common identity, purpose and strong in-group solidarity through a
constant search for unifying consensus.[43]

The Physician Leadership Development program gathers physicians from departments throughout the hospital into a collegial community, cultivating a spirit of
camaraderie and a shared mission to educate them for leadership within the current
healthcare environment. In this sense, the program very much represents a 'learning
community', centered on a monthly lecture series covering a variety of administrative,
industry and business skills and issues. Characteristic of a classic community of
practice, however, the educational program includes not only classroom instruction

– 'it's not just people taking classes and at the end filling out a survey whether they liked it or not' – but also an emphasis on tacit knowledge and experiential learning[47] by requiring all participants to complete a project intended to help develop their leadership skills.

The characteristic of a community of practice as an independent community that can span various organizational and institutional boundaries[45] is particularly applicable to engaging physicians in a medical center such as Cedars-Sinai, whose medical staff retain multiple affiliations with other practice and healthcare settings in the community. The gradual 'snowballing' in the growth of the program by 5 to 10 new physicians per year has utilized many of the same methods described earlier to engage physicians, such as enlisting physician champions and peer-to-peer interaction. The experience of the leadership program further emphasizes the emotional component of persuasion and forging commitments that this work entails:

> We create a community, and so when we try to change things, as far as philosophies and how you do it, you have to get the right people on board, that involves talking to the right individual . . . So I think that using present leadership is important. People who have credibility . . . but then it's the one on one . . . you've got to make the emotional connection . . . you had to create that sense of urgency. (Senior physician leader)

This community of practice is critically interrelated with the community represented by the wider quality infrastructure of the medical center. One of the other key functions of the program has been to develop leaders within the medical staff to populate the hospital governance and performance improvement structures:

> Because of this group . . . we have many chairs of these medical staff committees, people that have become members of the Medical Executive Committee and assumed leadership positions in their own departments. So we stimulated interest again . . . now we have a pool of individuals and that was the whole idea of that. (Senior physician leader)

At the same time, the medical center has increasingly moved to institutionalize this learning community by making the leadership development program a criterion for membership on the Medical Executive Committee and incorporating it within the MEC's general Performance Improvement Program along with the PICs, QICs and other elements of the improvement infrastructure.

The interplay of macro- and micro-systems

Up to this point this case study has delineated how key themes in the quality journey at Cedars-Sinai have played out similarly at various levels throughout the organization, such as the exploration and importation of new ideas by individuals at the micro- and macro-levels, bricolage and customization in both macro- and micro-level implementation processes, and engagement of physicians and other clinical staff in the quality agenda at multiple levels of the medical center. Yet there are also clear differences in the character of the quality journey between the macro- and micro-systems, implying differing sets of contributions, functions and even accommodations of each level in sustaining QI within the organization.

One of the unique contributions of the macro-system in this regard is creating a 'receptive context' for change and learning within the organization. This includes a number of features – such as strategic vision, good managerial relations, visionary staff in pivotal positions, a climate conducive to experimentation and risk taking, and effective data capture systems – associated with the capacity to embrace new ideas and implement innovations within and across units of an organizational system.[49,50,51] As discussed previously, a primary function of the improvement infrastructure at Cedars, and in particular the Quality Council comprising the top management and clinical leadership of the hospital, is setting a strategic direction for the quality agenda. This function involves formulating quality goals and priorities, incorporating the quality agenda into the mainstream strategic process of the hospital, and providing a framework or schema in which quality activities sum to a greater whole as opposed to languishing in disparate 'pockets' of innovation.

Macro-level actions to enhance trust

An equally important facet of creating this receptive context entails macro-level actions to enhance trust, which, as mentioned above, is an essential enabling condition for organizational learning and improvement. These actions include those designed to encourage trust and opportunities for co-operation among groups within the institution, for instance, through the hospital's code of conduct for clinical staff and the interdisciplinary meetings and joint grand rounds of Cedars-Sinai's MD/RN collaborative initiative. Others include those intended to build a trusting relationship between macro- and micro-levels of the organization, in which senior management feel confident in empowering lower levels, and frontline staff believe in the espoused motives of senior management with regard to the quality agenda:

> It's a longstanding relationship [with department-level leaders], and they know that what we [executive-level quality staff] are trying to do is for them and the patients. (QI director)

At Cedars-Sinai, trust of the macro-system has been greatly helped by stability at the top of the organization in both people and, notably, in direction over time:

> We have a benefit, actually a blessing, to have a CEO who . . . has . . . his career in this organization over 20 years . . . I think it's indicative of why this organization is where it is currently, because we have not had that kind of systematic change at the highest level. Organizations have changed too frequently, as a lot of them do. They are equally changing their course, and we haven't had to do that . . . (Senior vice president)

Likewise, senior management strives to develop a reputation for honest and direct communication:

> I think the . . . communication, effectiveness of communication, how issues are addressed, difficult as they may be . . . I think that they don't hide behind the issue, and they are very upfront about it, the communication is very open. (Senior vice president)

Macro-level resources for quality

Another fundamental role of the macro-system in creating a receptive context for change and learning is to provide the funding and resources required to support the QI process and to implement service improvements. Financial support for these activities are at a premium in healthcare, even in relatively well-endowed organizations such as Cedars-Sinai:

> One of the things that I think that we do well that other businesses don't do is we have to actually prove that something works because our margin as far as cash flow is so close in healthcare, there is no money for R&D . . . Every test of change has to be revenue-neutral, which puts some of them . . . I mean it won't work. You need to dedicate some resources . . . No one is giving away anything in healthcare right now. (ED physician leader)

Yet the allocation of funds often implicitly signals priorities within organizations.[52] Without sufficient resources, the macro-system compromises its credibility with regard to quality, individual units must rely on variable sources of support for improvement initiatives, and the quality agenda will be difficult to sustain against other, funded, priorities in the organization.

At Cedars-Sinai a good deal of this support for quality has taken the form of resources targeted at specific improvement initiatives at the micro-system level. For example, the ED petitioned, negotiated and received funding from the corporate level for the effort to increase the certification status of the nursing staff, the implementation of the internal training program, and the hiring of a dedicated pharmacist within the department, which emerged from the ED's participation in the IHI medication safety collaborative.

The institution has also expended substantial resources to support the quality infrastructure and improvement process across the organization. This level of resources includes QI training for staff throughout the institution, which has served to mobilize enthusiasm and provide a common 'working vocabulary' around quality, as much as to impart specific algorithms for process improvement.

Other institutional-level resources support the Performance Improvement Program structures, which include the central quality and performance improvement staff of co-ordinators and facilitators, headed by the quality and safety director. As described previously, this latter individual represents a unique position for visionary leadership and 'boundary spanning' within the organization:

> Really, what he does full time is focus on the quality initiatives of the institution. He doesn't have any other role basically, and he is a key figure and one of the ways that all the groups can get some direction ... having that type of designated protected physician ... a lot of facilities don't subsidize a protected physician like that. (Senior medical staff leader)

Individuals at the micro-system level also recognize and echo the value of this macro-level resource, both in terms of linkages externally and promoting change internally:

> [The QI director] is faculty there [IHI]. So that influence affects us heavily. I think it's very positive ... I think that having somebody in the key position to inculcate the rest of the physician group and medical staff was important. (ED physician leader)

A receptive, interactive context

The 'receptive context' for change that has resulted at Cedars-Sinai has generated much initiative and innovation for improvement from within departments and micro-systems in the medical center:

> Well, I would just say the rest of the organization provides direction, but a lot of the projects are self-initiatives. The core measures ... obviously have been hard-driven administratively, but individual efforts have actually been the brainchild of people from the respective departments. (Senior medical staff leader)

But this context also encourages interaction and mutual responsibility for quality between levels. As discussed above, the improvement infrastructure facilitates the flow of knowledge across the organization and, in particular, micro- to macro-level learning; i.e. the sharing and incorporation of micro-level innovations throughout the institution, as illustrated in the spread of the ED's quality process for aspirin related to chest pain:

> Five years ago, aspirin was introduced to the field for chest pain. Well, that obviously paralleled with what would become one of our core measures, which is aspirin to acute coronary syndrome. So we just paralleled that whole quality marker and of course, it went from our level to hospital-wide to make sure these people are discharged with aspirin. So you really see a continuum. I didn't sit here and design the process, it was happenstance that it all dovetailed together. It's kind of neat when that occurs. (ED physician leader)

The mix of top-down direction and bottom-up initiative (similar to what we observed at San Diego Children's, Peterborough and other case study sites) enables complementary roles and flexibility in leadership for quality across levels of the institution:

> I think you see more frontline behavior when you have champions . . . So in that environment, you can do different things. You can have a nurse that has great credibility and can start a hotline on safety and people will phone and give them information, and I might not be able to do that someplace else . . . But other places in the hospital I don't have that kind of physician leadership, other leadership, and so you do wind up with it being more top down. (QI director)

This interplay – in direction and flows of initiative, innovation, and leadership for quality – permits mutual adjustment between levels and the contribution of each in sustaining improvement and learning within the organization.

Conclusions

Although the link between continuous improvement and learning has been noted elsewhere,[12,53] the quality journey at Cedars-Sinai demonstrates the extent to which sustained QI depends on learning that is organizational as opposed to merely individual. That is, the lessons, habits and orientations of improvement become embedded in the culture, structures and routines of organizational life. This case study illustrates the processes by which this type of learning has unfolded over time in a large, complex medical center such as Cedars-Sinai, and how some of the pitfalls and dangers of organizational learning – such as inferring the wrong lessons, and blind or symbolic adoption of new practices – can be managed or overcome.

The detailed relating here of this quality journey highlights the role of boundary-spanners in exploring and exploiting new ideas, and of a learning infrastructure in sharing and vetting knowledge throughout the institution and supporting improvement activities through facilitation and expertise. This infrastructure has evolved through a pragmatic process of customization and bricolage, helping to ensure that new ideas and practices are relevant to the context at Cedars and suitably adapted over time by incorporating useful lessons from one experience (e.g. clinical pathways) into the next (e.g. key aspects of care and core measures). Indeed, the significance of this improvement infrastructure resides less in its particular features than in the process by which it was constructed and the functions that it serves:

> And whether or not our 'wiring diagram' is the right thing to do in every organization . . . may be a question. What we have done in this regard may not be right for everybody else. The important thing, the real important thing, is to have a wiring diagram, and a wiring diagram that works for your culture in your setting and that recognizes where the institution is in its quality journey and pushes that as far as it can. (Senior executive)

Another equally, if not more, fundamental process of embedding learning and improvement in the organization has been to anchor the quality agenda in the identity and culture of the institution. Every organization develops a distinctive identity[54,55] and culture[56,57] comprising organizational values, myths and self-images that accrue through the course of its particular history. At Cedars, twin pillars of these organizational attributes include a strong self-image of excellence and an ethos of striving towards that excellence. Over the years the institution, and those involved in shaping the quality agenda from across the medical center, have been able to refocus this striving for excellence towards a vision of QI:

> I think there's always been a culture here of striving for excellence. Whatever excellence meant at that time. So at a point in time in American healthcare, we had the luxury of being able to afford doing everything and anything we could do for everyone . . . In the 25 years that I've been here, public policy has evolved, medicine has evolved, the field of health service and research has evolved, and so quality has been redefined during this period with an emphasis on process measures, outcome measures, more quantification in general . . . (Senior executive)

This cultural rooting of QI is not as straightforward as the above quote might suggest. In particular, traditional notions of clinical excellence do not necessarily translate directly into an emphasis on service excellence and improvement. Over the course of its quality journey, Cedars-Sinai has consistently attempted to frame the quality agenda within the context of the institution's history, heritage and tradition (*see* Chapter 3 on Royal Devon and Exeter for a similar story). Champions of QI within the organization have also invested great effort in building learning environments and communities at both the macro- and micro-levels of the organization in which striving for excellence and improvement are co-articulated in practice. If successful, tapping into the innate understandings that various organizational constituents hold regarding the essence or character of the institution can present a formidable force to propel QI:

> One thing we have going for us in this organization – there's a certain amount of pride in the quality of the place, and this sort of excellence is important. I think most of the medical staff believe that. And that's something that we use a lot . . . (Senior director)

Despite the progress that Cedars-Sinai has made in embedding learning and improvement, both culturally and structurally over the past several decades, senior leaders still feel that the institution is far from fully making QI a routine part of organizational life within the medical center. These challenges include lingering tension between the quality agenda and traditional notions of medical practice:

> We're a long way, from my standpoint, a really long way from perfection . . . We've been at this a while, but I can tell you that today, it remains a struggle to really get this hardwired into the organization. Culturally, we're a little schizophrenic. We like and we do these [quality] things, but we're also dealing with the reality of a private attending staff as in every other institution who, number one, might not necessarily feel that way. And the medical staff governance process here and the culture here is still one that tilts towards the rights of the individual practitioner. So on the core measures, for example, our results are nowhere near where they should be. They're not. (Senior executive)

Likewise, there is a continuing perception of QI as 'add-on' work:

> We still struggle as an organization with people viewing this work as an add-on to their real job. I'd like to see us become more evolved, I guess, with a broader and deeper

number of people who truly understand and see it as part and parcel of their role, their leadership and management roles, in the organization. (Senior executive)

I think that for many people in the organization, they would perceive it in addition to, rather than part of or integral to, what they do. The sense is a distant throw-back to the early days of 'it's just an administrative requirement', something they're making us do, as opposed to doing this is [a] really crucial [part] of what we are. It's a far cry from that for sure, and we've made a lot of progress in that regard, but maybe it's my orientation that I want it to feel completely collegial and I don't know that I always do. (Senior medical administrator)

And the organization still experiences 'push-back' on the quality agenda from some quarters of the institution:

We're getting some push back from segments of the medical staff that I would describe as representing old line thinking. They're kind of organized to push back. And so we're trying to figure out how to break through on that. (Senior executive)

As part of the institution's culture of striving for excellence, individuals at Cedars tend to dwell less on previous progress than on these current challenges and hurdles. In a preliminary presentation of the case findings, participants in the study from both the macro- and micro-levels commented on the strangeness – as well as the usefulness – of reflecting on where they have come to at this point of their quality journey and the routes that have taken them there. It was also clear how much this ethic of striving has been integrated into the quality agenda and fuels its constant evolution; for example, the establishment after the end of our study at Cedars of health improvement teams (HITs) to supplement PICs and QICs as a new component of the Performance Improvement Program.

Deming discusses 'constancy of purpose' as one of the primary principles of quality management,[58] and striving and persistence have tellingly marked the quality journey at Cedars-Sinai:

When I started it was kind of like that . . . newscast, when they show the House of Commons [in the UK]. People grumble in the background . . . [The QI director would] get up and talk in this meeting of all the chairmen and vice-presidents . . . about quality stuff, and I thought, god, this guy's not getting very much respect. But he just stuck to it and pushed this agenda. Now I take it seriously. And I really think that was a big part of it. I saw the changes. It took years. And a lot of projects and a lot of education. (Senior director)

As the QI director himself notes, this persistence is a collective property, reinforced by advocates for quality in key positions throughout the medical center:

. . . bringing information in and publicizing it and not letting go. And introducing the concept of the dashboards and these other things; but then getting the co-operation from the CEO that yes, that's a good idea, let's do that, and making sure it gets on the agendas of the meetings. I can't do that stuff in a vacuum. (QI director)

However, in the context of Cedars-Sinai, this 'constancy of purpose' refers not only to a long-term commitment to providing value to a particular product niche or clientele, as often interpreted in the improvement literature,[59] nor even to a specific quality approach or paradigm, but to furthering the capacity of the organization to continually learn and improve itself.

5

Building a system of leadership for quality improvement: a Dutch hospital in pursuit of perfection

ORIGINAL CASE STUDY RESEARCHED BY MIRJAM VAN HET LOO AND TONY RILEY; NARRATIVE PREPARED BY MIRJAM VAN HET LOO, PAUL BATE AND TONY RILEY

Up until the 1990s there was an almost mythical preoccupation in management thought with the individual characteristics of leaders, with leadership being regarded as a quality of the person that was acquired or that one was born with. This view finally gave way to a more de-individualized concept of leadership as a system, 'distributed' between different layers and different parts and people within the organization: in other words, the notion of distributed,[1] multi-layered[2] and strategically collective[3] leadership.[4,5]

This case study of the Reinier de Graaf Groep (RdGG) hospital system in the Netherlands seeks to show that a preoccupation with an individual or a small group of leaders (usually at the top) may have led practitioners and researchers alike to overlook – or underestimate – the importance of multi-level systems-based leadership in quality improvement programs within healthcare organizations.

Gibb is credited with being the first to use the term 'dispersed leadership',[6] later elaborated by Gronn[1] in a series of statements about concerted (leadership) action.

❏ Spontaneous collaboration occurs through the interactions of the many leaders.
❏ Intuitive understanding is developed through close leader relationships or network partnerships (co-leadership).
❏ Formal leadership structures are predicated on a first-among-equals, rather than a hierarchical, basis.

For Gronn, distributed leadership possesses properties of interdependence and co-ordination. Interdependence produces complementarities and occurs when leaders' roles overlap, thus reducing the likelihood of errors and encouraging mutual support for decisions. The second property is co-ordination, which involves managing interdependencies and ensuring that people and resources are all synchronized to achieve the required performance. This modern concept of distributed leadership only recently entered the field of local government and healthcare, although it remains a minority view.

BOX 5.1 Case profile: Reinier de Graaf Groep

CASE PROFILE

Type of Organization:	One of the oldest hospitals in the Netherlands, dating from 1252. In 1982 several separate hospital facilities merged to form the Reinier de Graaf Groep, named after a famous local physician.
Focal Micro-System:	Varicose (vascular) surgery
Size:	A hospital system employing 3000 people, including 165 medical specialists.
Location:	Centered in Delft, the hospital has sites in Voorburg (for elective procedures), Westland, Ypenburg, and Naaldwijk (an outpatient clinic), serving a general population of approximately 250 000 residents.
Country:	The Netherlands
Awards and Recognitions:	One of the first sites selected in Europe in 2002 for the Pursuing Perfection initiative sponsored by the Institute for Healthcare Improvement and Robert Wood Johnson Foundation. Also received the European Gold Helix for its 'mamma' (breast) policlinics (1996), the Dutch national award for 'Best Annual Quality Report' (1997), and the Gold Helix for its 'flow varices' project (1998).

KEY CONCEPTS

Multi-Level Leadership: recognizing the strength of leadership for quality improvement that is 'distributed', 'multi-layered', and 'strategically collective' across different parts and people within the organization, in contrast to a preoccupation with an individual or small group of leaders, typically at the top.

Focused-Factory Design: an approach to service design based on the assumption that routine actions positively affect outcomes, and which attempts to improve efficiency by limiting packages of services to sets of standard procedures that can be planned and scheduled, while triaging patients requiring non-routine treatment to separate trajectories of care.

Denis *et al.* have similarly defined strategic leadership in the specific context of healthcare organizations ('a classic pluralistic domain involving divergent objectives and multiple actors linked together in fluid and ambiguous power relationships') as a collective phenomenon in which leadership is shared, with no single individual having complete authority over all others.[3] The power of the senior executive is further reduced by the influence of other professionals or external supra-organizational agencies (e.g. regulatory bodies, professional associations, third-party insurers, and various organized interest groups). In their eight-year study of five Canadian healthcare organizations, the researchers explored how leaders can achieve deliberate strategic change in organizations where leadership roles are shared, objectives are divergent and power is diffuse. They concluded that the 'creation of a collective leadership group in which members play complementary roles appears critical in achieving change'.

In this case study we contend that RdGG displayed strong characteristics of this type of multi-level distributed leadership, and that these were core to their pursuit of quality and service improvement. Decision lines were shortened and managers empowered at various levels to exercise influence in the decision-making process, not least around quality matters. Leadership and structure were closely aligned, allowing the joint leadership of quality through RdGG's quality steering group, and the vertical and horizontal integration of different quality projects and roles across levels of the organization.

This system of leadership extends from the top of the institution to the level of clinical 'micro-systems',[7,8] which are seen as fundamental to change at RdGG. The implication for quality endeavours is that they require a concept of leadership as depersonalized, collectivized and dispersed between the micro-and macro-systems, and aligned and co-ordinated through a networked structure both horizontally and verti-cally in the organization. On a broader front, this case lends further support to the 'meso' perspective in which the micro- and macro-system serve complementary functions in supporting quality (*see* the San Diego Children's case study, Chapter 2), comple-mentarity being very much the concern of the organizational leadership system.

RdGG's route to high-quality healthcare

RdGG began as a guesthouse for the sick in Delft, and is said to originate from one of the oldest hospitals in the Netherlands that was first mentioned in 1252. In 1982 separate hospital facilities in and around Delft merged to form the Reinier de Graaf Groep, which was named after a famous local physician.

Around the same time, quality had started to gain increased emphasis within Dutch healthcare policy, with the introduction of national practice guidelines for medical specialists from 1982 onwards and general practitioners (GPs) from 1987,[9] and the spread of peer review site visits and audits to all specialties by 1998. The 1990s also brought several notable regulatory developments concerning healthcare quality, including the Quality of Health Institutions Act of 1996, which required healthcare providers to develop quality norms, procedures, and certifications; as well as the Dutch government's 1999 annual budget document, which presented steps to strengthen collaboration and integration at the regional level around quality issues.[10] These policies were intended to encourage healthcare providers to pay more attention to quality of care and to develop integrated quality strategies and measurement systems. At the same time, authorities attempted to provide support and resources towards these ends. For example, the Dutch Ministry of Health granted a subsidy for RdGG to join the Pursuing Perfection initiative (described below, and in which the RD&E also participated, *see* Chapter 3), which enabled the hospital to participate in the program.

RdGG was one of the first hospitals in the Netherlands to respond to these appeals with a systematic focus on quality, beginning with an important transformation initiated by the chief executive at the time. As indicated by the following quote from an executive member of the board of directors, as well as other events described below, this transformation and RdGG's ensuing agenda of quality improvement have been closely intertwined with – both encouraged by and helping to shape – the wider changes in Dutch healthcare.

> We have a long history of quality in this hospital. One of the previous directors of RdGG is one of the leading people in the field of healthcare quality improvement in the Netherlands, and he did a great deal to stimulate quality improvement initiatives in RdGG.

During this time staff became increasingly engaged with quality issues. A number of master classes were held in Delft in 1990 and members of the organization, such as the quality advisor, pathology lead and specialist advisor for quality, began to champion quality locally. This period is credited as being the 'start of quality improvement in the hospital' (Senior manager).

The next distinguishable phase in the organization's journey came a few years later, when external guidance was sought from the Juran Institute in the US. This was shortly after the Institute, founded by the legendary pioneer in quality improvement Dr Joseph Juran, began applying their well-known improvement philosophies and methods (such as the define-measure-analyze-improve-control cycle) to healthcare.[11] The approach, designed to produce improvements in quality while lowering costs and maintaining a focus on the needs and expectations of patients, was considered an important foundation to the development of quality improvement in the institution:

> It uses a medical thinking model that focuses on the analysis of the causes of complaints. It became clear that merely treating a complaint is not sufficient and that one needs to identify the cause of the complaint. Another strong point of Juran's method is its focus on employees; for instance, the recognition that it is important to be sensitive to the people on the work floor, and the need to identify 'champions of change'. Further, the method indicates that 'success leads to success', meaning that it is important to disseminate information on one's successes. This was done through presentations and education and development programs, at which the basic principles of Juran's method were explored. It provided a good start for the quality improvement process in the hospital. (Quality Department member)

In addition to the Juran Institute's approach, RdGG has utilized a number of other existing quality improvement methods and techniques, including Deming's quality improvement principals, the rapid cycle method to improve care processes, and business process redesign to guide large-scale change projects.[12]

In 1996 RdGG decided to merge with a hospital in Voorburg that had recently failed in a merger attempt with another hospital in The Hague. The motivation behind the reorganization came from the fear that the hospital in Delft would 'become too small'; which is to say, it was realized that a hospital in the Netherlands requires a certain scale in order to be able to deliver the volume and breadth of services that are necessary to survive in the current healthcare environment.

The hospital's quality agenda temporarily stalled during this period because of the turmoil surrounding the merger:

> The main challenge of the merger was merging the various specialist groups working in the two hospitals. The CEO's predecessor had done this in a relatively short time. He started as CEO in 1999 . . . with the main objective of creating a better working atmosphere. At the moment he took over, staff turnover, especially among nurses, was high and morale was low, because of the turbulence caused by the merger. (Board executive)

However, the previous momentum that had built up was sufficient for work on individual quality projects to continue, led by quality champions who had emerged during the initial era of quality improvement at RdGG. Thus, despite the organizational disruption, it was not long after the merger that the seeds sown in the early 1990s began to bear fruit, a mark of recognition coming in the form of a number of national and international quality awards. In 1996 RdGG was awarded the European Golden Helix for its project 'Mamma [breast] Policlinics'. This came as no surprise to the manager of the department, who stressed that they 'had been doing it (quality) for many years', albeit in isolation:

> Mamma [breast] care was the first. After that we did other projects but I think the problem was that these projects were islands, silos in the organization, and what you see with Pursuing Perfection [see below] is that you have more connection between them, more learning moments. This was not so in the beginning. (Member nursing staff)

This was, nevertheless, the first major quality award RdGG had received. The hospital did not have to wait long for further recognition, achieving a creditable second place in the annual Golden Helix awards for its project Wheel-chair, as well as a Dutch award for the Best Annual Quality Report in 1997.[12] The following year the team that manages the veinal (vascular) surgery and what would be known as the Flow Varices project also entered into the act:

> We were trying to reorganize the vascular outpatient service, and for that we got a Dutch Golden Helix Award in 1998. (Medical staff member, Flow Varicose service)

The next significant phase in the organization's development occurred when the current chief executive was appointed in 1999, and the former chief executive went on to direct the Dutch Institute for Healthcare Improvement, an indication of RdGG's reputation and leading role in Dutch healthcare QI.

In the meantime the number of individual quality projects grew rapidly, but still in the context of the lack of any wider strategy for quality, this being partly due to the continued distractions caused by the merger:

> In the beginning we only did individual projects. It was only later on that we realized we had jumped into the water and wanted – needed – to swim but didn't know where to swim – the direction. (Executive management team member)

The chief executive, the chief financial officer, and key staff such as the internal quality advisor, the specialist manager for quality and the manager for pathology (among others) came to the conclusion that the organization needed to alter its underlying approach to quality if it was ever to achieve its potential as a quality system:

> Currently it is realized that Juran's method is like a car that is broken for which no spare parts are available any more . . . The weaknesses were now being recognized: there was too little time on the work floor to focus on quality. Projects lasted too long, and it took too long before success occurred. At any one time RdGG was trying to implement 90 projects; as a consequence of which there was a lack of short-term successes. Problems were identified and explained, but no solutions to these problems were found, and in some cases people did not even determine the source of the problems. (Quality Department member)

Still, the organization continued to mark up individual project successes. For example, in 1999 it established a Transmural Care working group to improve care for stroke patients, with wider key stakeholder involvement including local GPs, nursing homes, health insurance companies and the Ministry for Health. Research revealed that the earlier that diagnosis and possible accompanying complications are known, the better the outcome for patients. Co-ordination of medical and nursing care for stroke patients within RdGG contributed to a better prognosis, a higher quality of life and fewer limitations compared to other stroke patients elsewhere in the Netherlands. The probability of dying of stroke in RdGG itself declined by 11%.[12]

A year later, a management development program was implemented at RdGG, which led to the first fully stated formulation of the mission, vision and values of the organization – a major step towards healing the fragmentation that had developed within the quality agenda. Moving words were used to capture the imagination of staff in the form of the motto 'Ever better care,' and the needs and wishes of patients were recognized as the priority concern. By adopting a common language, the leadership was assisting integration and making transformation more readily acceptable to staff in the organization (*see also* Stahr[13]). Table 5.1 lists the organization's core values that were articulated during this process and which have subsequently become integral to the organization's quality strategy.

Table 5.1 Core values of RdGG

VALUE	WHAT DOES IT MEAN?
Trustworthiness	Patients and employees can trust us; we do as we say.
Co-operation	We cherish teamwork inside and outside our organization.
Result-oriented	We strive to achieve the best results for our patients.
Discovering new horizons	We introduce new strategies and techniques.
Involvement	Respect for patients and colleagues is the basis of our actions.

Source: Realization of Pursuing Perfection, 2002[12]

To help the organization maintain accountability to these values, RdGG has subscribed to a number of external systems of quality standards and accreditation. These systems include the ISO 9000 international management standards, the management model of the Dutch Institute for Quality (INK-model), the guidelines of the Dutch Institute for the Accreditation of Hospitals (NIAZ), and the Balanced Scorecard system.

- ❒ *ISO 9000:* The ISO 9000 family of standards represents an international consensus on good management practices with the aim of ensuring the organization can consistently document and follow procedures to deliver products or services meeting pre-specified requirements.[14]
- ❒ *INK-model:* This model, promoted by the Netherlands Quality Institute (or INK), seeks to improve the quality of management by focusing on appropriate organizational structure and outcomes.[15]
- ❒ *NIAZ:* This quality system, developed by the Netherlands Institute for Accreditation of Hospitals, outlines the organizational requirements applicable to a hospital as a whole which must be met to assure healthcare quality.[16]
- ❒ *Balanced Scorecard:* The Balanced Scorecard, as used by RdGG, is a set of critical success factors and performance indicators related to five domains: finance, customers, internal processes, innovation and personnel.

The effects of these quality frameworks related to performance standards and measurement, combined with the various methodologies mentioned above for implementing change in services and organizational process to achieve desired outcomes (e.g. Juran, Deming, rapid-cycle improvement), have been reflected in the overall reduction of admissions and lengths of stay within the institution between 1998 and 2002.

In sum, in the space of two decades 'quality' moved – despite some bumps in the road, such as the merger – from hardly being taken seriously to a key strategic focus of the hospital and a normalized means of conceptualizing and managing routine care processes and clinical practice. Yet there was to be one defining moment that would serve to draw together the assorted strands of RdGG's quality journey, and which warrants particular attention.

A defining moment: Pursuing Perfection at RdGG

Many of those interviewed, particularly in the upper echelons of the organization, believed that the 2001 Institute for Healthcare Improvement (IHI) conference in Bologna was *the* critical moment in the development of the organization's quality agenda, which did more than anything else to propel RdGG forward in the quality direction. This conference introduced the idea of the Pursuing Perfection (PP) initiative to senior leaders.* As a leading internal quality advisor put it, becoming part of the PP initiative 'was the big next step . . . it felt like "growing up"'. A member of the senior executive team takes up the story:

> So, [the CEO], my colleague, brought it home as an idea and we discussed it and he said it needs a lot of work and our first impulse was, 'Let's forget it, and get on with our daily work.' But then we started talking with a lot of people in the organization, and they kept saying, 'Why not?' We have some ambitions, we have some dreams, we aren't there yet, so this could give our organization a new impulse. That and the fact that there were ideas in our minds . . . It was very important for us to think about patient flows. So that was something that had to be done.

The leadership of RdGG decided to submit a proposal, and were successful, having the privilege of being the only organization in mainland Europe selected to take part in the PP initiative.

The introduction of PP at the end of 2001 led to a new emphasis and a shift in responsibilities for quality care and quality policy. Basically, the locus of responsibility in these areas was to shift substantially to the line organization, to the extent that quality would no longer be a 'project' but an integral part of the work of clinical and other departments throughout the organization.

The leadership at RdGG saw the PP initiative as an exceptional opportunity to develop what they termed 'co-operative medical care', improving collaboration and joint working among GPs and other healthcare providers, such as nursing homes and tertiary care. In the classic mold of the IHI's change strategy, the leadership began with two projects, closely followed by a further five projects which would take forward the lessons and experiences into organizational-wide change – the 'two to five to all' principle.

Hospital leaders considered one of the strengths of PP to be that it set highly ambitious objectives that would force the organization to innovate. Whereas previous quality models employed in RdGG (such as NIAZ and ISO 9000) had also been aimed at improving (though mostly assuring) quality, innovation and radical improvements of the kind now being pursued had not been on the agenda before.[17]

A unique feature of RdGG's plan for the PP initiative was that typical vertical projects (organized through the clinical micro-systems within the organization's departmental clusters) would be supported by logistical and operational 'horizontal' projects, such as information technology, human resources (HR), medication supply and safety, and reductions in bureaucracy – in other words, a quality matrix.

Take HR as an example of one of these horizontal dimensions:

---

* Two other case sites in this study, the Royal Devon and Exeter and the Kings College Hospital NHS Trusts in the UK, are also participants in the PP initiative.

> Quality has different components. In the first instance, it is important that the Human Resource Department itself is well-organized, and that quality is assured. Further, the department supports quality management in other parts of the organization by analyzing and improving work processes, and by recruiting high-quality personnel. It is very important in recruiting to determine which quality and competencies are needed in the organization. Herein lies an important task for the Human Resource Department. (Member HR Department)

Figure 5.1 provides an overview of the matrix. Vertical projects focus on the patient pathway itself, concentrating on designing and improving the various care processes associated with it, while the horizontal projects seek to ensure the pathways and care processes are properly supported and have optimal and receptive social, technical and clinical contexts in which to flourish. Projects give focus, and support programs give spread and context:

> The main aim of the horizontal programs is to transfer lessons to the whole organization. All projects are owned by people from the management team. As a result of the horizontal and vertical projects, the organizational structure can now be described as a 'quality matrix'. (Chief executive)

This matrix concept also reflects a degree of 'systems thinking' – identifying core processes and functions of the organization, where they interface, and how they interact as a system – which provides a perspective indispensable to managing and co-ordinating QI efforts across the institution (*see also* the Luther Midelfort case study,

Support	Care processes							
	Varices, gall bladder	ENT, inguinal hernia	Gastro-enterology	COPD	Heart failure	Diabetes mellitus	Hip fracture	Neonatology
Patient logistics								
Patient safety								
Transmural care								
Medication safety								
Evidence-based medicine								
Good logistics								
Care pathways								
ICT								
Quality assurance								
HRM & leadership								
Mortality								

FIGURE 5.1 Vertical and horizontal matrix of Pursuing Perfection projects

Chapter 6).

The priorities of the PP agenda and the goals of specific projects have been centered, as comprehensively as possible, on the Institute of Medicine's six dimensions of quality care:[18] safety, effectiveness, patient-centeredness, timeliness, efficiency and equity:

> Two years ago when it started off we brought in the initiative to help us to think about quality in all of its dimensions. It's a philosophy ... Now, we're trying not to skip things anymore, it's about '360 degree quality'. We're now trying to use better people, and be more holistic in the way we do things. (Member top management team)

To ensure continuity in the transformation effort, new staff are socialized into the PP way of working and introduced to the six dimensions early in their induction. The aim is to make quality culturally embedded from the outset in norms and values that relate 'the way we do things around here':[19]

> Quality is defined by the six Pursuing Perfection dimensions. In the induction course for new employees, these dimensions are [introduced], with people split into small teams to discuss them. This is a good way to get them familiar with the Pursuing Perfection idea, and when the new people start working, they instantly recognize these dimensions in their daily practice. We are farther on with some dimensions than others; for example patient safety still needs more attention, but are pleased with the progress that has been made. (Quality Department member)

RdGG has gone even further, aligning the objectives of the organization as a whole, as well as the objectives of the quality agenda, with the six dimensions, 'translating' them into a formal set of promises to patients.

- ☐ *Safety:* We promise you an integrated care plan, and will ensure that all information is available to all care providers when they need it.
- ☐ *Effectiveness:* We promise you that the care you receive is based on the best, most recent medical evidence.
- ☐ *Patient-centeredness:* We promise you that you will have the opportunity to add personal information, to express your needs and to remove duplications.
- ☐ *Timeliness:* We will do as well as or better than the access requirements set by government.
- ☐ *Efficiency:* We promise you that we will liaise with your general practitioner to prevent repeat visits, and arrange a consultation with an anesthetist. We promise that you will know what will be happening to you.
- ☐ *Equity:* We promise you no variation in care resulting from [unwarranted] professional discretion. All patients will receive similar care independent of the provider who is giving the care and the location at which it is given.

The first two pilot projects chosen to begin the organization's quality transformation under PP were the Diabetes Care and Flow Varices (Varicose Flow) initiatives. Diabetes Care links RdGG's outpatient services with inpatient wards, GPs and governmental services, in order to more effectively manage patients with chronic illness. Chronic obstructive pulmonary disease (such as emphysema, chronic bronchitis and chronic asthma) and heart failure were selected in the second phase as a natural extension of the work in chronic diabetes care, again in the 'two to five to all' fashion. However, in an overall evaluation of PP, it was concluded that establishing the vertical and horizontal projects had not led to the desired acceleration of organization-wide healthcare improvement. Currently the focus is on better integration of PP in the strategy, the line responsibilities, and the daily activities rather than on pursuing perfect care through separate projects.[20]

Of these initial efforts, the Flow Varices project has been the longest-running and sustained clinical-level PP project, and one mentioned by several interview respondents as highly successful in terms of improvements achieved in quality, which prompted the selection of the team providing these services as the focus for the micro-system portion of this case study.

Pursuing perfection at the micro-system: the Flow Varices project

As we have seen, following the merger in 1996 the central administration of the organization was consolidated on the Delft site, allowing the hospital at Voorburg to be reserved solely for elective surgery. Improved quality was one of the main driving forces behind this strategic decision. The reasoning was that admission of high-urgency, high-risk patients produces disturbances in otherwise stable flows of care, and the efficiency of the care process can be dramatically improved by limiting the package of services provided to interventions that can be planned and scheduled, and by triaging patients requiring more variegated treatment into separate trajectories of care.[21]

Based on the assumption that routine actions positively affect outcomes, the Flow Varices project at the hospital in Voorburg was the first in the Netherlands to apply this so-called 'focused-factory' approach.[21] Admitting patients with similar medical conditions, and without comorbidities, allowed a certain amount of production-line automation to be introduced, and the Flow Varices project for non-complicated varicose veins was a case in point. By organizing the care process more efficiently in this way, the length of the process is reduced, the burden of work on medical specialists is lowered, and unnecessary visits to the hospital are avoided.

Applying the focused-factory approach has changed the nature of the contact with the patient, but, counter to what one might expect, the medical specialists themselves do not see this as a problem. Despite the fact that the care delivered has in a number of respects been routinized, they report that their own work has become less boring and administratively burdensome because all standard information is now collected and made available electronically. In effect, the automation of mundane tasks and standard data requirements allows clinicians to concentrate on the more professionally challenging aspects of varicose surgery and treating patients.

For example, a computer program has been developed to follow the patient from referral by the GP up until several weeks after surgery. The program enables patients to fill out the anamnesis (a medical or psychiatric patient case history based primarily on the patient's recollections) at home and email it to the hospital. When a medical specialist sees a patient for the first time, he or she can bring up all the important information on the computer screen immediately. Additional diagnostic tests can also be requested digitally.[21]

The project operates on a one-day-per-week basis in Voorburg, with varicose surgery taking place in the morning and the clinics in the afternoon of the same day. Effectively, the varicose vein directorate acts as a one-stop clinic. All patients scheduled for operative appointments must see the surgeon within a designated time from GP referral. On the same day of the GP consultation, if the patient is required to have surgery it is booked there and then, and the patient then proceeds to see the nurse and anesthetist for preoperative assessment.

This so-called 'combination visit' (in which anamnesis, diagnosis and treatment are combined into one visit) was introduced in 2002, and has continued ever since, despite the pressures of an increased number of patients, which has often made it difficult to offer the complete combination visit. By the end of 2003 a number of steps had been taken to make the combination visits easier: a varices 'marathon' was organized to cut the waiting list,* electronic patient files were introduced, and information provision to patients improved. To avoid unnecessary repeat visits, a survey was developed for patients to complete and return six weeks after surgery.

As with other PP projects at RdGG, the progress of the Flow Varices effort was defined and tracked from the very first initiation meetings using a variety of indicators along each of the six dimensions of care. According to these predefined indicators, the project has been generally successful in meeting its objectives, particularly in terms of reducing unnecessary post-operative assessments and enhancing the efficiency of the operating theaters and clinics. The most important indicators specified for these dimensions by the hospital were the percentage of realized one-stop visits (target = 100%), the period between the first contact with the hospital and the first visit (target ≤ 3 weeks), and the period between the first visit and the operation (target ≤ 4 weeks). The objective of 100% one-stop visits had almost been achieved by the time of this case study. The current waiting list for varicose vein surgery had dropped to approximately two weeks, one week shorter than the targeted three weeks. However, the average waiting time between the first visit and surgery was still two weeks longer than the three-week target.[22]

Further benefits relating to safety and patient information were reported as a result of advanced operative screening. In addition, anesthetists in the micro-system claimed that their work in the theater and the clinic in Voorburg had earned them greater esteem and professional respect among their clinical colleagues in the hospital and improved their relationships with surgeons.

Leadership at every level

The structure of leadership at RdGG – which defies the typical labels of either 'top-down' or 'bottom-up' – has played a crucial role in driving the quality agenda and journey described above. Leadership at RdGG is shaped by an underlying principle that people in the best position to make a decision should be empowered to do so, while carrying responsibility for that decision and its consequences. This has allowed the organization to operate in an increasingly decentralized way. RdGG also has a dual leadership structure in which various medical clusters are managed jointly by a general manager and a medical specialist. Key to RdGG's vision is the notion of 'supporting' leadership,[17] this being a good example.

'Quality' leadership starts with the executive board at the top of the organization – the chief executive and chief financial officer – but may also be found at all tiers, from cluster level (administration and specialist), through the departmental level, down to the micro-system level on the clinic floor. As a result, leadership for quality at RdGG is built into the main body of the organization, as well as being reflected in specific infrastructures – such as the hospital's Quality Steering Committee and Quality Department – to guide and support execution of the quality agenda at the strategic and operational levels, respectively.

It is our contention that this multi-level, dispersed but integrated system of leadership (*see* Figure 5.2) holds many of the keys to RdGG's 'whole systems' approach

---

* During this event in April 2003, which took place over the course of a weekend (a time when the Voorburg site is normally closed), a team of 75 surgeons, anesthesiologists, nurses, and other clinical staff operated on 76 patients, with the effect of shortening the waiting list for varicose vein surgery from 4 months to 4–6 weeks.

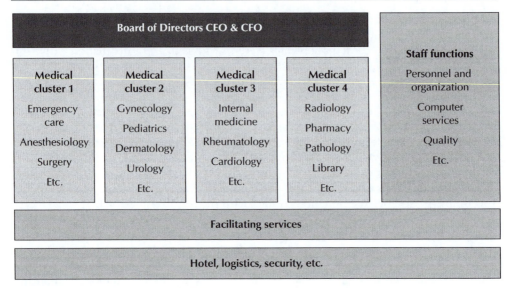

FIGURE 5.2 Organogram of RdGG

to quality, with the main focus resting at the departmental head level (note the parallels with Figure 5.1, which also reflects an advanced degree of 'systems thinking'). Denis *et al.* have an apt term to describe what we found at RdGG: 'constellations' of leadership,[3] 'constellation' (based on Hodgson *et al.*[23]) suggesting not only multiple actors but also a certain division of roles among them.

Executive board

The executive board of directors at RdGG has represented the equivalent of Kotter's 'guiding coalition' for change[24] or, in this case, quality. They were described to us by people in the interviews as 'very enthusiastic' about quality, 'enormously committed to quality in both words and deeds'.

More specifically, the role they play involves formulating, actioning and promoting the overall vision of quality for the organization (*see* Ferlie and Shortell[2]), providing a kind of road map for quality efforts, maintaining a sense of urgency around the need for continuous improvement, and providing both moral and practical support for local initiatives:

> Quality is something that needs to be seen as important at all levels of the organization. The employees who are working in their own micro-system in the organization, they all have ideas about their work, how they can do it better, smarter, how can they reduce red tape. But in a lot of situations, they cannot make it happen, and to make it happen the higher management levels in the organization must be open for this kind of improvement. They must believe in their employees, they must stimulate them, and from that perspective my colleagues and I believe that we can bring something to the organization. (Board executive)

Formulating a clear but simple vision and strategy is seen as a prerequisite for successful quality improvement,[25] as is providing the necessary inspiration for change.[26] In this regard, an important role of the executive board at RdGG is to 'spread the word' across and down the organization to raise levels of awareness and debate around quality, using

PP as the motive and focus:

> My colleague and I started with some lunchtime sessions organized by the nurses, and they invited us to come and tell them something about Pursuing Perfection; and so we started a dialogue with them. We're saying, 'What does quality mean for you? How do you experience quality or "not-quality"?' And then they started talking, and they began to address many of the issues around our six dimensions. So they start to *think* quality, and then they try to *act* out quality in their work. (Board executive)

The executive board also sees an important role for itself in promoting cultural change that will enhance quality; for example, supporting the development of a 'no-blame' culture in which people who make mistakes 'should not be afraid to tell it'. Respect for each other is also considered critical to organizational success. This 'cultural' vision is widely shared by the leaders at all levels:

> It is only possible to improve the care process if staff are willing to openly discuss what goes wrong. A couple of weeks ago, when a medical error was made, the CEO and another member of the management team spoke to all those and together they discussed in a blame-free way what went wrong and what could be done to prevent such mistakes happening in the future. (Board executive)

On the 'harder' side, executive board members use every opportunity to press the 'business case' for quality – the thesis that high-quality healthcare reduces costs:

> My goals are to make quality work. We have to keep saying that in the end quality costs less, because there are still a lot of people who think and say 'It costs us a lot of time, a lot of energy, so where are the results?' (Board executive)

The board sees its leadership role as extending outside the organization, with the promotion of the quality message at the 'supra-organizational' level:[3]

> [The chief executive] and I are doing a lot of that stuff. We are, in a way, the eyes and ears of the organization. We have to go and tell those outside about what we are doing in the organization and why we are doing it. For example, last year I gave a presentation to a large group of general practitioners and I told them about Pursuing Perfection and how it connects with them. We have to get them to care about quality management too. That's a very important part of our job. (Board executive)

Members of the executive board are kept regularly informed about the progress of the PP project by the secretary to the board, who is responsible for liaising with IHI and ensuring that new developments in the PP initiative are taken up locally.

The board also seeks to encourage clinical leadership of quality at the micro-level by providing the necessary financial and resource, as well as moral, support:

> Quality is something that must be very important at all the levels of the organization. The employees who are working in their own micro-system . . . when there are good ideas, proposals, we will support them. I will support them. When it costs money, you could say, 'Ah, not possible because it costs money, and money is a scarce commodity in a hospital so forget it.' But no, I try to run it a bit like a private company, so we see it as an investment, not as a cost. (Board executive)

Cluster leaders
Cluster leaders make up the next level of this multi-layered leadership system at RdGG. The eight cluster leaders come together with the two highest ranking executive board

members and the specialist quality manager in a linked system of leadership. The chief executive described the management structure and team composition:

> The management structure is divided into four [medical] clusters. Each cluster is managed by a full-time general manager and a part-time [one day a week] medical doctor. Additionally, there is a medical specialist responsible for quality on a two-days-a-week basis. In total, the leadership team consists of 10 to 15 people – CEO, CFO, eight managers for the clusters, and a specialist manager for quality.

To ensure the involvement of clinicians in the decision-making process, part-time medical leaders are situated alongside the full-time managers as co-heads of each medical cluster, working two days a week on management and leadership issues. 'This way physicians can exert strong influence on the medical organization.'[12]

In addition, several staff members are involved in both quality improvement initiatives and daily medical practice:

> I work in the outpatient clinic for two-thirds of my working hours here. I'm on call every two weeks through the weekends, so there's a lot of work. On the other hand, I'm part of the Quality Management Department for the rest of my time. So I support them and help to improve the quality, [and help promote] the ideas of quality. (Management team member)

This interaction between clinical and management leaders is also credited with improving understanding and relationships between the two cultures on a wider and deeper basis. Llewellan talks about the 'two-way windows' that are opened up as a result of clinicians taking on quality leadership roles, and the breaking down of the professional barriers that once separated them:[27]

> If a two-way vision is enhanced, this suggests that differences in meaning between medicine and management may be becoming less marked and, therefore, mutual understanding is promoted.

Certainly it is the opinion of a number of those we interviewed at RdGG that the view through the windows has been improved – from both directions.

This dual system of leadership involving clinicians and managers is acknowledged by many in the research literature as one of the prerequisites for successful quality initiatives.[3,28] Weber *et al.* in particular write about the value of having the right physician leaders in such 'boundary-spanners' roles and their ability to generate the positive involvement of clinical staff necessary to successfully implement quality initiatives.[26]

It can therefore be seen that clinicians at RdGG have a strong presence at a number of levels of the organization, and together with the professional managers they can be said to make up a powerful 'coalition for quality'. It is this coalition of clinicians and managers that underpins the PP initiative at RdGG, and which has arguably been as or more important than the method itself in bringing about improvement and change:

> We are going on the PP road, we have a coalition of people ... and we have a motto and that's what we want to do, we really want to do it from the Board of Directors to the professionals. (Member senior management team)

The approach to making quality work at RdGG is therefore to build coalitions of people committed to quality and who will enable it to spread across and through the organization. Such coalitions can also reduce the bureaucracy in the organization and shorten decision lines.

Cluster leaders are also allowed to initiate and implement their own quality improvement projects, and do not have to wait for permission from the center to do so:

> Quality improvement processes are sometimes initiated by the cluster and department managers, and not necessarily the Board of Directors or the Quality Department. The Quality Department does not even have to be aware of these initiatives and only gets involved if the managers approach the department for support. (Cluster lead)

Micro-system leaders

The Flow Varices project is run by a project management group comprising, among others, the clinical lead for this area and the surgical department manager. This is another example of the dual leadership at RdGG, the 'clinician innovator' and the manager of the surgery department sharing the leadership responsibility but both playing different roles. The guiding ethos is one of partnership in quality:

> The Flow Varices project team is rather enthusiastic and everybody feels engaged in the project. One of the main reasons for this is that all stakeholders were involved from the beginning . . . There is a lot of mutual understanding, and team members discuss with each other how things can be improved . . . All people in the project team are equal; and I believe there is no barrier for people to introduce new ideas or to approach people when something goes wrong. (Member nursing staff)

The clinical lead on the Flow Varices project was mentioned by all interviewees in the micro-system as the individual who takes a leading role in initiating quality improvement initiatives.

> He usually generates ideas and asks others to figure out whether it would be possible to implement these ideas.

> He is the clear leader of the project. He is very enthusiastic, and more a visionary than a manager.

During one of the Flow Varices project team meetings we observed, the clinical lead clearly acted as the visionary of the group, offering his views on how the care should be delivered, what should be done to improve quality, and how to evaluate the care that had been delivered. In these discussions the doctor's assistants played the role of the pragmatists, trying to apply the acid test of practice to the ideas he was putting forward. At the same time, representatives from the quality department offered support and assistance in resolving the mismatches between desires and constraints.

Flexibility and teamwork – both considered essential to quality work in micro-systems[2,29] – were, therefore, much in evidence in the meetings we observed, reminding us again that these organizational issues are as or more important than the PP method itself in bringing about improvement. Certainly it is hard to see how PP could have been successful without them.

With such considerable sources of leadership around quality across levels of the organization, the threat of entropy and fragmentation of the quality agenda at RdGG is especially acute. The hospital has reduced this risk through two specific mechanisms to co-ordinate the quality agenda at the strategic and operational levels: the Quality Steering Committee and the Quality Department.

Quality Steering Committee: strategic leadership for quality

The Quality Steering Committee at RdGG is an excellent example of institutionalized collective leadership.[3] This group is responsible for the organization's quality vision and strategy, and for the co-ordination of the various quality initiatives within the hospital.[30] The Committee consists of all the cluster managers, the executive board members, their secretary, and the specialist manager for quality, and meets for two hours every two weeks. Members of the executive board attend all of these meetings, sending a visible signal to the staff of the hospital's commitment to quality:

> The steering committee on quality is seriously committed to quality. They were the ones who chose to go for Pursuing Perfection. They are accustomed to having long meetings, yet members of the committee are almost always present. This shows how important quality is to them. (Senior member, Flow Varices project)

Quality Department: implementation and dispersal

Practical support for change at the micro-system level is provided by the Quality Department. Its members provide the necessary professional direction, in terms of technical assistance and co-ordination, to those pursuing the quality agenda locally. This department, which has the equivalent of approximately seven full-time staff, works very much like the transformation teams found in many health and hospital systems, including the other case sites in this study. Its role is not to direct centrally but to resource locally:

> The role of the Quality Department within Reinier de Graaf is not to initiate and manage projects, but to offer support and information to ongoing projects. (Quality Department member)

Despite the diminishing size of RdGG's overall budget, the number of staff within the Quality Department has increased, again demonstrating the priority the organization places on quality:

> Concrete indicators of the commitment to quality are the fact that the number of staff working on quality has actually increased [in number of FTEs], whilst at the same time the purse strings of the hospital have needed to be tightened. Another indicator that is highly symbolic is the fact that the Quality Department is located next to the offices of the Board of Directors. (Quality Department member)

One of the roles of the Quality Department is to help gather data for the PP project. Its other role is linking the macro- to the micro-system. As part of the PP initiative, project teams are formally charged with co-operating in specific projects such as Varicose Flow and Diabetes Care. Progress is monitored and used to gauge outcomes and levels of success, and performance indicators are used to check whether various standards have been met.

The head of the Quality Department likened its current stage of development to 'walking on a bridge while we are still building it': on the one hand the department is continually learning the best way to introduce quality into the hospital, and on the other hand they have to offer practical support to the many projects that are underway. These cross-linking functions and structures for introducing and supporting QI across the organization also play prominent roles in many of our other case studies (*see*, in particular, Cedars-Sinai Medical Center in the US, Chapter 8, and Peterborough and Stamford Hospitals Trust in the UK, Chapter 7).

Conclusions: rethinking the leadership of quality

In this case study we have seen how a great number of factors have contributed to RdGG's growing success and reputation in the service improvement field over the past decade: an integrated organizational structure, strong teamwork, a strong clinician–management relationship, outstanding individual leaders, a clear mission and core values, a supportive culture, the learning and adoption of formal quality management and improvement methods, and not least the IHI's Pursuing Perfection method itself, which has brought focus, discipline and an added impetus to the internal quality drive. Some of these elements have been planned and strategic, while others – including PP itself – have been more the result of serendipity and good fortune.

A case could probably be made for holding up any one of these for special attention, but we have chosen instead to highlight one factor on which all of the others seemed to rest: the leadership system. Following the trend in leadership writings over the past 10 years or so,[1,4,31] but one that with certain exceptions[3] has remained stubbornly absent from healthcare research until very recently, we wish to propose a view of leadership that is more depersonalized, de-individualized, more collective and systems-based than the one that is normally associated with the organization and quality literatures.

At a time when there is a strong 'cult of the leader' in the wider society and a tendency to lionize individual corporate leaders in the popular business press, it is important to dwell on the main finding of this research that leadership is a collective, not an individual, activity. The idea of a single leader bringing about quality improvement is a nonsense, especially in a professional 'inverted pyramid' organization such as a hospital, where power tends to be concentrated in the 'expert' operating core (the clinical interface, where care is delivered) rather than in the upper echelons of the formal hierarchy, and where it is widely dispersed among a plurality of professional groups. Despite the impression they frequently give or like to give, individual leaders do not – indeed can not – 'make it happen'; the RdGG story shows that it is groups, networks or constellations of leaders that do. As another of our case sites that is participating in the PP initiative (RD&E, Chapter 3) has also shown, like RdGG, there were important leaders who preceded PP, and those who came after it, each of them individually and in concert with others bringing a particular set of 'helping hands' to the evolving improvement process.

In their study of Canadian hospitals, Denis *et al.*[3] make a number of observations on how leaders achieve strategic change in organizations, such as hospitals, where strategic leadership roles are shared, objectives are divergent, and power is diffuse. For example, in such 'pluralistic' organizations, change is:

- more likely when members of the leadership 'constellation' play distinct roles
- tends to occur in a cyclical manner, in which opposing pressures are reconciled sequentially rather than simultaneously
- is strongly facilitated by conditions of slack resources, strong social ties among coalition leaders, and a focus on creative win-win solutions, which allow diverse interests to reach agreement and maintain a common focus.

However, Denis *et al.* also concluded that as they focused mainly on fairly narrow leadership élites in the hospitals they studied, there is a vital need to extend the collective leadership perspective vertically to people and processes at other levels who are crucial to stimulating and implementing substantive change[3] (i.e. down to the meso- and micro-system levels).

The RdGG account offers broad support for their propositions, demonstrating that a quality process needs leaders at many levels of the organization, not just at the top. This does not, of course, rule out individualism, but simply makes it part of a larger joint endeavour. As Krantz puts it in a phrase that might well have been written for RdGG:

> In systems terms, leadership is a property of the overall system and stems from the ongoing process of interaction among the important elements of the system. From this perspective, leaders and followers mutually co-produce overall system leadership.[31]

Of course systems do not form and maintain themselves, nor does co-design and production work according to some natural harmonious principle that can be left to its own devices. The co-ordinated quality system found at RdGG, with its complex connections between different levels of leadership, had to be created by particular individuals, most likely within (or at least with the support of) the senior management team. As we have found elsewhere (e.g. the Cedars-Sinai Medical Center case study, Chapter 4), possibly the most important role of upper echelon leadership is to initiate, and then maintain, the management and leadership system upon which the quality process is founded, and through which it is sustained, so long as the emphasis of this is confined to 'initiate' and 'maintain', since networks and systems, particularly in healthcare organizations, are not conducive to hierarchical command and control.

The evolution of a 'quality' leadership system at RdGG is still in its formative years, and arguably never found its true energy or direction until the PP initiative came along and breathed life into it. As this initiative loses its initial flush, the only question that remains is whether its legacy in terms of improvement knowledge and skills will be sufficient for it to continue to progress in the future. Certainly the strong, integrated and multi-level system of leadership it has managed to construct makes that a strong possibility.

6

Smart socio-technical design in healthcare organizations: sustaining quality improvement at the Luther Midelfort Mayo Health System

ORIGINAL CASE STUDY RESEARCHED BY GLENN ROBERT AND JIM ZAZZALI; NARRATIVE PREPARED BY PETER MENDEL, GLENN ROBERT AND JIM ZAZZALI

The goal of this case study is to understand how the Luther Midelfort Mayo Health System in Eau Claire, Wisconsin (*see* Box 6.1), a healthcare organization serving a relatively small, rural community, has become a nationally recognized leader in sustained QI.

The analysis here points to the character of Luther Midelfort as a smartly designed socio-technical system, attending equally to the social aspects of the organization (its culture, the commitments and motivations of staff, the formal roles and informal patterns of relationships among groups), *and* to the technical aspects of its work systems (the transformation of effort and resources into products and services, the transfer of information, and the use of technologies). All organizations, to varying degrees, need to maintain this dual focus, but Luther Midelfort is distinguished in the extent to which the interactions between the two dimensions in different areas and levels of the organization have been deliberately cultivated to achieve a synergy that furthers the organization's goals, particularly with regard to quality of care.

The inter-relationship between the social and technical aspects of organizations has been the explicit concern of socio-technical systems (STS) theory, an approach to conceptualizing and designing work systems that dates from the early 1950s.[1,2,3] Born out of mid-twentieth century experiences with the effects of advances in manufacturing technologies on people and productivity, STS theory offered the rather radical insight (especially in light of the dominant management paradigms of the times) that production processes are open systems fundamentally composed of human and technological elements that must be considered as symbiotic and interdependent.[4,5] Since arrangements that are optimal for one element may not be optimal for the other, trade-offs are often required between the social system – defined as the structure of occupational roles and the mechanisms for controlling and co-ordinating effort – and the technical system – defined as the materials, territory and processes used to convert work inputs into outputs. As a result, the overarching emphasis of STS theory and those practising organizational design within this tradition has been to jointly optimize the social and technical aspects of work systems, with the aim of maximizing both efficiency and quality of work life.[6,7]

BOX 6.1 Case profile: Luther Midelfort Mayo Health System

CASE PROFILE

Type of Organization:	A combined hospital and multi-specialty medical group system, formed by the merger of Luther Hospital and the Midelfort Clinic in 1992, and affiliated with the world-renowned Mayo Health System the same year.
Focal Micro-System:	Critical care unit
Size:	A full-service acute care hospital with 310 beds, and a multi-specialty group practice with 200 physicians offering more than 40 medical specialty services. The combined system includes 3600 employees.
Location:	Centered in Eau Claire, Wisconsin, a relatively small, rural community in the mid-Western region of the US. The health system is the main provider of primary and acute care services for residents in the local area through the hospital and main clinic campus in Eau Claire, as well as a network of community-based satellite clinics throughout the Chippewa Valley.
Country:	United States
Awards and Recognitions:	Governor's Forward Award of Excellence 2006 (the highest category of Wisconsin state's equivalent of the national Baldrige Quality Award; also received Mastery level in 2005 and Proficiency level in 2004); Acclaim Award 2005 in recognition of the system's chronic disease management program (the American Medical Group Association's most prestigious award conferred to only one recipient per year).

KEY CONCEPTS

Socio-Technical System Design: an approach to the conceptualizing and design of work systems that emphasizes the *joint optimization* of the social and technical aspects of an organization, with the objective of maximizing both productivity and quality of work life.

Organizational Slack: a 'cushion' of resources within an organization that facilitates innovation and change by providing crucial time and support for learning and creativity to occur.

Although direct applications of the STS design tradition, which encompasses a specific body of principles and methods for work redesign,[8,9] have tended to be limited to isolated 'field experiments',[5] accumulated evidence indicates positive results of such interventions on productivity and job satisfaction.[7] Perhaps more significantly, STS theory has come to underlie many of the innovative work designs and team-based structures now prevalent in organizations.[10]

STS theory and design have also been applied on occasion to health services. A variety of examples have been recorded from the 1970s to more recently,[11–13] but these efforts have typically yielded mixed results at best.[14] Some reasons for this less-than-dramatic success in 'non-linear' service settings are related generally to the approaches taken in conventional STS design, such as a complicated and lengthy design process, unconventional work designs that have proven difficult to sustain or spread, and, despite the theory, a tendency in practice to focus on primary work units or clusters of units rather than the organization as a whole.[5,6,10] Other reasons appear to be associated with the unique features of healthcare organizations, including the high degree of both technical complexity (e.g. the range of simple to highly advanced clinical and therapeutic technologies; the high inter-dependence and risk of tasks; and the intricacy of the human body itself) and social complexity (e.g. the unique role and autonomy of professional workers; the sheer number, variety and fragmentation of producers, regulators, and intermediaries involved in the delivery of care; and the human implications and unpredictability of treating patients as 'objects' of the work process) that characterize the delivery of health services.[14] These features of healthcare organizations as complex adaptive systems have long proven daunting to organization development, and change efforts of all stripes[11,15] and have only become exacerbated over time.[16,17]

Interestingly, the trajectory of change and QI at Luther Midelfort has proceeded without reference to STS theory *per se* or the involvement of self-described STS consultants. Indeed, it is highly unlikely that leaders or others in the organization would describe their approach to achieving synergy between the social and technical processes supporting improvement with any label resembling 'socio-technical design'. Rather, this notion is embodied in their own lexicon through the term 'integration', a phrase often repeated to the point that it almost represents a habit of mind or, as one physician put it, 'a culture that is integrated'. It is variously used to refer to the two milestone mergers the institution has experienced (between the Luther Hospital and Midelfort Clinic, and with the Mayo Health System), the unified identity of the current organization, and the joint physician–administrative roles that have persisted from the previous separate organizations to the new system.

The merger between the Luther Hospital and Midelfort Clinic, in particular, freed up resources in the form of 'organizational slack' that was pivotal in enabling innovation, not only for individual change efforts but also for a quality infrastructure and a 'process management' framework for understanding system-wide change. This framework is exemplified in the organization's 'high-level system map' that incorporates the technical flow of work, processes of organizational culture and leadership, and a patient-centered perspective on the system of care. Luther Midelfort's approach is similarly manifested in a formal physician compact that attends to the mutual task and citizenship obligations between the institution and its medical staff.

It is also interesting to note that this 'systems thinking' at Luther Midelfort developed out of the organization's frustration with incremental improvement methods and subsequent experimentation with Six Sigma, a set of quality practices commonly associated with 'lean production' techniques. While STS theory shares a number of similarities with lean production and other process improvement techniques (such as a focus on multi-skilling, teamwork, a committed workforce, and continuous improvement or redesign), it also differs markedly in its emphasis on strong work group boundaries (versus interchangeability of people across units), control of work through decentralization and self-regulation within work groups (versus standardization of work processes and direct supervision), and the value it places on improving the quality of work life and intrinsic satisfaction of jobs in addition to productivity and efficiency.[5,18,19]

In essence, Luther Midelfort has translated and transformed Six Sigma and its 'basket' of other QI methods in practice to an extent that their approach may be said to truly reflect the essential insights of the STS perspective. As such, it illustrates an instance of successfully implementing and combining intelligent socio-technical design with many of the benefits of a lean production paradigm, such as flexibility across units of the organization, perspective on the production process as a whole, and mechanisms for communicating across organizational boundaries.[18,20]

The following case study examines the roles of senior leaders at the macro-level of the institution and of units at the micro-level, illustrated by one particular clinical department, the critical care unit (CCU), in attaining this level of socio-technical 'integration' that marks out Luther Midelfort's journey of improvement from the others related in this book.

The (pre-)history of quality improvement at Luther Midelfort

The Luther Midelfort Mayo Health System consists of the Luther Hospital, founded in 1905 by a group of Norwegian Lutheran clergymen, and the Midelfort Clinic, which was opened in 1927 by Dr Hans Christian Midelfart, a Norwegian immigrant, and five colleagues. The two merged in 1992, and the main clinic expanded significantly in 1995 when it opened a five-floor medical office building attached to the Luther Hospital.

Centered in Eau Claire, Wisconsin, a relatively small city in the mid-western region of the United States, this healthcare organization now comprises the hospital and a multi-specialty physician group that operates across 10 different sites, including the main clinic. It is notable that Luther Midelfort is located in a predominantly rural community, with no academic medical center in the nearby area and few competitors for its services. Thus one cannot point to the effects of strong local competition or influence as driving forces behind the rise of Luther Midelfort as a place known for delivering high-quality healthcare. Yet it was clear from our purposive sampling for this study that the Luther Midelfort health system had attained standing among a number of national experts for being at the forefront of QI in healthcare, a reputation that has since been borne out not only in our fieldwork, but also in formal recognitions received after the site visits for this case study were completed (*see* case profile, Box 6.1).

The focal micro-system for this case was the CCU in the Luther Midelfort hospital. At the time of our fieldwork the CCU included 60 staff (49 nurses working 12-hour shifts and 11 ancillary staff), in addition to the physicians who worked in the unit. The CCU was selected because of the very strong team-based collaboration within the department and its known proficiency with quality measurement, tracking and improvement. The depth of collaboration was most apparent in the daily multi-disciplinary care rounds, which we observed. Although increasingly common in intensive and critical care units, the rounds in this department had an especially interdisciplinary and patient-centered character, with the team responsible for each patient – including physician, pharmacist, nurse, social worker, respiratory therapist, physical therapist, chaplain and dietician – co-ordinating care among team members, the patient, and his or her family. The department had also undergone something of a change in culture during the 1990s with regard to QI, as staff throughout the CCU became attuned to learning from quality data and (as described in more detail below) adept at using this information to improve patient care and service.

Two key events, described by the CEO as 'two simultaneous mergers', both occurring in 1992, were largely responsible for putting in motion Luther Midelfort's current journey towards a systematic approach to quality and improvement. The first was when the Luther Hospital became part of the world-renowned Mayo Health System (another mid-western institution based in Rochester, Minnesota), and the second was the merger of the Luther Hospital with the Midelfort Clinic, which came about because of 'some very forward thinking' by members of the boards of the two organizations and staff from the Mayo Health System. The merger of the hospital and the clinic has resulted in a very close-knit organizational structure, with one chief executive for both entities and boards of directors that meet jointly. These arrangements have allowed for an unusual level of strategic co-ordination across units of the organization.

The combined institutions are and always have been led by a physician, a fact that senior members of the organization felt was important in securing the 'hearts, souls and minds' of the medical staff for the health system's improvement efforts. This joint physician–administrative leadership is replicated throughout the organization, including initiatives relating to quality:

> . . . in terms of our leadership model we actively tend to put the non-physician and physician leadership together and jointly manage most of the initiatives . . . from day one the physicians and the traditional non-physician administrative management roles are together. (Chief executive)

The strong history of physician leadership was maintained with the appointment of the current chief executive, who explained the deliberate planning for succession involved and the stability this has lent to the organization as a whole:

> We actually had a year's transition . . . I was named in the position a year before I actually took up the post. So it was a fairly programed, orchestrated sort of leadership transition and we did that purposely. It helped add stability to the organization. (Chief executive)

Joint ownership of leadership and quality by physicians within the organization, and the 'level playing field' it puts them on vis-à-vis professional managers, was also emphasized by rank-and-file members of the medical staff:

> . . . you have to have ownership and that means you have to have physicians as they matriculate through their careers become involved in this specific organization . . . and they are pretty good about that here in terms of involving younger physicians in their careers and into the central nuts and bolts of what we do and what administration does and is . . . very much a level playing field where all of us are working with administration; it's not this sort of pyramid . . . (Comment during focus group with physicians)

A senior vice president described this as 'needing both sides of the same coin – clinical and managerial expertise'.

These facets of joint governance (between the hospital and clinic), leadership (between physicians and administrators), as well as physical location of the hospital and main clinic sites, have all contributed to a closely knit organizational identity in which individuals feel part of the merged institution as one entity, rather than harbouring divided loyalties. Another benefit of this integration, with both social and technical implications (as we shall discuss in more detail later), is that it:

> . . . liberated and freed up a tremendous amount of energy in the organization . . . things don't tend to happen in an organization unless you create some sort of slack, and integration really did that for us. (Chief executive)

The joining with the Mayo Health System was presaged by a historical connection stretching back to the beginning of the Midelfort physician group. The founder of the Midelfort Clinic, Dr Hans Christian Midelfart (the organization's name was later changed to Midelfort), was a protégé of the Mayo brothers and was greatly influenced by their philosophies regarding group practice and clinical innovations. This early 'imprinting' of organizational values and culture[21] would predispose both institutions towards a shared emphasis on high-quality care over half a century later.

Since 1992 the formal affiliation with the Mayo Health System has provided patients with the opportunity to receive care from visiting specialists and seamless access to specialty services at the Mayo Clinic, when appropriate. The professional relationships between physicians and other clinical providers have allowed staff at Luther Midelfort to benefit from what one interviewee termed the Mayo medical education 'machine'. This education machine quickly extended to issues of QI, for example through a global training contract that Mayo established shortly after the merger with the Juran Institute.

Prior to these two milestone events, interviewees variously described the quality activities at Luther Midelfort as 'traditional quality assurance' activities, 'hiring good people, putting them out there and letting them go to work', and 'mediocre with just a few little things going on just like everybody else'. Although attempts at formal measurement and improvement of quality had occurred earlier, these efforts were greatly accelerated and systematized after the 'two simultaneous mergers'. In 1992, the same year as the mergers, Luther Midelfort became affiliated with the IHI, and later became affiliated with the Juran Institute as well through the relationship with Mayo.

Through these and other intentionally cultivated affiliations, Luther Midelfort was able to connect with organizations and resources in the wider QI community. These activities supported and were mirrored by efforts within the organization to develop an infrastructure for quality (such as their Quality Resources and Education Departments), a framework for understanding and managing the movement of patients and system-wide change in the organization, and an explicit agreement or 'compact' of mutual expectations between physicians and the organization, including issues of leadership and improvement (*see also* the Cedars-Sinai case, Chapter 4).

Just as social and technical systems are inherently intertwined, these events and processes are similarly inter-related. For example, the merger of the hospital and clinic produced economies of scale, and much of the 'slack resources' generated were reinvested into the organization's quality improvement endeavours, resulting in greater involvement with IHI. This led to submitting a grant and links with other healthcare organizations in IHI's Pursuing Perfection initiative, which in turn allowed for increased opportunities for 'knowledge harvesting'. We touch on all of these themes but organize our discussion around three milestones in Luther Midelfort's quality journey: the hospital–clinic integration and its consequences, the 'process management' framework and development of 'systems thinking' within the organization, and the institution's 'physician compact' with its medical staff.

Hospital–clinic integration, organizational slack and the enabling of improvement

As mentioned above, the integration of the Luther Hospital and the Midelfort Clinic had both social and technical implications. From a technical systems standpoint, integration provided a greater degree of clinical co-ordination for delivering a continuum of care, and also freed up considerable resources due to economies of scale, which were subsequently directed at building the organization's quality infrastructure.

As part of the integrated structure of the merged organization, the board of directors contains three oversight committees: Teaching and Planning, Business Performance and the Practice Committee. This latter committee is where strategic direction and responsibility rests for clinical quality and physician personnel matters, thus integrating quality improvement within clinical oversight, as opposed to having separate governance of QI. This committee is also responsible for developing and monitoring departmental and physician specialty sets of quality and related measures.

From a social systems vantage, this integration resulted in a highly unified identity among members of both the Luther Hospital and the Midelfort Clinic. The level of integration within the merged institution remarked on previously is notable because many integrated delivery systems have found it immensely difficult to achieve co-ordination across the continuum of care, and are often integrated in name only. Consolidation of healthcare organizations without at least a degree of actual service integration typically fails to yield the efficiency and other benefits expected of integrated systems,[22,23] particularly in the case of combined physician–hospital organizations.[24]

Organizational slack

Considerations of organizational 'slack' have long been a topic of interest to management researchers,[25,26] being first defined by Bourgeois[27] as the 'cushion of excess resources' that are essential to the safeguarding of organizational quality and effectiveness. Lawson makes the case for the 'value of slack' in modern organizations, this being important for organizational adaptation and innovation, and for allowing time for learning and creativity around new forms of service delivery to occur.[28] In short, slack is not a 'surplus' or a 'luxury' but something that needs to be built into an organization for it to continually support innovation and improvement.

The medical director (who had worked at Luther Hospital since 1976) recounted how, when Everett Rogers, author of the classic text on diffusion of innovations,[29] was asked the one thing he would do 'to get innovation going', Rogers' reply was 'quite simply to create slack'. Thus, the creation and use of 'slack resources' – a concept referred to by several other executives as well – was a purposeful strategy that permitted the merged organizations to pursue a quality agenda and set of activities otherwise not possible:

> ... it was a conscious decision to integrate; it wasn't a passive decision ... things [like integration] don't help unless you create some sort of slack [resources], and integration really did that for us ... It frees up a tremendous amount of energy in an organization ... That's a very liberating effect ... [A]s we freed up our energies, the timing was right [to have] filled that up in many ways with the commitment to quality and quality efforts, because if we had been busy doing lots of other things, I'm not sure we would have literally found time in the day to be able to do [many] other things ... (Chief executive)

But merely freeing up slack resources will not result in a commitment to quality on the part of the larger organizational entity that is produced from such a merger; the fact that both organizations had such an orientation before the merger was a critical precondition. The medical director commented that prior to the merger both organizations were moving ahead in terms of their quality journeys. When asked whether QI was the impetus behind the merger, he replied, 'We were on our way on that before [the merger] ... for sure.' But once the merger was accomplished and the initial 'shake-down' period passed, the additional slack resources allowed the combined organization to build on this original commitment to quality in ways that the two separate organizations could not have accomplished on their own.

Once the merger was completed, Luther Midelfort pursued two sets of activities that have been central to its quality journey: 'knowledge harvesting' from the broader quality improvement community, and the development of an internal quality infrastructure in the form of its Quality Resources and Education Departments.

Knowledge harvesting and exploitation

Luther Midelfort put these 'slack' resources to good use, pursuing a prolonged strategy of 'knowledge harvesting' (i.e. exploring and importing information from a wide variety of external sources) with regard to QI principles and techniques. As a result, Luther Midelfort was able to render its rural location and relative geographic isolation moot in terms of hindering its ability to stay abreast of the state of the art of healthcare improvement, and it has excelled at linking itself to national sources of information and expertise regarding QI.

One of the most important relationships in this regard (like so many other of our cases) is the close tie with the IHI. The CEO recalled the advice that Luther Midelfort received from IHI at an early stage of their collaboration, 'to get out, to find out what is going on in other places', which led to a number of important connections with innovative thinking elsewhere. The initial involvement with IHI began in 1990, and continued in earnest after the series of mergers, with several teams receiving training in QI principles and techniques and 'seeding' this knowledge within the organization on their return. One of the senior physician leaders at Luther Midelfort, who would eventually be designated as an internal improvement consultant (and assume the job title, 'agent of change'), became an instructor with IHI and has functioned as a central link between the two organizations ever since.

The involvement with IHI has resulted in sharing and acquiring specific tools and improvement ideas. For example, the CCU participated in an IHI improvement collaborative with the ICU at Johns Hopkins, from which they acquired a daily goal sheet. This sheet was further adapted by the CCU into a series of templates of issues for each discipline to address during daily rounds. On a broader level, the involvement with IHI has led to engagement with organizations involved with the IHI's Pursuing Perfection initiative, and other significant improvement activities, including the Six Sigma movement.

In addition to the relationship with the IHI, the affiliation with the Mayo Clinic in 1992 also served as a rich source of knowledge and expertise. In fact, even at the micro-level in the organization there was a keen awareness of the impact the Mayo affiliation had on Luther Midelfort's access to knowledge and expertise. One CCU nurse commented that as a result of the merger:

> I think we saw more innovative thinking. And I also think we were looking at a broader area of hospitals to benchmark against. We were always benchmarked against . . . hospitals [of a] similar size, [in] similar towns, [and with] similar clientele . . . But now we're looking at big organizations and who is doing things well and how can we mimic some of those things so that we can do as well even though we're a small organization. (CCU nurse)

The Mayo affiliation has likewise had a direct effect on improving the clinical expertise of physicians at Luther Midelfort. According to a vice president of the organization:

> . . . the Mayo Clinic is like an education machine, a medical education machine . . . We have specialists [from Mayo] come over here on different days for different things. We have a flow of physicians that go over there to get updates on things . . . there's plenty of influence, not isolation. (Vice president)

Again, 'organizational slack' was essential in providing the organization with resources that could be targeted at acquiring knowledge from the broader external environment. Some individuals in the organization, such as the designated internal QI consultant mentioned above, were actively engaged in this endeavour. This leader and others cited 'buying plane tickets' as a specific example of dedicating resources to this activity, referring to a call by the head of IHI, Don Berwick, for increases in cross-organizational networking, benchmarking, and knowledge exchange relating to QI techniques.

But merely going out and harvesting knowledge is not enough to initiate change: the knowledge must be successfully integrated into the organization, or sufficiently 'exploited' in order for the organization to learn and benefit from its newly acquired information (*see*, in particular, the Cedars-Sinai case, Chapter 4). This process also requires the provision of 'slack time' on the part of various champions of change in the organization. Such a philosophy underpinned the initial approach taken at Luther Midelfort:

> The definition of slack time is not 'I am going to give you 30% of your salary and I want you to work on these two projects.' That is not the definition of slack time. Slack time is 'I am giving you 30% of your time and you really do not have to account for it but I want you to work on improvement.' (Internal QI consultant)

The medical director described this as involving trust in staff and some 'leap of faith' based on the premise that 'if you dedicate some physician time then you will get something back'. The internal QI consultant expanded on this notion in recounting how the strategy has developed at Luther Midelfort from his perspective:

> In the early 1990s the CEO and the medical director ... recognized the concept that slack time is required to work on ideas and innovations. I was that slack time, or part of it, that was created. My job was to go out there and change things. They didn't specifically give me a road map on what to change. They said go out and change things. One of the arenas I was pointed to was medication safety, but otherwise there was no restriction on what I could or I couldn't work on. In fact, looking back at it, whether it was by design or by chance, it's difficult to tell, but the concept that slack time was necessary and you gave it to someone to work on things, ends up being a way that this organization actually learned about how to do improvement ... [T]hey no longer send people at all stages to work on anything, it's very directive and very organized, but the principal that's behind it is people are given time to work on innovation and change. It becomes part of their work. They get paid for it; it's done during what I like to call the shank of the day, which means it's done during working hours, not done early in the morning and late at night and noontime. If you value change in an organization then you put it right up with everything else you do and it doesn't take second place. (Internal QI consultant)

Although the approach has therefore changed over time, 'slack' has been retained within the evolving quality structures and resources at Luther Midelfort, as this same physician leader described in terms of his ongoing role:

> ... the way the organization keeps being able to change how it looks at talent and resources and moves them around for their best benefit ... [the amount of time] is not spelled out but it is enough that I can still move around the organization. (Internal QI consultant)

Indeed, his role has become not only one of change agent, but also one of boundary-spanner, having split his time equally between Luther Midelfort and IHI. This arrangement has helped institutionalize Luther Midelfort's ability to ascertain the state of the art in QI by 'bringing new ideas from outside continually into the organization'.

Developing the organization's infrastructure and capacity for improvement

The slack resources that resulted from the merger of the hospital and clinic were not only directed at knowledge harvesting and implementation, but also at building the organization's infrastructure for QI and organizational development (OD). A year or two after the mergers in 1992 the Quality Committee that had previously overseen QI activities at Luther was thrown out:

> There is no Quality Committee at Luther Midelfort, but you go to 90% of other organizations in the country and there is a Quality Committee. So that milestone was that quality will be dealt with at every aspect of every committee, every department, everything that is being done in the organization. So that was a very major milestone because now quality is not separate from everything else . . . it is not a separate function . . .

Central resources for improvement

A number of individuals we interviewed also mentioned the allocation of resources for the development of the Education Department and, in particular, the Quality Resources Department, as another example of the use to which 'slack' resources were put. The Quality Resources Department comprises nine full-time staff, who are responsible for the technical support for measurement and improvement activities. The staff maintain clinical registries, and educate, coach and facilitate others in the organization regarding QI techniques and activities. The medical director recalled how, at first, these staff would visit a clinical department and say, 'You need to work on this and by the way we will help you.' But that proved to be a 'faulty strategy because they didn't have the organizational credibility and it is hard to be directive and a helper'. Over time this approach had therefore changed:

> In a lot of organizations quality resources are the people who try to push the improvement projects out there. Here [at Luther] the QR department is a resource; they are not responsible for improvement – they are responsible in part for measurement – but what happens is that everyone is responsible for measurement.

The Practice Committee and the Quality Resources Department now set the general direction and expectations and then make it possible for frontline teams to 'get there'. The medical director succinctly summed up the approach as: 'If there is improvement going on and we do not know about it, then that is the best problem we can have.'

A 'whole basket of methods'

In our interview with the director of the Quality Resources Department, she commented that there is a repertoire of QI techniques used in the organization and that 'a whole basket of methods was needed'. Indeed, the staff at Luther Midelfort seem adept at using – and continuously reflecting upon – a variety of QI tools and techniques, including Juran ('too long and arduous for some projects'), rapid-cycle plan-do-study-act methods ('doesn't work for everything . . . never find root causes'), as well as Six Sigma (there were 11 Six Sigma projects ongoing at the time of our first visit). In fact, the conference room next to the chief executive's office contained several books on various QI techniques and principles. Such a repertoire indicates a degree of technological sophistication with regard to QI in terms of the organization being able to select the most appropriate QI method for the issue at hand.

Despite the wide range of approaches to improvement employed at Luther Midelfort, a number of those interviewed commented on the deliberate strategy of using a 'common' language and curriculum for staff. As part of this strategy, each employee at Luther attends a primer educational session that focuses on quality and serves to reinforce collective understandings. This orientation is led by the director of the Quality Resources Department and the chief executive (prompting the observation from one interviewee that 'Quality is always led by the most senior managers here'). In this regard, the institution was also greatly aided by the highly publicized report from the Institute of Medicine in 2001, *Crossing the Quality Chasm*. The chief executive described this as having had a 'significant impact on us' and 'a major gift to us as an organization and to me in a leadership position'. As a senior vice president commented, the report had 'put words to our thoughts' about quality.

Availability and use of data

The work of the dedicated internal QI consultant and boundary-spanner to IHI in importing improvement techniques and orienting the organization towards a QI perspective, coupled with the work of those in the Quality Resources Department, seems to have made a range of staff at Luther Midelfort better at dealing with data measurement, reporting and interpretation. The organization, both at the macro- and micro-levels, has focused on handling and using data for the reason that 'good measurement drives improvement' (medical director). The bulk of senior management are trained in QI principles and techniques, including using data to monitor clinical and administrative processes over time. The general audience for the training sessions held by the Quality Resources Department is middle management, so they too are quite comfortable in this regard. In fact, the director of the Quality Resources Department, who runs a four-day class on basic data analysis for healthcare, stated that although the training had been initially targeted at middle managers, it had now worked its way down the organization and was now aimed at leaders on the 'frontline' ('third genera-tion training', as she referred to it). This general trend was confirmed in the CCU by two of the nurses, who indicated they no longer needed 'hand-holding' and that capability for data measurement and interpretation now rested at the departmental level.

Anecdotal but nonetheless telling, we recall that during one of our site visits we overheard a conversation in the hospital cafeteria among a small group of frontline staff, who were discussing data from a QI project in which they were engaged and generating ideas to explain the patterns they were observing. Such a conversation appeared to reflect a skill, willingness and excitement at learning from quality data and an investment in changing the way that work is carried out and care is delivered.

Management within the CCU similarly appeared adept at using quality data. The demands of the work in the CCU require the line staff to monitor and apply a large amount of clinical information about their patients within a very tight timeframe. However, using clinical data for the care of one patient is quite different from using aggregate data to understand patient care processes and outcomes. In the CCU there was a bulletin board with run charts indicating the discharge data over time, mechanical ventilation rates over time, and other quality indicators. Staff in the CCU said they were not initially comfortable with such quality data being posted in the unit for patients and staff to see, but that their attitudes changed over time, and so has their use of such data. CCU staff on the whole were genuinely interested in these data, and some expressed pride at minimizing variation in rates over time.

A 'unified' identity

As we have seen, a final impact of the merger between the hospital and the clinic relates to the identity of the organization (*see also* the RD&E case for a detailed description of this concept and its role in sustaining quality, Chapter 3). In the case of Luther, aside from the significant economies of scale and the technical efficiencies that were realized, the merger between the Hospital and the Midelfort clinic also resulted in the development and reinforcement of a strong and highly unified organizational identity among those with whom we spoke. Although legally two separate entities, the high degree of integration has resulted in those in the organization perceiving themselves as working for Luther Midelfort, not just the hospital or the clinic.

At the macro-level the extent to which people identified with the overall organization was particularly high. This was reinforced by the institution's small number of senior managers* and the ability of the organization to effectively screen potential candidates to make sure there is a good 'fit', or to promote from within only those who have a high degree of identification, with the organization. The 'physician compact' (discussed below), which outlines the values of the organization and the expectations of prospective medical staff, represents one important tool for such screening of physician recruits.

Systems thinking: mapping how patients move through the organization

Another noted key milestone in the organization's quality journey was the development of a Patient-centered Process Inventory, High Level System Map, (*see* Figure 6.1) also known as 'process management.'

This map was mentioned by a number of individuals at the macro-system level as a turning point in the organization's understanding of how patients move through the various systems of care and the development of a more patient-centered approach to overall improvement. It covers how patients access the system at Luther Midelfort, what happens to them once they enter or engage with the system (assessment, treatment and follow-up), and the factors that influence what happens to the patients (e.g. organizational culture as well as leadership and support processes).

The driving force behind the development of this map was the organization's involvement in Six Sigma, which Luther first began experimenting with in 2000 and which has subsequently become a 'huge educational component' within the organization, co-ordinated by the Quality Resources Department. Luther's widespread adoption of Six Sigma came about partly through frustration with other, more incremental improvement techniques they had employed:

> [We used] Juran and rapid-cycle improvement through much of the mid to late 1990s and we really became disenchanted with both. You can do Juran and never get anything done if that is the only piece and then you go to rapid-cycle improvement and we have done lots of it and it is done very, very well but it can't always take you to large-scale organizational change. (Chief executive)

As part of their frustration with these other techniques, the chief executive rejected the notion of the 'two to five to all' model of spreading improvement within an

---

* Luther Midelfort has a relatively flat organizational structure, with six vice presidents heading up the clinical services reporting to the senior vice president, and three other vice presidents heading up the corporate functions reporting directly to the chief executive.

organization:

> So we know how to do projects and we were convinced that we could do a project pretty well . . . we can isolate and we optimize one sub-process of the organization to world-class performance but it might bring everything else to a standstill – to compromise it. (Chief executive)

Senior management at Luther came to recognize that they could only go so far with QI techniques before they hit cultural barriers, which explains – as well as the Systems map – the development of the physician compact and the use of a common language and understandings about quality already referred to in this chapter.

The search for these different solutions was driven by a culture of very high expectations:

> . . . we are not just training for the local 10 km race here; we are training for the Olympics. That is the kind of performance that we are talking about and what would it take to do that . . . this whole concept of organizational transformation is a very, very big piece and part of the approach that we have taken now. (Chief executive)

As the chief executive also explained, Six Sigma is 'a broader system of thinking' and 'really a philosophical approach to understanding your processes . . . One of the first things you need to know is what the core processes are.' To understand the core processes:

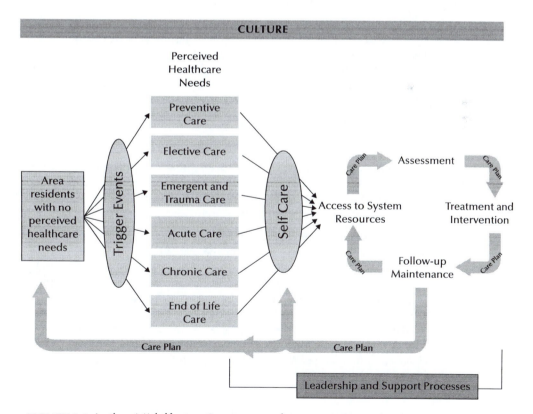

FIGURE 6.1 Luther Midelfort patient-centered system map

... we divided [into] two groups and we gave them the same assignment and said we
want you to do it independently, but ultimately, in the end, you need to come together
to have a single product.

The product of these two groups is a patient-centered understanding of core organizational processes, a rather refined analysis of the technical elements of the direct work
of the organization and how various social elements, like culture (which runs across
the whole system in Figure 6.1), are related to this. This analysis includes the structure
of the organization itself:

It has been very helpful in terms of changing our thinking about how we view ourselves
as an organization, and the concept right now is if we really want to be able to move to
a significant higher level of quality, then we need to look at the real nitty-gritty guts of
our organization about how we are set up and managed. (Chief executive)

In short, it is a mapping of their socio-technical system from the patients' perspective.

A permanent management team (each with a vice president and a process manager)
is in charge of each of the four core processes shown in Figure 6.1: access to system
resources, assessment, treatment and intervention, and follow-up maintenance. These
four horizontal management teams are responsible for the 'dashboard of measures'
used across the organization, which often lead to QI projects. Once a month these four
groups come together in what is called the Process Management Forum to resolve any
issues that may have arisen. The chief executive further explained how the vertical and
horizontal management of the organization fits together:

... what we are doing is laying on top of our traditional organizational chart this
process management structure which is a much more horizontal approach ... we are
not throwing out the vertical relationships; we are too big not to have those kinds of
relationships – and we are not adding any new people – but what is starting to happen
is that people are spending part of their day in the vertical world on the organizational
chart and part of their time looking horizontally. (Chief executive)

The dedicated internal QI consultant saw the development of these groups and the
system map as the start of Luther building a real, lasting structure for improvement,
rather 'than having this band of brothers out there doing things'.

The senior management had a strong grasp of this map, what it was and what it was
not, and how it could be used to understand what actually happens to patients. In the
opinion of the chief executive, this patient-centered dimension sets Luther Midelfort's
approach apart from typical efforts at such 'system maps':

[T]his is very important to remember [that] this is patient centered, because there're
lots of places that have put together system maps and that in itself isn't terribly unusual.
... [T]he whole issue [is] about patient-centeredness. I'm not sure that happens just by
putting some patients on an advisory group or putting patients on a committee. I think
it has to fundamentally strike at how you view, how you deliver care, how you organize
yourselves. So this comes from the patient's viewpoint, how do they experience their care
... it's an incredibly simple model. Basically, people need access, they need some sort of
assessment, they're using some sort of treatment and that might be a single trip or you
might get referred to another specialist in primary care and you go through it again, you
might get kicked back out. This just tries to recognize that there're lots of things that
patients experience in their care ... (Chief executive)

This understanding of how patients move through the healthcare system was likewise present among the physicians and other staff within the CCU, albeit at a different level of understanding. Related to the development of the systems map, one of the physicians credited this and the senior management at Luther with the cultural change he had observed during his time with the organization:

> I think part of it is from the top – administration makes the assumption that you have very good people doing their best and it's a matter of finding the things to support that and that is ultimately where technology can help. If there are 30 things you have to remember and you are under a lot of pressure and it is two in the morning and you have just remembered 29 of them, it's not because you're a bad person, it's because the system needs to be changed. I think the focus on system improvement shifts away from blaming the individuals and just finding ways to make it work. (CCU physician)

Another physician drew on an example from his own practice to illustrate how such an 'integrated' systems framework has contributed to 'breaking down silos':

> Nowhere else are you going to find cardiology really trying to open up beds for trauma surgeons in the unit because they are short. They will say, 'We have got to get the people processed through the system', and it is not only on a day to day basis; it's the strategy, it's the strategic view of how we do this . . . you are just not going to find that where you don't have an integrated system that breaks down your silos.

The CCU staff we spoke to were also able to identify their piece of the system map, how patients get to them and what happens to them after they leave the CCU. In fact one of the QI projects in the CCU was a Six Sigma-related initiative to improve the patient discharge process, which took up a large portion of the department's QI / data bulletin board. As part of our site visit we observed a meeting of the CCU discharge redesign team, where representatives from several departments that were part of the patient care process discussed various cultural barriers among professionals in reaching consensus on when a patient might be discharged.

The physician compact

Among the set of tools senior managers use to develop a high degree of organizational identity among physicians working in the organization, one of the most significant is the 'physician compact' (see Figure 6.2 overleaf). This compact consists of a standardized presentation to physicians interviewing at Luther Midelfort about the goals, mission, vision of the organization, and, just as important, what the physicians can expect of the organization and what the organization expects of the physicians:

> . . . in a very simplistic sense it is just really trying to define mutual expectations between physicians and the group that they work with. It's a sort of 'give' and a 'get'. If I come here what should I expect . . . (Chief executive)

This not only acts as a screening tool but also a method of socialization and acculturation into the ways of the organization and, no doubt, reinforces the strong organizational identity we observed. The CEO described the wording of the compact as 'part of our common language as an organization'. In many respects this can be seen as a form of social as well as technical engineering:

> If we want to truly improve the quality of care and what we are doing, you need to move much more to a compact concept that encourages things such as inter-dependence, delegated authority, ownership of issues . . . (Chief executive)

The compact spells out the behavioral expectations on the part of clinicians with respect to clinical proficiency, the particular approach to patient care (i.e. multi-disciplinary), as well as how to treat others in the organization. Although the compact does not explicitly set a figure for how much time each physician is expected to devote to QI work, the senior physician internal QI consultant stated that 'every physician has an obligation to do about 10% of their time on continuous improvement. That's built into expectations'.

This obligation was accompanied by due recompense:

> We recognized that commitment to quality and working on it was work, and we recognized it as work, and by recognizing that it was legitimate work it also meant that we would compensate physicians for their time and allow them to spend time and energies working on it. (Chief executive)

One supporting document produced by the organization provides examples of how one can understand and apply various components of the physician compact. For example, in the portion of the compact that relates to a team approach, the document specifies that 'Solutions to issues are usually best achieved by the involvement of individuals from a wide variety of disciplines.' This spells out how the organization wants patient care to be organized, acknowledging that from a strictly technical standpoint there are numerous providers aside from physicians who deliver care and whose contributions are essential.

The impact of these expectations for patients was made clear by one of the physicians we spoke with:

> One of the things that comes up frequently, and we see this in day-to-day rounds, is that when you have a culture that is integrated like ours is and mutually supported for quality, lots of the 'grey zone' variables surface. Nurses are very willing to tell doctors about smaller things . . . and so patients actually get better care because the nurses are

---

The Luther Midelfort Compact

What can you expect from our group?
1. A physician led organization that manages with integrity, honesty and open communication
2. A commitment to recruit and retain superior physicians and staff
3. Provide support to physicians and departments as they strive to accomplish organizational goals
4. A commitment to make the changes needed to ensure future success.

What can our group expect from you?
1. A focus on decision making that serves the needs of our patients and their families
2. A commitment to treat all members of Luther Midelfort with respect and embrace a team approach to achieving optimal patient care
3. A commitment to professional development including:
   • current knowledge within an individual's area of expertise
   • use of objective measures of clinical outcome to improve the care given to our patients
4. A recognition that personal change will be needed to accomplish organizational goals.

FIGURE 6.2 The physician compact

more willing to say, 'Mr Smith just looks funny to me – I don't really know what it is.' And the doctor is now aware of it and looking, and it's surprising how often in day-to-day things those are very early signs of something that is wrong. The nurse is experienced – she just can't put her finger on it. If you can't have that kind of [communication], it often slips beyond your screen or your horizon.

The document also specifies expectations that have implications for the social aspects of the organization as well: 'All providers (including PA [physician assistant], NP [nurse practitioner], etc.) are recognized as important, knowledgeable members of LM' and 'Verbal abuse or belittlement of staff is not acceptable.'

In relation to the physician compact, several members of the senior management indicated that the organization would not tolerate physicians who were 'cowboys' and did not abide by the compact:

> The expectation on the part of the physicians is that autonomy will not trump quality. That's a real big issue and it is one that the organization is constantly working on . . . there's no room for cowboys. Quality comes first.

The effect of the compact and other steps to increase teamwork in the organization has been marked:

> There is a general culture change that has occurred in this organization in the last six to seven years and that culture change is very dramatic; there is a tremendous amount of movement from physician autonomy to teamwork. (Internal QI consultant)

One of the stories recounted during several macro-system interviews was how the organization has asked a number of physicians to leave, even those who were very productive and big generators of revenue for the organization. Letting such individuals go is a very visible and powerful statement of organizational values and the identity projected by the organization and accepted by members. Interestingly, firing the 'cowboys' did not seem to create a fearful environment, nor did it seem to lead to 'false' organizational identity (i.e. people espousing an identity with the organization out of fear of losing their jobs). Instead, it positively reinforced the values of the organization. These accounts, and their significance, were repeated by nursing staff in the CCU:

> Their [i.e. the administration's] big thing was they didn't want any cowboys . . . there have been physicians who are excellent physicians that took very good care of their patients, but there were a lot of issues . . . where they wanted to do their own thing and could have some conflicts with nurses. And we really have felt . . . that the administration is supportive of nursing in that way, and that these kinds of things weren't . . . tolerated. [Two CCU nurses]

An integrated socio-technical perspective on healthcare improvement

Viewing organizations as socio-technical systems implies recognizing the interdependence between the social and technical aspects of organization. The other cases in this study have attended in depth to both the technical and social aspects of organizing for quality, both the 'hard' and 'soft' sides of improvement (a feature of virtually all the cases, but *see* especially San Diego Children's Hospital, Chapter 2). Even so, Luther Midelfort is distinguished by the degree of joint optimization, synergy, or – to use their own terminology – 'integration' that has been deliberately sought, and is continually strived for between the two elements of organization.

The use of organizational slack to support knowledge harvesting and a quality infrastructure, the development of whole systems thinking to map the various processes involved in patient care, the joint physician–administrative leadership roles and the physician compact between the institution and its medical staff, all incorporate careful insight into the inter-relation between the organization's social and technical systems, serving to strengthen and enhance their interaction. This strategy of organizational design and change has been fundamental to Luther Midelfort's journey of improvement.

The socio-technical perspective also emphasizes the nature of an organization as an open system, interacting and interdependent with its broader environment. In conventional STS theory and design, this broader environment has typically been interpreted in the form of general technological and competitive features of industries or general societal values.[4] The case of Luther Midelfort illustrates how such values, as well as mindsets and technical know-how on improvement, are imported into and can influence organizations through specific connections to other organizations, networks and communities in the external world.

Previous work on STS has argued for the potential utility of socio-technical design in healthcare organizations and similar types of 'non-linear' services that differ from traditional manufacturing,[5,6] yet has noted a need to modify conventional STS approaches for greater success and relevance in these settings.[14,30] The journey of Luther Midelfort represents one instance of how this can be done, including meaningfully incorporating the unique roles of patients and healthcare professionals in the quality improvement process. A likely contributing factor in this case has been Luther Midelfort's synthesis of socio-technical insights (if not an explicit STS approach) with lean production and other conventional QI techniques. As some authors have observed, realizing the combined advantages of both approaches cannot be achieved through mixing and matching their different features on paper, but only through thoughtful application in practice of organizational design.[18] Here, too, Luther Midelfort affords a unique example.

To some, the ability of Luther Midelfort to achieve this level of integration and viable socio-technical design may appear atypical, a function of its relatively small size and isolated locale with little competition. However, it is clear that geography was not a significant deterrent to making connections to the larger community of healthcare improvement, and 85% of hospital facilities in the US are community hospitals,[31] many not much larger than Luther Midelfort. The Luther Midelfort Mayo Health System may provide inspiration to such organizations that high levels of quality and service improvement are a real – if not easy – possibility, and an example of the usefulness of a socio-technical perspective for sustaining QI in healthcare organizations.

7

Empowering quality: demonstration and democratization at the Peterborough and Stamford Hospitals NHS Foundation Trust

ORIGINAL CASE STUDY RESEARCHED BY GLENN ROBERT, LOUISE LOCOCK AND TONY RILEY;
NARRATIVE PREPARED BY GLENN ROBERT, LOUISE LOCOCK AND PAUL BATE

The main theme for this case study came clearly to the fore during the fieldwork at the Peterborough and Stamford Hospitals NHS Foundation Trust and the radiology department within that organization (*see* Box 7.1). During this time we were repeatedly told about a myriad of factors associated with quality, including:

❑ the role of a central change team in facilitating service improvement (by others throughout the organization)
❑ the non-hierarchical structure, which encouraged strong links between the 'top' and 'bottom' of the organization
❑ the emphasis placed on 'local solutions' and networking with external stake-holders
❑ the inclusive culture of the organization.

These features and the constant references in the interviews to 'openness', being 'supportive', and even the specific terms 'empower' and 'empowerment', all pointed us to the notion of an empowered culture and the implications this has for healthcare quality.

Empowerment involves the generation, distribution and use of power, including formal authority and more informal control over organizational resources and decisions.[1] The concept, as used in research and practice, is typically given one of two faces, being broadly defined either as a relational construct (the granting of power to someone) or as a motivational construct (giving someone a sense of confidence or self-esteem).[2] Empowerment is therefore both a process and a description of a relationship between people.[3] Various authors have suggested key organizational practices[4,5] or organizational characteristics[6] that are associated with empowerment.

However, in the management literature the term itself has tended to become an overworked and narrowly defined word (albeit still an under-worked activity), often having 'delegation' and 'accountability' at its core. As Conger and Kanungo[7] and others[3] argue, delegating or resource sharing is only one set of conditions that may (but not necessarily) empower subordinates. Rather, empowerment in the context of this case study should be seen as an enabling rather than a delegating process,[3,8] about trust rather than accountability, and about creating a new, ongoing relationship between members at all levels of an organization.

BOX 7.1 Case profile: Peterborough and Stamford Hospitals NHS Foundation Trust

---

CASE PROFILE

Type of Organization:	A regional National Health Service (NHS) trust that includes a full range of acute care services, complemented by a college of health studies and postgraduate medical education center.
Focal Micro-System:	Radiology department
Size:	The primary provider of acute health services for a surrounding community of 280 000 persons, with nearly 600 total hospital beds and 2300 whole-time equivalent staff.
Location:	Centered in Peterborough in the east of England (80 miles due north of London), the Trust operates three main sites: Peterborough District, Edith Cavell, and Stamford and Rutland Hospitals.
Country:	United Kingdom
Awards and Recognitions:	Top-ranked '3 star' rating in NHS performance tables several years running; one of the first 10 trusts in the UK to be granted Foundation Trust status, which permits greater independence in managing local budgets and services; received the Health Services Journal Award and first ever Prime Minister's Award for Excellence in Healthcare Management (for cataract services, 2002), and the Health and Social Care Award for improving patient choices (2003).

KEY CONCEPTS

Empowerment: both the process of granting power over decisions and resources to members at various levels of an organization and, as or more important, a relationship with formal leadership that infuses those members with a sense of confidence, self-esteem and trust to exercise that power.

Demonstration: motivating support and ownership of improvement through demonstrating (rather than dictating or pontificating) the viability and value of an organization's quality and change strategy and participation in it.

Democratization: instituting formal organizational structures, policies, and procedures that provide opportunities and supports for empowering members at various levels of an organization.

The notion of creating conditions is one that particularly resonated with the findings from our research at the Peterborough and Stamford Hospitals NHS Foundation Trust. Consequently, we rely on the broader, deeper sense of the term, one akin to Quinn's[9] distinction between an organic as opposed to a simply mechanistic view of empowerment. The former concept injects a more realistic and powerful perspective into the tired literature and management-speak on empowerment. Here we examine the impact empowerment as a process and a relationship has for employees, and its consequences for organizational creativity, flexibility, learning and effectiveness.[1]

Empowerment, organizational effectiveness and improvement

As 'empirical support [has] begun to accumulate regarding the link between employee empowerment and important work-related outcomes',[10] it seems that empowerment may prove to be a vital strategic process for leaders attempting to induce and manage organizational change.[7] Although limited, this empirical support includes Spreitzer's[11,12] survey of a Fortune 500 company, which found that empowered staff are more innovative, effective and influential in their organizations; and Koberg et al.'s[2] quantitative study of the US healthcare sector, which found that:

> . . . workers who feel empowered have beneficial effects for both organizations and individuals through increased job satisfaction and work productivity/effectiveness and a decreased propensity to leave the organization.

However, there have been few systematic attempts and only anecdotal evidence to indicate how empowerment and quality may be related, particularly in the context of healthcare. This case study directly addresses this topic, reflecting, first, on how upper echelon (macro) leaders at Peterborough and Stamford Hospitals NHS Foundation Trust have attempted to empower staff in their organization (through what we term 'demonstration' and 'democratization'); and, second, the meaning of these managerial structures, policies and practices to micro-system staff and the impact on the quality of the services provided.

This case study is also significant in that often when a central transformation or change team exists – and as at Peterborough has a key role over a sustained period of time – it usually results in ownership being held centrally and not being transferred to the front lines. As a consequence, skills and activities remain locked up in the change team and quality is something that is 'done to' the frontline departments. In contrast, an empowerment perspective means that the central team remains, but its role changes from direction to steering, co-ordinating, facilitating and supporting, and above all imparting skills (and allocating resources) to those involved so that they can do it themselves: acting as a server (in service) or supply line to the clinical departments. This is another example of the complex and subtle interactions between micro- and macro-systems; if too 'micro', improvement attempts are piecemeal, fragmented and patchy (the '6 West' problem[13]) and do not blend or come together in any kind of system; but if too 'macro', they are selective and uneven (because of having to prioritize limited central resources), and too distant to get local buy-in and ownership. In the language of empowerment, we ask whether and to what extent senior management efforts, including the transformation team, at Peterborough have increased 'people's belief in their capabilities to mobilize the motivation, cognitive resources, and course of action needed to exercise control over given events'? (Ozer and Bandura 1990, as cited in Koberg et al.[2]).

So, while it is often assumed, as we have seen, that empowerment is the same as delegating or sharing power with subordinates,[1] this case study follows recent discussions on the nature of empowerment[10,14] in conceptualizing 'empowerment not simply as a set of external actions [but] as a process of changing the internal beliefs of people'. Echoing this distinction, Seibert et al.[10] point out (citing Liden and Arad[15]) that the literature on empowerment 'has developed both a macro perspective that focuses on organizational structures and policies, and a micro perspective that focuses on empowerment as intrinsic motivation'. We attempt here to capture – and reconcile – both these perspectives in examining the journey to quality made by the Peterborough and Stamford Hospitals NHS Foundation Trust and its Radiology Department over the course of more than a decade.

The macro-system

Peterborough's 'journey to quality' covers a period of three chief executives with differing leadership styles over a 10-year period, of early experience with piloting business process re-engineering as a radical change management technique, and of the ongoing role of a central change team. The macro-system story which follows traces the role these milestones have played in the development of three key organizational practices and processes: senior leadership, demonstration and democratization, each of which has sought to empower staff at all levels of the Trust.

Senior leadership

As Randolph states,[16] 'empowerment clearly involves a high form of leadership', or what Manz and Sims[17] call 'superleadership', one which is all about 'facilitating the self-leadership of others'. Weiss[18] suggests that senior leaders can empower staff in a variety of ways, such as by providing direction through ideals and vision, rewarding formally and informally, using involvement and feedback to further staff development, and appealing to the aspirations of staff for autonomy and independence.

However, empowerment in practice poses an intrinsic paradox which can spell the success or failure of empowerment efforts: there is an inevitable tension between the potential loss of control inherent in empowering individual groups and members and the organizational need for goal congruence and co-ordinated action.[14] For example, McDonald[19] describes how an empowerment 'program' in a primary care trust in the NHS resulted in outcomes at odds with the chief executive's original intentions for the program. Such experiences are not uncommon and can militate against the adoption of an empowerment strategy by leaders who are reluctant to relinquish any form of 'real power' or degree of influence in decision-making. This section aims to map out the efforts made by senior leaders at Peterborough to solve this paradox.

The recent history of senior management at Peterborough revolves around what were described to us as three very different management styles at the chief executive level, which moved through what might be termed an aggressive to a more conciliative and ultimately progressive leadership approach.[20] The general feeling was that the 'radical' approach of the chief executive prior to 1995 was initially a necessary shock to the system but that, in time, it became damaging to the organization (phrases such as 'a culture of fear and intimidation', 'macho management', 'a sledgehammer to crack nuts', 'a reign of the long knives', and 'carrying on knocking down the wall' were commonly applied to his tenure).

The appointment of his successor, the second chief executive in this line of succession, brought with it a more 'honest and open' approach and a much more 'hands-off' style, as indicated by the frequent use of the word 'empowerment' by many of those we interviewed:

> [The previous (i.e. second) chief executive's] style is still very much across this organization. Not knowing him beforehand, I don't know how much of it was there already, but certainly his approach and style – the level of empowerment here – people are not only interested in the results, they're totally supportive of good things. (General manager, service unit)

> I think that tone was set by my predecessor [i.e. the second chief executive]. [He] was always very straight and told things as they were, and that was quite empowering for the top team. Certainly in the first press conference, sitting alongside him, I found his honesty quite disarming. I think the press did. But it was very liberating because it meant you could say it as it was, and I've always done that and my colleagues do that, so there's no sort of side when you're talking to staff groups. If you don't know an answer, you just say so, and all that lowers suspicion. (Current chief executive)

This style of leadership has been continued by the current chief executive, who held the position of director of finance under his predecessor. Although seen as more focused on operational concerns than the previous chief executive, he is viewed as very approachable, described in a recent external review as 'highly visible and enthusiastic',[21] and similarly lends support to staff development even when resources are scarce:

> We've got a financial crisis at present – trying to pull back a million quid – and very quietly the chief exec's saying, 'I don't want to squash this empowerment workshop that's taking people away.' It's going to cost us four grand, but I said that's building for the future, that's getting a new level of understanding of how the Trust and team work and we shouldn't stop doing that. Quietly, he's saying, 'Well, there might be a kick back but I can sense what you're doing', so there's that trust about if you are firmly committed and believe it, then you go with it. (General manager, service unit)

Note the reference in the quotation above to the high levels of trust between individuals at different levels within the organization, something we will encounter repeatedly in this chapter and a feature of empowered relationships that can emerge only over time. Organizational trust has been defined as the extent to which one is willing to ascribe good intentions to, and have confidence in, the work and actions of other people (Cook and Wall[22] as cited in Firth-Cozens[23]). As Quinn[9] and others[24,25] suggest, an empowered organization needs high levels of trust to underpin the new relationships between staff members. At Peterborough the origins of the development of a culture of authenticity and trust were consistently ascribed by interviewees to the previous chief executive ('he was extremely laid back, he had a very open-door mentality and that broke down barriers').

Also contributing to the high levels of trust and openness (or 'low levels of suspicion' – see quotation below) within the organization are the relatively high levels of stability and cohesion among the senior leadership team. For example, as noted above, the current chief executive was previously the director of finance (from 1993 onwards), the director of organizational change was referred to as 'Mr Peterborough' and had worked in the organization for 26 years, and the medical director (who joined the organization in 1980 and had been medical director for 11 years) was highly respected and very important in securing clinical support for the senior management team's strategy. This stability has the attendant benefit of encouraging clinicians to invest in senior managers who are seen to be credible and 'in it' for the long term.

> I don't think I am deluding myself, I think that levels of suspicion are a lot lower than elsewhere because by and large there is a recognition around here that people are batting for the same side. The other absolutely key thing is how long people have been here – that is number one on our Foundation Trust application statement for quality of management: longevity. Not getting in a rut but basically people not coming here to just do a couple of years and then go off saying they have done this and that. We have come here, changed some things, messed some things up, lived through our mistakes and tried to correct them. There is ownership; management own the problem as much as the

clinicians. If you are constantly changing a team, where does the sense of leadership and culture emanate from? It just dumbs down without that stability. (Chief executive)

The current chief executive was also very conscious of the need to bring everyone along together, and that this could only be achieved over the long term:

> If we are on a rollercoaster, I am at the front and I think I can see where it can go but someone else is over the hump, on the other side, looking the other way and having a different view of life, and we have to get everybody lined up, and that takes some time. (Chief executive)

In terms of what members of the top team themselves thought they brought to the micro-systems' efforts to improve services within the organization, the director of organizational change highlighted 'support, interest and making things happen', while the chief executive said that:

> ... we do try and we are supportive and facilitative. If you take issues like expenditure on equipment, for a long time we have not been into this 'lowest price equals better value' thinking, so we would generally try and get the best thing we can for the department. We are open door – accessible – and we do listen. (Chief executive)

Here again we find facilitation and an inclusive culture to the fore. In this sense, the Trust's executive team, in line with the role of leaders proposed by Seibert et al.[10] and Connor,[3] have served to 'create a climate' and 'build an environment' where employees can help shape the organization's course in those areas in which they possess special expertise and/or insight.

To sum up, although Peterborough has seen very different styles and personalities among its senior leaders, not least its chief executives, the stability and cohesion of the senior leadership team over recent times and their long-term strategy of building a culture of trust, openness and inclusiveness have helped to balance the need for local ownership of change with the organization's need for coherence and performance across micro-system boundaries. In essence, they have created the necessary conditions for an empowered organization. The next two sections highlight how, through demonstration and democratization, these leaders have sought to further deepen relationships with frontline staff.

Demonstration

One of the key elements of the senior leadership's long-term approach to enabling quality to happen at Peterborough has been its internal 'change' (or 'transformation') team, whose role has been to facilitate and support – rather than lead – the improvement efforts of frontline clinical teams:

> ... it's the way the transformation team integrates and works with others. It's not about the transformation team itself, but the fact that we have got a team like this helps in oiling or facilitating and supporting the process of change. (Member of transformation team)

The origins of the team lay with the last chief executive's experience of using business process re-engineering (BPR)[26] at his previous hospital. This experience, and a series of discussions between different stakeholders involved in the Trust, shaped the 'transformation' project that he subsequently initiated at Peterborough. The then chief executive saw the primary objective of the project as the development of a better relationship between primary and secondary healthcare in the Trust, specifically to cope with a pressing increase in demand for emergency and planned admissions, but which he also saw as vital to better overall patient care. The broad aim of the Peterborough project was therefore to re-engineer the way these patient processes take place.

Writing with others in a review of the early successful experiences of the project, the director of organizational change gave two examples: the re-engineering of the patient admissions process in collaboration with nine general practices in the community, which resulted in substantial reductions in inpatient admissions; and the re-engineering of the dermatology referral process, which used new information technology (IT) to allow dermatology consultants (the equivalent of 'medical specialists' in the US) to prioritize cases by receiving pictures of patients' conditions before they arrived at hospital, enable community GPs to make more effective recommendations to patients, and provide patients with greater information and certainty about their condition before visiting the hospital.[27]

The relationship building that was necessary to re-engineer the primary and secondary care interface was achieved in a number of ways, one of which was by what the chief executive terms 'Bill's parties' (Bill being the director of organizational change). These were organized to allow people to get to know each other on a personal level and to start people talking about improvement and change.

The program initially recruited about 25 staff from across the organization, of whom 12 to 15 would work on specific 'transformation' projects at any one time. The staff were seconded to the project for periods of up to six months or a year, with a guarantee that they could return to their normal jobs at the end. Nonetheless, there was an acknowledgement that through the process they might themselves be 'transformed' and might not wish to go back to their old jobs.[28] Over time, the Human Resources (HR) department began to be more systematic and careful in who it recruited to the transformation team and how they were deployed, building in-house capacity and drawing on local knowledge:

> HR helped when it came to selecting the people for the transformation team. We did it on merit and we offered it to anyone in local health service, whether it's primary/ secondary care or social services, and anyone interested could apply for secondment to this type of work. So it's broad based. Other places have said, 'Well, have so-and-so because s/he doesn't fit this department.' We have based it on quite detailed selection work. (Director of organizational change)

Both the previous chief executive and the director of organizational change were 'students of the business process re-engineering guru Michael Hammer' and saw 'his vision as something they want[ed] to bring to the NHS'.[27] However, acknowledgement of the limits of imposing industrial change techniques in a professionalized organization such as the NHS led to the original top-down re-engineering strategy being adapted in favor of a more long-term, bottom-up, negotiated approach to change:[29]

> Yeah, he always did say that it was a difficult job to do – it was very difficult to measure cultural changes – but I think he was very clever in the way that he fostered what was being done in the beginning. He said it would be hard but it was like the relationship building; suddenly it was a slow cultural change – it wasn't something that was imposed, it was almost a mild osmosis I suppose. That was why, I think, it's probably sustained because I think people have become familiar with it; it wasn't going and giving them a load of jargon in a different language about how things should be done. I think we did it in a very practical way. (Member of transformation team)

When contrasting the approach of the transformation team at Peterborough with that of central change teams in other UK hospitals, interviewees would highlight the bottom-up nature of their work and emphasize the importance placed on 'building relationships' over time:

> . . . [hospital x] and [hospital y] had a transformation team, but they went down a different route to us. We see this bottom-up approach – right in the beginning it wasn't like an advertised thing. We almost went in quite quietly and worked, and built up the relationships with the people to move things along and it wasn't until we actually looked back, you could see the improvement and we'd sustained this here more than in other places . . . it is the building of the relationships – that's been the biggest part. (Member of transformation team)

The style of implementation of the transformation project also reveals the strong reflective side to senior leaders within the organization. In addition to the previous chief executive tailoring the re-engineering approach based on his prior experiences, the current director of organizational change and chief executive have both written extensively on the experiences with re-engineering at Peterborough, the former in the published article mentioned above,[27] the latter in a Master's dissertation completed during his time as finance director of the Trust.[28]

During and beyond the early re-engineering initiatives, the formation of the transformation team has had a key role to play in demonstrating to staff, especially clinicians, the value of participating in QI efforts:

> When we started, we had to convince a sceptical clinical audience and, again, I remember the first presentation we gave to the consultant executive body, one of the senior surgeons turned round saying, 'Well, what you're saying is we've been working in a naff way for years . . .' We had to persuade and change and demonstrate, above all else demonstrate, that (a) we can do it, and (b) it's worth doing and that the people doing it know what they're talking about. I've had to develop credibility for the team and protect it and protect its reputation and you can't afford a mistake because that costs you a couple of years. There were a whole lot of factors but the culture has changed . . . Yeah, it's because we try and do it, and the other consultants watching in other specialities, see what's going on. That encourages change. (Director of organizational change)

> The transformation project would have open days and put notices up in fact sheets and try and get the word around. It's a bit like the fly wheel – it takes some time to get the momentum going but once you get it spinning it gets a bit easier, which is probably the culture changing. It then gets easier to praise people. I am very conscious since I became chief executive that whenever I have a forum of people to take the opportunity to tell them how good this organization is and how good they are. I do that in public as well. Perhaps it's persistence? Maybe it's about playing a good percentage game. (Chief executive)

Conger[5] suggests that empowerment information can 'come from the vicarious experiences of observing similar others (i.e. co-workers) who perform successfully on the job'. Note the emphasis in the quotations above on the need to demonstrate the benefits of the transformation team and the projects they undertook (e.g. 'convince a sceptical clinical audience', 'persuade and change and demonstrate', 'develop credibility for the [change] team', 'try to get the word around'). Much of this resonates with the discussion in a number of our other case studies of the importance of homophily as a mechanism by which to spread and sustain quality improvement efforts throughout a healthcare organization. As individuals see their peers improving their services – and gaining recognition for their efforts – so they too take ownership ('it's not our project;

it's whatever project comes up from within the organization') and begin to draw on the resources made available to them by the organization:

> ... more and more people are approaching us and saying 'Can you come and help us map something that we're doing or developing ourselves?'; so we will go and facilitate and give advice and provide the tools and techniques. Then often they'll go away and actually do it themselves. But if they do need us for anything they will come back. (Member of transformation team)

Consistent with encouraging such bottom-up initiative for improvement – and as the Commission for Health Improvement noted in its external review of the Trust[21] – the transformation team prefers to use flexible target dates, placing frontline ownership of projects before timescales to facilitate effective change management (note again the emphasis on 'demonstration'):

> Somebody is more or less seconded to the change of work program, working with diabetes, for example, and also monitoring other change programs for them ... there's maximum devolved responsibility; that's because everything you do has to be a demonstration to other people that they can change and they don't need a standard, structured way of doing things. (Director of organizational change)

More generally, the work of the transformation team, and the strong support given to it by senior leaders in the organization ('part of the success is that there is clear under-standing and support in the organization that's led by the top team' – Director of HR), played an important role in getting clinician engagement and mobilization. Those involved with leading the work observed how resistance has moved down through the organizational levels over time and that the organization was no longer reliant on just transformation team-led change:

> They will also use us as an advice mechanism in the sense that recently we have had some specialist nurses, for instance, that are working on their own projects or developments and they have come along and said, 'What do you think about this' or 'Could you add some advice on some set of guidelines or protocols' or 'What else do we need to draw into this to make it work?' (Member of transformation team)

As well as its 'soft', cultural impact on the organization, the transformation team also provides 'harder' forms of support. For example, training in quality tools and techniques is provided on an 'as required' basis by the team:

> We don't do a kind of a systematic sheep dip approach ... but for example, when we had a clinical governance workshop a few months ago, we had the transformation team there just simply talking about some of the basic processes in change management, and then running some groups and workshops. I didn't quite know how that would go down because we had quite a few consultants, medical staff, and a real mixture – and actually, it went down very well. (Director of human resources)

By learning from their experiences and 'bumps in the road', such as with staffing of the transformation team,[28] and to some degree by revising their expectations, the senior leadership team began to see significant improvements in terms of organizational performance:

> I don't think it was necessarily disillusionment with transformation, but [the director of organizational change] found the first two years really hard going and, I suppose, we got to a point where we had to change our expectations a bit and focus it on projects

which were perhaps a little less ambitious in terms of quantitative change but actually, if you got them right, could deliver quite a lot. Then what we found is that if you string two or three or four of those together, you actually had changed quite dramatically. (Chief executive)

Beyond the benefits realized from specific projects completed, there were knock-on effects throughout the organization, not least the emerging sense of empowerment and dispersed decision-making. The following example cited in the article co-authored by the director of organizational change relates directly to the micro-system – and major innovation in role redesign – that we focus on later in this case study:

Re-engineering has also opened the way for many more avenues of change throughout the organization . . . [and] has led to an influx of new ways to facilitate training and development. Whilst Peterborough has deliberately moved away from creating new roles in the hospitals to support process re-engineering, they have empowered staff to a degree that autonomy exists at levels never previously thought possible. Ward managers for example are now more empowered than ever before; radiographers now write reports and have multi-skilled roles.[27]

Anecdotally, one of the service unit general managers we interviewed described how, during this period, she had been an outpatients manager and 'I altered something small in one clinic which demonstrated change and before I knew it my title was swiftly changed to service improvement manager!'

At the time of our fieldwork, the transformation team had 11 full-time staff who were acting as project managers/brokers/facilitators of 'modernization' initiatives, and nine local service redesign projects were ongoing. Although some of those interviewed felt that the direct impact of the team may not be as evident as it once was, its indirect influence was still being felt across the organization:

. . . a lot of the time in the NHS there is enthusiasm, plateau, enthusiasm, plateau, and I think that to some extent the transformation team has plateaued. But there are lots of people still coming and saying 'Can we do this . . . can we do that . . . I'd like to think about putting this in.' Not necessarily with the transformation team but with some of the principles that they've seen being used in different units [that have worked with the transformation team]. (Medical director)

The transformation team has nonetheless retained a high profile, both inside and outside the Trust, as illustrated by receipt of the prestigious national Health Services Journal Award and first-ever Prime Minister's Award for Excellence in Healthcare Management for their redesign of Peterborough's cataract service in 2002. This redesign initiative, which allows for patients to be referred directly from optometrists to the hospital for day surgery without the need for outpatient or GP appointments, reduced waiting times for cataract procedures from 1 to 1½ years to six to eight weeks, and the proportion of cataract patients treated as day cases from 8% to 96%.

The work of the transformation team was also included as one of six examples of 'notable practice' identified in the Commission for Health Improvement's May 2002 assessment of clinical governance at Peterborough, which was conducted as part of the Commission's rolling program to review organizational processes for accountability, monitoring and improvement of services in all NHS facilities:

The work of the transformation team [is notable], and its structures and systems should be shared with other trusts as a possible way of helping others to drive the modernization agenda forward for the benefit of patients.[21]

Reflecting on the process, the current chief executive, who in his Master's thesis described becoming at one stage 'increasingly frustrated with the transformation project',[28] stated:

> Having . . . a strong sense that my own organization was going soft on its re-engineering efforts I have changed my view and feel more relaxed about the process . . . Some writers might classify us as being one of the 70% of BPR failures but even the literature has mellowed in recent years . . . I also sense that this is only the start and that if we move into a period of incremental improvement we are likely to be improving considerably more than if we had not got the program in place. Cultural change takes many years and we have only been doing this for two . . . The degree of expertise and specialization within the clinical professions make it unlikely that a hospital could ever be defined by two or three main processes. So it is almost inevitable that we are constrained to tinkering at the edges, but if we tinker enough we can change the whole organization.

In fact, the trade-off for switching from a radical re-engineering to a more incremental approach is that Peterborough has not yet been able to complete organization-wide 'transformation':

> It was set up to promote change but to capitalize on existing champions for change, and what you end up with is a situation where maybe you've got 65% of the system has changed or people willing to change, but you're still running two systems because the 35% don't change and you've extracted no efficiencies whatsoever and parties get confused and the GPs don't know how to refer. (General manager, service unit)

It is a widely recognized concern that a proliferation of smaller-scale redesign projects, while increasing ownership and sustainability in various organizational pockets, may make no difference to the organization's performance as a whole.[29] Against this is the experience of re-engineering as a brutal top-down imposed solution which, while successful in challenging accepted norms in the short term, often fails to bring about significant long-term improvement. Peterborough, like many other organizations in the public sector, has been striving to find the elusive middle way, and the path they have chosen is to invest in additional dedicated resources outside direct operations, or 'organizational slack' (*see* the Luther Midelfort case, Chapter 6, for discussion of this concept) in the form of a small central team to support ownership of the improvement process throughout the organization.

In parallel with the role of the transformation team, and as a further example of how a central function of the organization has been deployed as a service to frontline departments, Peterborough has also used its IT staff and systems to help demonstrate improvement. Again, this has been supported by senior managers ('we've had two chief execs that have supported information, which has been a godsend' – Information services manager). So, underpinning the work of the transformation team and supporting demonstration is the fact that the organization has a very good performance monitoring system, although, like the rest of the NHS, good quality clinical information is still mostly lacking. As noted in the Commission for Health Improvement review, the Trust is 'an excellent provider of quality data on performance management information', including access for executives and all unit managers to live waiting-time lists and other performance targets:[21]

> I can tell you the trolley weights in Accident and Emergency, I can tell you our waiting lists position, when patients are coming, in real time, which has been developed internally . . . so really good information systems (Director of organizational change)

Furthermore, the information systems were developed in-house and not by a commercial partner:

> We have just agreed for one of my members of staff to develop an audit tool for orthopedics. We were looking outside to buy in something that would be quite costly and didn't do very much. I decided it was worth engaging the orthopods to persuade them of the benefits of developing a local database which was specific to their needs in dialogue with us – a winning cause. We have achieved that now . . . Through that route we are hoping to have on board one of the toughest groups of consultants in the organization. If we can get them on board in terms of the data quality, etc then we feel we can get others cracked as well. It's resourcing things for specific reasons. (Information services manager)

The head of information has taken on a broader role in the organization, including aspects of operational support, principally around performance management, and has been chairing various waiting list and winter planning groups. This has led to what he refers to as a 'skills-based service' (or what we would characterize as central functions being services to frontline teams) with in-house IT experts taking responsibility for specific operational areas.

Mirroring the senior leadership team, the Information Services department has also been able to build on the stability of its core staff:

> The second arm of the success is [our] stability. I don't think that is fortuitous, however, because what we've tried to do is a virtuous circle to push our service as being at the forefront all the way along the line. 'It'll do' isn't an approach that we take, certainly in the time that I've been doing this. It's very much pushing the boundaries, which means that we've been fortunate to engage, retain people who have got an interest in and are quite skilled, and we have retained their interest by a number of things, one is by giving them the flexibility, so that they are not stagnating. Based on promotions and staff development I have been able to retain key people because of that. (Information services manager)

As with the staffing of the transformation team the values of the Trust therefore lead it to recruit and develop IT specialists in-house.

All the central services mentioned above (the transformation team, IT and HR) appear to be providing specialist *support* services for local redesign, not trying to direct or control the work hierarchically or in a command-control kind of way. Tellingly, one member of the transformation team described themselves as 'a resource – and we think of ourselves that way: helping to oil the machine'. Such an approach brings to mind the notion of the inverted pyramid organization,[30] which places the clinical professionals at the top of an inverted pyramid and the chief executive at the bottom to ensure the organization provides support for their professionals and maintains them and the organization at the forefront of their fields. This structure is suited to an organization that builds expertise by providing frontline professional staff with ongoing training and support to enable them to constantly update themselves on the latest and best practices to meet customer needs. Inverted pyramids are organizational designs that allow those closer to the core activities to bring their expertise to solve customer requirements and thereby create a competitive advantage through knowledge in action.[31] This appears to be the ambition – if not the complete reality – at Peterborough.

Democratization
Running alongside the 'demonstration' ethos of the Trust described above is its

'democratic' structure and processes. Taken together, the two serve to empower staff in decision-making in relation to quality and service improvement.

Indeed, Seibert *et al.*[10] highlight the important role that organizational structures, policies and practices play in bringing about high levels of intrinsic motivation; empowering structures and practices are seen as contextual variables affecting employee feelings of empowerment. However, structuring for empowerment, like the trust that underlies it, has to be a gradual process.[16] In the case under study here, Peterborough has been refining its approach for at least eight years. Now, the organization has a relatively flat matrix structure and has increasingly widened the participation of its staff, including the clinicians, in senior decision-making meetings and processes.

> We started changing the structure; we got general managers elevated up to Trust executive, so instead of having it through the director of ops, we had a greater spread of people around the table which we found gave us better information, and that's really improved the quality of discussion. Then, more recently — in the last about three or four years — we got senior clinicians on to the top table as well, and I felt the quality of the discussion improved immeasurably at that point and got it less 'businessy'. (Chief executive)

In terms of formal quality structures and systems within Peterborough, the Trust has pursued a service unit structure as opposed to the traditional clinical directorate model.[21] Not that the term 'quality' is commonly used. As with a number of our other case studies, most notably in the UK (e.g. Royal Devon and Exeter), the term by itself has a sullied connotation and the Trust has preferred to make the quality construct integral to wider issues rather than have it stand as a formal definition in its own right:

> I don't think you could sell it on 'quality'; I don't think you could sell that quality ethos now anyway. (Director of organizational change)

> We try to build it up with the clinical governance agenda, we try to build it up through service improvement, we try to build it up through things like patient experience. To say 'quality' isn't used would be wrong, but we don't go down the line of quality improvement circles or a director of quality. I think 'quality' was the big push in the early to mid-1980s and was boredom personified. Because it was a concept that sounded great but was difficult to bed down. Sadly a lot of directors of nursing had to become directors of quality as well. A lot of the time it didn't mean anything. 'Quality' as far as a lot of medical staff were concerned was, 'Are you comfortable in bed . . . did you get your tea on time?' (Medical director)

The organizational structure at Peterborough is atypical among NHS hospitals. The Trust has one medical director who has responsibility for clinical governance, clinical risk management and disciplinary procedures, and four 'service units': surgery, medicine, women and children, and clinical and high support. Each unit has a senior lead clinician and a clinical management team, and is shadowed by one non-executive director. A general manager working in partnership with the senior lead clinician heads each service unit. The result is a form of clinical–managerial collaboration that aims to ensure clinical quality and effective resource management. As one of the general managers explained:

> I have a responsibility for ensuring both the quality and quantity of surgical services so that's broadly seven specialities: urology, ENT [ear, nose and throat], ophthalmology, all surgery including orthodontics, general surgery, orthopedics, urology . . . I have to have

my eye on the total volume of work and the quality issues. Below me I have a structure of three assistant general managers. One general manager has a focus on performance, a second one is involved with theatres and a third is in quality. It's a matrix model. They also have their own specialities that they manage in a first-case way, so they're operationally responsible, but that theme generates a level of overlap in our team which is quite helpful. (General manager, service unit)

Significantly, the general managers sit on the Trust board, allowing staff within the service units to have access to the board via an appropriate representative. The Trust board monitors clinical and non-clinical performance through information received from a clinical management board, a clinical governance committee and a conformance committee.

The Trust's 'hierarchical structures are somewhat flatter than in many trusts',[21] having the advantage of making it easier for staff to access the Trust board. However, any structure will only work if it is underpinned by a culture that reinforces and puts meanings around the various roles and relationships, and clearly there was a strong sense of alignment between the two at Peterborough:

I think our culture here is quite open, with the willingness to look at things and develop ... It's still not easy, but with the willingness to do that, and we've got support of the chief executive and the trust executive, etcetera, and it's quite a flat structuring, this Trust, in the sense that, in my opinion, I think it's quite open, that anybody can approach anybody about anything, if you like, to work on whatever development or any problem that you feel needs to be managed. (Member of transformation team)

For example, senior staff who have worked in other hospitals are struck by the honesty at all levels of the organization and the fact that 'everyone has a voice':

The way the porters speak to you, the look of the reception, whether staff have eye contact in the corridor, and that sort of thing. Peterborough is a special place. I've worked in lots and lots of hospitals and I know them well and I've studied them as well. There's a culture here which is big on consensus, big on openness, asking people to do all they possibly can to help but being reasonable at the same time. This thing about communication, the one sin in Peterborough is you do something without telling people. (General manager, service unit)

We have had really good feedback from staff surveys and other people, recognizing that there is a lot of honesty around the place. There is not too much internal politicking around, you can have pretty adult dialogues with any group of staff . . . (Chief executive)

When the Trust received an additional £1 million in capital funding, the staff were asked what they thought the funding should be spent on – another example of the commitment to a culture of participative and democratic decision-making:

And they responded with things that were on the softer side, [but] arguably important things, like improving the bed stock. Well, we had a bed replacement plan that was going to take about four or five years, and I think we allocated 25% – £250,000 – to it in one chunk, which means we can replace a heck of a lot of beds straight off; and £200,000 on security, which again, was something that meant a lot to the staff; but also has patient benefits; and probably we would have been a little less adventurous . . . if we hadn't had the money. So that was trying to put that back to people and say, 'That's really good.' (Chief executive)

Consultation with staff with regard to this additional capital funding was not an isolated example:

> We also put an awful lot of emphasis on communication, real communication, up and down the organization, and listening as well as speaking. We are very inclusive and very involving, I believe, and the way that we've done our health investment planning, which is in our super new hospital, intermediate care centers, and things like that, was right out there. So the requirements for the physical buildings, the clinical protocols, the key issues, have all been identified by the teams [in these facilities], such as the things that are a problem now compared to what you would see as the desired state, the best environment to care for your patients . . . And there is a mixture of different ways in the organization where I think people feel free and confident now to contribute. (Director of human resources)

Many organizations espouse democratic ideals, but the practice can often fall far short, resulting in pseudo- or quasi-participation, which has the effect of undermining and inhibiting trust. The view at Peterborough, however, was widespread among those interviewed from all levels that the reality reflected the rhetoric, with a sense of ease in relationships and an opportunity for real involvement in decision-making as part of the organizational community. Indeed, the restructuring of the Trust described above is very much in keeping with contemporary thinking in organizational design 'to minimize hierarchy and introduce simpler structures in which there are opportunities for bottom-up initiatives, more open and wide-ranging communication, and the greater involvement of all staff'.[32]

As the organization has matured, another important element of an increasingly open communication strategy – which has aimed, in part, at 'getting a name for Peterborough' – has been to celebrate the work of the transformation team more openly. As the director of organizational change put it, when talking about the Health Services Journal Award in 2002, 'We started to publicize what we were doing rather than quietly getting on with it':

> I like to be the best. I'd like this hospital to be the best. I like to be a winner. I like this hospital to have the national reputation and the recognition and the public like it. The people of Peterborough like it. That's what keeps me going. (Director of organizational change)

The chief executive traced his own 'emotional journey' to quality, offering a reminder that most organizational development processes are also personal development processes for those involved, requiring constant reassurance, recognition and confidence-building activities:[3,33]

> We started the transformation project in 1996 and struggled with that for a couple of years – really just understanding its potential and the limitations to it. Over that time we have just got rather more confident; we have started getting better results but actually started talking ourselves up a bit. I was reflecting on the importance of the talking up because it is quite difficult to get positive stroking as individuals and as an organization, especially when the NHS is almost perpetually being depicted as failing. So if you start getting confidence and you can somehow start engineering some positive stroking, which is partly by people like [the director of organizational change] pushing it a bit and saying, 'Hey look, this is what we are doing.' Then you start getting recognized, and the trick is to retain a high degree of humility about it all and not start thinking for a minute that you are particularly spectacular at anything necessarily. (Chief executive)

Just as internal relationships have been characterized by participation and involvement of staff at all levels, so, too, have key external relationships with primary care trusts and local social services departments been characterized by a similar inclusive, participative, trust-based relationship. This point was picked up by the Commission for Healthcare Improvement in its external review, with the observation that:

> ... the work of the Trust in close partnership with other NHS and local authority organizations, as part of the Greater Peterborough Health Investment Pan, is notable. It is an extensive whole-health system capital investment and clinical change strategy.[21]

The director of organizational change laid the foundation for these partnerships, starting in the mid-1990s, by spending approximately 18 months meeting with every GP practice in the area, explaining what the transformation project was all about and trying to enlist their support for it. He explained how he had 60 local GPs working in different groups with consultants in different specialities, believing that 'if you get them to agree how to practise medicine, then the patients will get a better outcome – that was the nuts and bolts of it'. Partnership then began to spread to other parts of the health community:

> We got incredible support from PCTs [primary care trusts] ... suddenly there was an air of trust and the feeling that we really could work closer together on everything and we could get a better result all round. I think that changed some of the dynamics within our own top team, and we started getting more confident about boundaries or not having boundaries around our organization. (Chief executive)

Enabling quality to happen

If we return to where we began this description of the macro-system, it would appear that another key point at which the paradox of empowerment – the only way to retain control is to share it – is being most successfully managed and resolved is at the general manager / clinical director level of the organization (one tier below the top team). In this regard, many general managers seemed well aware of the idea of sharing power in order to gain a deeper influence:

> Within each of the specialities, there's also a lead clinician and broadly speaking I have a fair say in who those people are, and one of my primary jobs is the developmental role in getting those guys to understand the principles of leadership, the ways to generate multi-disciplinary decision-making, planning, organizing, and so my model on the surface is giving away power. That's encouraging, giving away responsibility and autonomy. In fact, it's one of those paradoxical situations that the more you invest time and energy in other people to feed their own patch, the more you are able to influence and support them. (General manager, service unit)

The key point here is that middle to senior managers genuinely felt empowered, otherwise what would have been the point of considering and deploying strategies to empower others, as described above? Hence, one of the impressive achievements of the macro-system was that it had enabled the initiative for 'quality' work to be grasped and taken at this level of the organization, this being experienced in the true sense of feeling enabled rather than 'delegated to', or even, as may often be the case, 'dumped on':

> I've worked at a lot of hospitals but I've never stayed as long as I have here. The reputation of the Trust is that we have can-do culture. You feel empowered to get on and change things yourself ... (General manager)

Yet connections between levels are retained. So instead of being a culture that says, 'Get on with it and get back to me when you've done it,' it is more a case of 'Get as far as you can on your own and when you've got as far as you can, then you can get support from the chief executive to do the rest. It encourages local solutions, not solutions imposed from above' (General manager – service unit).

> The culture here is bottom-up. We discuss with patients and with GPs. We try not to say 'thou shalt do'; we try and bring it up from below and encourage people from below. (Medical director)

But it does not exclude a contribution from higher up, as we have clearly seen with the important roles played by support services, such as the transformation team, IT and HR. For instance, one of the general managers we interviewed described how the multi-level participative process worked around an issue such as improving health records:

> The health records manager is drawing up a paper with the staff so there is already ownership of the problem and the solutions. They say what their preferred solution is and why. Occasionally the Trust might overrule something – if they had good reasons – but it's a rarity. So when you come to implement the change it's already owned. (General manager)

This emphasis on consultation and involvement is an aspect of the culture at Peterborough that we shall see more of in our study of the micro-system.

In summary, at the macro-system level Peterborough appears to have adopted the ethos and many of the organizational practices and processes found to be associated with empowerment. For instance, Kanter[34] suggests that organizations that (a) provide multiple sources of loosely committed resources at decentralized or local levels, (b) structure open communication systems, and (c) create extensive network-forming devices, all of which might be descriptions of what was found at Peterborough, are more likely to be empowering. Such features as the mixed transformation team, the emphasis on 'local solutions centrally supported' (including HR and IT support), the flat/matrix structure of the organization, and the emphasis placed on establishing 'inclusive' relationships both within (IT staff, the transformation team) and outside (PCTs, GPs) the Trust, all lead us to suggest that senior leaders at Peterborough have put in place the enabling conditions for quality to happen in a collaborative, shared and empowered way.

Greenhalgh et al.[35] talk about a continuum of change, with 'make it happen' at one end, 'let it happen' at the other end, and 'help it happen' somewhere in the middle. Peterborough's approach to quality and service improvement lies very much in the 'help it happen' middle zone, spurning both coerciveness and laissez-faire-ism to the right and left of the spectrum. Equally, one could describe this approach, in Dunphy and Stace's[36] terms, as 'collaborative' rather than 'coercive'; 'tender-minded' and trust-based rather than 'tough-minded' and manipulative.

At the same time, realism and hard-headedness rather than idealism or even 'niceness' seemed to be the main driving forces behind this particular approach to service and organizational development. One of the main reasons why leaders adopt such an approach is that they do not feel omniscient and do not believe they can actually compel anyone to do anything,[20] particularly in the healthcare quality arena, which has much more to do with professionalism and professional concerns than hierarchical or corporate concerns. The leadership at Peterborough (and especially the director of organizational change, who had a strong industrial relations background) seemed to belong to that camp of real-world pluralists who believe that a command-and-control approach to change will never be successful, especially in professional organizations where the pyramid of formal authority and the pyramid of 'real' informal power are often the exact opposite of each other, and where senior managers may often find themselves in positions of 'high' authority but with little power to make it happen on the ground. The chief executive, medical director, director of organizational change and other members of the top team (past and present) seemed to know only too well that they did not have the 'luxury of the imposed solution' in matters of quality and service improvement, and could never impose their will unilaterally on the rest of the organization, or be able to count on undivided loyalty to its agenda.

Faced with this 'dilemma' (some would say deeply insightful and realistic reading of the situation), empowerment, and the parallel humility and trust this called for were not just one option: they were the only way of getting the required level of engagement and mobilization around the improvement agenda, thus the paradoxical but pragmatic view that the only way to regain control was to share it.[20] Far from abdicating on the quality agenda, the 'macro-system' at Peterborough were merely recognizing the limits to their influence and using whatever means they could to deploy and exercise whatever influence they had. As Child states:

> What pays off is adopting the mutually supporting aspects of new organizations *together*: fewer hierarchical layers, devolved initiative, teamwork, helpful human resource policies and ICT support – rather than just bits and pieces.[32]

The skill and effectiveness of the macro-levels at Peterborough in doing this are evident in the successes they have achieved, and offer food for thought for those organizations both at the coercive, command control and at the laissez-faire ends of the influence spectrum. We now turn to see what all this actually means for staff in the micro-system under study, the Radiology Department, and the implications for the quality of service provided in that unit.

The micro-system: the Radiology Department

The Radiology Department was selected as the micro-system to study at Peterborough for a number of reasons. First, it is central to the successful functioning of many areas of the Trust:

> They underpin [nearly] every clinical activity in the hospital. They're usually funda-mental to diagnosis for something... They're at the core of emergency care and elective, and they're a good team that's worked together through the most difficult circumstances imaginable, with several radiologists leaving in one go for a whole host of different reasons. But they've pulled round, gelled together, they've got some good leadership in there. The radiology services manager is exceptional – he's a radiographer by profession – and they're absolutely at the forefront in terms of extended roles, new roles, advance practitioner roles, and for years we've had our radiographers doing things that are still only done by consultant radiologists in other organizations. And they impact everywhere in the organization. (Director of human resources)

Second, the department has not had much direct involvement with the transformation team. Many of the projects the transformation team has been closely involved with have been studied and described previously,[27,37] so we anticipated that we were unlikely to find much mention of the team (or indeed BPR) in the Radiology Department. However, the department would offer an opportunity to discover what has gone on in other parts of the organization, away from the spotlight, and to assess how the 'knock-on' effects of the empowering practices implemented by the macro-system have manifested themselves by influencing other teams at the front line of the organization.

Third, as the chief executive observed, the department has seen a remarkable turnaround in its fortunes in the past several years:

> I couldn't praise that department enough, they're an absolute bunch of stars, and that is the department that was on the brink of collapse about two or three years ago, or less even, and they are just a shining example. Virtually all of it has been bottom-up from the department. (Chief executive)

Such a change of fortunes in itself offered a highly attractive opportunity for us to explore how and why the turnaround had occurred, and to what extent the story of what had happened fitted with the wider organizational narrative for improvement or was simply a one-off, purely local phenomenon.

Structure of the micro-system

The Radiology Department is spread across two sites: Edith Cavell Hospital houses magnetic resonance imaging (MRI), ultrasound, breast care and general x-ray for outpatients, GP patients and elective surgery; while Peterborough District Hospital (PDH) has trauma / accident and emergency (which includes a brand new casualty x-ray room with state-of-the art digital imaging equipment), computed tomography (CT) nuclear medicine, radiotherapy and general x-ray. There are also outposts at the maternity unit and Stamford Hospital. The clinical director for radiology and other senior staff are based at Edith Cavell Hospital.

As described in the macro-system section, there are no clinical directorates within Peterborough, only four service units. Radiology is part of the clinical and life support service unit (the other three being surgery, medicine and women and children). The general manager of this service unit has been at the Trust since 1992, originally as a ward nurse, and has been general manager of this unit since January 2002. She reports directly to the chief executive. Each section the general manager is responsible for has a professional head of service, referred to as a clinical director.

All the service units are trying to involve a wider group of people: 'We're trying to move away from the model of one or two powerful people and get groups meeting together, but it gets unwieldy.' This process was described as 'democratizing' by the general manager and was also driven by the perception that:

> The [existing] structure is not right to cure the problems. The structure is too lean. We need more time for development and learning . . . There is not enough apprenticeship for succession planning, freeing people up to go for the ride, sit in, learn. (Clinical director, radiology services)

The flat organizational structure of the Trust as a whole is mirrored in the Radiology Department:

> When I first came to Peterborough, one of the things that really hit me was that it's not a very hierarchical place. As doctors, at some point in our careers we've been through teaching hospitals, and certainly the teaching hospital environment I came from was a very hierarchical environment . . . (Lead clinician in radiology)

The radiology services clinical director oversees approximately 140 staff in 16 sub-sections, some of whom report directly to him while others report through the deputy clinical director (based at PDH). A senior manager oversees capital projects (of which there were eight major ones ongoing during our fieldwork), and there is a local quality assurance manager. None of these post holders are physicians, but rather, like the clinical director himself, are trained radiographers.

The clinical director drew a picture (*see* Figure 7.1) to explain the dynamics of the micro-system and micro–macro relationships, adding the caution, 'It's not three circles, it's more like frog spawn. Everyone has loads of their own bubbles: including their family, home, colleagues, friends.' The three 'overlapping sets of dynamics' identified in the figure are: (a) operational and professional (led by the clinical director and his deputy), (b) Trust-level issues of finance and targets (led by the clinical director), and (c) environment and equipment (led by the clinical director and the senior manager responsible for capital projects).

The clinical director argues that it is invaluable to have clinically trained radiographers filling managerial roles in order to manage these overlapping areas of responsibility:

> The dilemma is that some people believe you can manage a unit professionally and not have any clinical knowledge, and that a good manager will be able to manage that, but I'm still convinced that a hybrid manager – someone with a clinical background going into management, management skills – is the sort of person that is going to take people forward into modernization. And I think we've started to prove that. A lot of my colleagues are the same sort of person. (Clinical director, radiology services)

Comments such as this underline once again the importance of peer-to-peer homophilous relationships, with clinicians invariably in the best position to manage their colleagues (*see* the San Diego Children's Hospital case, Chapter 2), the hybrid clinician–management roles where a single person can 'walk both sides of the street' (*see* the Cedars-Sinai case, Chapter 4), and the notion of better understanding by clinicians and managers of each other's perspectives as a result of the 'two-way

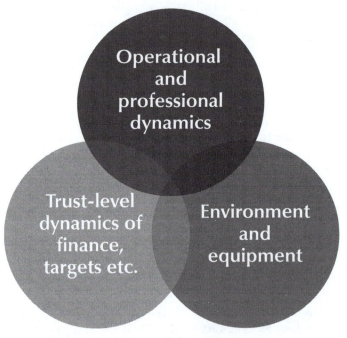

FIGURE 7.1 Overlapping areas of responsibility, from the micro-system perspective

window' that enables them to see into each other's life worlds (*see* the Reinier de Graaf case, Chapter 5). Apart from seeing this as giving clinicians greater credibility and authority over their staff, the clinical director added that they were also in the best position to know, and argue for, what was technically possible or safe – a major issue in such a technology-driven service as radiology. This allows them to avoid suggesting unreasonable changes but still to know when to challenge:

> As a clinician you know the limits, you can challenge resistance, you can push change but you can also then keep the management hat on and say, 'Right, in order to do that in a safe way, we're going to do this, this and this professionally.' (Clinical director, radiology services)

In the clinical director's view, the fact that they have clinician managers within the department has helped them design their service effectively, although it may not have been 'trumpeted' in the same way that prize-winning redesign (transformation team) successes in ophthalmology have been:

> We were doing these things before the transformation team was ever thought of. Our Early Pregnancy Unit has direct patient referral, where we actually allow our patients to ring us without going through everybody, they come straight to us. Long before ophthalmology ever thought of it but we've been doing it for 11 years . . . before ophthalmology even got on the map. (Clinical director, radiology services)

The department has a new quality assurance / clinical governance lead post which was also created out of a clinical role (a senior radiographer) to give some 'organizational slack' for improvement at the department level: 'it's seen as so important' said the clinical director, who meets with the post holder on a weekly basis.

BOX 7.2 Local clinicians' definition of quality in the Radiology Department

Access:	access is about getting patients x-rayed or scanned as soon as possible to aid further diagnosis and treatment. Referring GPs and consultants need quick access to appointments or unscheduled slots; patients need this too. Access is also about waiting time once someone is in the department, ensuring machines are used at maximum capacity, previous records can be retrieved quickly, and patients are distributed efficiently through the day.
Safety:	for both patients and staff, this involves ensuring radiation doses are not excessive, ensuring patients are not subjected to unnecessary procedures and are not harmed by procedures, and ensuring needle biopsies are carried out safely. Wherever possible a non-radiating technique should be substituted for a radiating one if it is possible to obtain the same or better results.
Accuracy:	encompasses accuracy of film-reading/diagnosis, to ensure the patient gets the most appropriate treatment, and also accuracy of film-taking (or accuracy of needle biopsies). Poor-quality film-taking reduces the chance of accurate diagnosis and results in repeat films being taken. This both exposes patients to further procedures (affecting safety) and results in wasted films (affecting efficiency).

According to those involved, the dual clinician/manager role in radiology has raised the profile of and improved clinicians' understanding and commitment to quality. One of the consultant radiologists we interviewed was particularly eloquent in explaining the nature of quality in relation to his area, stating that the ultimate goal of an x-ray department is to get as many patients x-rayed or scanned as quickly, correctly and safely as possible, and to ensure the results are made available quickly to other clinical teams involved in the patients' care. Other clinical staff drew our attention to three main areas of quality as it related to radiological services: access, safety and accuracy (summarized in Box 7.2).

Averting the 'precipice'

Several years before this case study the department had been faced with a sudden shortage of consultant radiologists. From having 11, three left and two retired:

> We came to a precipice. We either fell over or fought back . . . We really did come to the brink . . . There was a risk of becoming 'bog-standard'. (Clinical director, radiology services)

Although they had been working on developing extended roles for radiographers before this point, the crisis of a shortage of radiologists forced this upon them and accelerated the process of adoption: 'simply, the service would have collapsed without them' (Clinical director). The Trust, realizing that if radiology fell apart the impact on the rest of the hospital would be devastating, gave the department freedom to do whatever it thought was needed to 'pull the necessary rabbits out of the hat', which they agreed hinged on rapid adoption of the extended role. The crisis combined with top management support for this course of action achieved the desired effect:

> Suddenly people could see the scope for radiographers to extend their role. I don't think they would have tolerated it when we had 11 radiologists. (Manager of specialist unit)

There is much in common here with the literature on business process re-engineering, which argues that radical remedies such as these are more likely to work where there is no choice but to undertake some second-order change – 'radical times, radical remedies'.[36] Although extended role development is happening nationally in the UK, given the local crisis it is now more advanced at Peterborough than at many other places. It will be recalled that this notion of 'crisis as a turning point' is also a central feature of another story in our overall study (see the RD&E case, Chapter 3).

To implement these new extended roles it was vital to demonstrate that they were safe. The different teams within radiology were 'given ownership' (empowerment again) to develop the scope of the extended roles. Extended-role radiographers are now known as 'advanced practitioners', and in ultrasound, where 40 to 60% of the work used to be done by radiographers, it is now 85 to 90%. Radiologists only carry out the highly specialized work and they are 'comfortable' with this, or at least there is 'acceptance of reality [and] tacit acceptance by the doctors that they needed [the new roles] to survive'. Not everything has been fully accepted as yet, and some concern remains about the possible loss of 'bread and butter' skills by radiologists and the de-skilling of specialist consultant roles.

Such 'job crafting' as developing the extended-role radiographers involves shaping the 'task boundaries'[38] of a job by altering the form or number of activities the post-holder engages in while doing the job. This links closely with the notion of empowerment, in that the perceived opportunity to job-craft refers to the sense of freedom or discretion employees have in what they do in their job and how they do it. In the case of the radiology department at Peterborough, this discretion came about as a result of a potential crisis in the service, but, as already highlighted, the chief executive nonetheless felt that 'virtually all [of the improvements] have been bottom-up from the department'.

'Allowing it to happen' at the micro-system level

Within this micro-system we found a consistent emphasis on empowering staff and giving people autonomy to 'just get on and do good things':

> Quality must come from within: there must be an inner desire to go forward. It gives you headaches but it also gives you an empowered workforce who enjoy their work and feel integrated into the department. (General manager)

> We have built-in peer review. Quality from individual to individual: are you doing it right? We've been doing that for five years already. Our working practice has got that built-in without anyone telling me to do it . . . We've also been consulting patients about what they think of us for years. I personally for the last six years have been asking 100 patients every year to tell me what they think of me as a person; this is before patient involvement was even thought of. (Consultant radiologist)

One good example of how staff at the departmental level feel empowered to push for things they believe are essential and to find creative ways to get around problems is the way in which the clinical director of this particular micro-system had to 'fight and fudge the budget' to get a full-time personal assistant. Initially, he used some vacancy money to buy in some support and then the 'new role became indispensable'. He described his approach as 'risk-taking, lying through your teeth, getting a criminal record!'

Staff in the radiology department told us that they could come to the clinical director with any problem to 'get it off their chest in a safe environment', although the clinical director himself stated that people should not keep coming to him because it may be a sign that they weren't managing their situation. He could give them advice, but it should be up to them to find solutions and sort out their own problems as far as they were able. This he felt was 'encouraging people to grow and take on responsibility'. Such an approach fits well with the notion of managers assuming empowering roles as 'coach, mentor and team leader' rather than relying on hierarchical power.[16]

The clinical director's leadership style had clearly played a key role in shaping the department's particular kind of open, democratic culture:

> He's very well respected and I think this is because he stands back and lets every head of department deal with their own bits, and then if he needs to step in, then he would do and if they need to go [to] him, then they would and he would step in. (Clerical co-ordinator)

> [The clinical director] has been instrumental in leading. He's the sort of person who pulls the team together. I have enormous respect for him. He's very open, democratic, transformational, very hard working. (General manager)

Finally, and relating back to our earlier discussion on the creation of 'organizational slack' for staff members to review their working processes, the clinical director said that if he were to send two people to a conference or on a hospital visit to look at equipment, then he would often end up sending four, 'two for the ride'. Doing so gave them 'responsibility and ownership' for choosing equipment or redesigning space utilization, but it also demonstrated to his staff that it was hard work traveling and writing up a report, and better still that it was 'nicer at Peterborough!'

Conclusions: real empowerment and the quest for quality in healthcare

In the management literature, empowerment is commonly associated with a set of management techniques or the act of the more powerful sharing some of their power with others who have less. For example, the ideas of delegation or devolution and the decentralization of decision-making power have long been equated with the empowerment notion. Historically we also find that much of the literature on empowerment deals with participative management techniques such as goal-setting by subordinates, management by objectives, and quality circles as the means of sharing power or delegating authority, and increasing involvement.

The limitation of this line of reasoning is that it does not adequately address the nature of empowerment as it is actually experienced by the recipients themselves (or, for that matter, the 'empowerers'). Empowerment is not something an organization grants to its staff or can transfer to them through training. It is 'a special status that is merited by building credibility through previous interactions'.[3] It is in this sense that empowerment and trust go hand in hand; the one underpins the other and it is therefore not surprising to find that the conditions commonly cited to promote trust within organizations – the need to be less bureaucratic, high levels of staff participation in decision-making and openness of communication[23] – are similar to those we found at Peterborough.

By focusing on the experience of empowerment in this case study, we have discovered that it involves a good deal more than being, or even feeling, 'more powerful' or 'more involved'. Real empowerment is this and much more: it is about relationships, trust, motivation, and about feeling more valued. On the motivational aspect, for example, Seibert *et al.* observe that empowerment at its core 'involves increased individual motivation at work through the delegation of authority to the lowest level in an organization where a competent decision can be made'.[10]

This was certainly the case at Peterborough, although it went even wider to include the feeling of being trusted and respected: 'if you can prove competence, credibility and security, people trust you to offer solutions' (Clinical director). 'Empowerment' described not so much a power transaction but a whole relationship, signifying that one was regarded by one's colleagues – especially senior colleagues – as professional, reliable, adult, equal, competent and best placed to make decisions. This is important for, as Quinn[9] points out, 'ultimately, each of us has exactly as much power as we really want', and being in a relationship where one's contribution is valued and opinions respected is much more conducive to staff wanting to take on more power. In this sense, Connor[3] uses the notion of an empowered relationship, based on trust, as something new between people rather than something that is passed on from someone (usually at the top) to someone else (usually at the bottom). So rather than formal contracts (as seen in the form of the physician compacts in some of our US case study sites), trust at Peterborough was more traditional in nature and based on personal relationships, strengthened by a positive experience of those relationships.[32]

Not that this was always straightforward or comfortable in an organization where hierarchy and dependency relationships were never that far away from established mindsets and practices. For example, one of the senior nurses told us how, in a previous post as a ward nurse, she had been shocked to find that some building work that had partially closed her ward had not been completed, leaving her unable to re-open the beds for the busy Easter period. Her natural reaction was to telephone the director of operations in the expectation that he would authorize the completion of the work. In the event, she said, this did not happen. His reply to her was, 'If you weren't happy with this standard of work at home you would sort it out, therefore why not do the same here and sort it out for yourself?' She said that her first reaction had been to think he had just been trying to offload responsibility back on to her. However, on reflection she felt like she had been supported in finding the solution for herself.

At Peterborough, the executive team and the transformation team were widely credited with resisting this tendency to fall back on hierarchy and quasi- or pseudo-participation techniques, realizing that they had only limited powers to influence what was actually done on the frontline service provision (*see* the earlier discussion on the pluralism of healthcare settings), a point that had not escaped the attention of the frontlines themselves:

> I suppose the thing that has the most impact is them allowing people at [clinical director] level to manage how he wants to manage . . . in the sense that the Trust's chief executive recognizes he can't affect people individually at the bottom. (Manager of specialist unit)

So there was no option other than to redefine the role as support rather than direction, at the same time as accepting that the responsibility for mistakes still rests formally 'at the top':

> Having seen other hospital Trusts, the way they work, the direct systems and the way of the management, allowing the managers to work, not independently but they have a certain amount of freedom has certainly contributed a lot to innovation through this Trust, I'm sure. People are being given the support and the chance to make mistakes. (Clinical director)

Acceptance of the limitations of one's powers to direct and control from the top (as opposed to formal authority) had shaped not only the way the senior team managed and led the organization generally, but more specifically the way it went about the whole issue of quality and service improvement. This may be characterized as:

❏ *demonstrating* rather than dictating (letting service improvement achievements speak for themselves; helping the word to spread), and
❏ *creating the conditions* for people to seek empowerment for themselves, rather than espousing it as some kind of top-down ideology or strategy (by resisting dependency and 'upward delegation' of decision making by others; focusing on building trust, confidence and the inner motivation for people to take ownership for local service development for themselves).

This case study and recent literature on empowerment provide strong evidence for the need to adopt a wider conception of the term than has been the case up until now, one that embraces not only the usual power and control issues, but also issues of organizational style, relationships, motivation and culture. Modern writers on the subject, such as Feldman and Khademian,[1] reveal just how broad-ranging and potent these issues are. They suggest that empowered employees are able to develop new understandings of the work of the organization and their individual role in that effort. These new understandings lead to new ways of approaching work and the ability to engage in 'job-crafting' issues, exemplified by the extended radiographer's role in the micro-system described above.

Employees who are empowered to 'leave their desks' are able to make new connections with people who do work that is relevant to theirs. If accomplishing the goals will be better served by connecting with others outside of their unit but within the same organization, across other organizations or with members of the public, they have the freedom to make these connections. Finally, empowered staff are able to utilize new sources and types of information in the pursuit of their work.

Just as empowerment affects values, attitudes and behaviors in general,[16] so, as we have seen, it has a similar impact on improvement values, improvement attitudes and improvement practices in particular. Empowerment and improvement have not been explored in any level of detail in healthcare and quality research up until now, and only Seibert *et al.*'s[10] study of a Fortune 100 company in the US has sought to integrate macro- and micro-system approaches to empowerment. The fact that the close connection between them accounts for so much of the success of the Peterborough and Stamford NHS Foundation Trust in the quality domain may now encourage others to examine this relationship more closely.

8

Mobilizing for quality: the case of an HIV/AIDS treatment center in Albany, New York

ORIGINAL CASE STUDY RESEARCHED BY KEITH MCINNES AND TONY RILEY; NARRATIVE PREPARED BY KEITH MCINNES, TONY RILEY AND PETER MENDEL

Many people living with HIV not only must manage a chronic and, in numerous quarters, still highly stigmatized disease, but also suffer from a range of other medical, mental and social conditions that they and their care providers must struggle to address. These include various other physical ailments, as well as behavioral and social disorders, such as mental illness, substance abuse and homelessness, that interfere with both HIV treatment and meaningful improvement in their quality of life.

Despite these challenges, individuals with HIV in north-eastern New York State, regardless of health or social status, have access to high-quality HIV care because of the AIDS Treatment Center (ATC) in Albany New York (*see* Box 8.1). People who come to the ATC are assured state-of-the-art clinical therapies, appropriate support services, compassionate and dignified treatment, and an approach to care that allows and encourages the patient to be a participant in the care process.

If one were to list the key features of service provision that have been associated with such high quality, the list would include items such as top-level support for quality and service improvement,[1] use of multi-disciplinary teams,[2] clinical specialization,[3] use of data systems,[4] customer-centered practices, and involvement of staff in the development of work and care standards,[5] among others, many of them covered elsewhere in this volume. A striking characteristic of the ATC is that it excels in so many of these areas. What is it that enables this HIV/AIDS center to succeed in so many areas, even in light of the complexities of treating clients with a chronic stigmatized disease, a substantial number of whom belong to vulnerable populations?

This case study of the ATC identifies four dimensions on which the ATC as an organization stands out and that have been central to its ability to achieve key aspects of service excellence and high levels of performance: balanced leadership, staff commitment and work ethic, a patient-centered focus, and a proactive approach to quality and service improvement.

Unlike other cases in this study, which give fairly equal weight to the analysis of the macro-system and the micro-system, our focus here is primarily on the micro-system: the AIDS Treatment Center (ATC). This is because the factors that have led to its high performance are attributable as much to the internal characteristics of the micro-system and the wider contextual nature of AIDS care in the United States as to the direct influence of the larger medical center of which it is a part. Thus, although the Albany Medical Center (AMC), as described below, has clearly created a receptive context for the micro-system's pursuit of quality, the case pays special attention to the broader macro-influences of the ATC's environment.

BOX 8.1 Case profile: AIDS Treatment Center (ATC), Albany, New York

CASE PROFILE

Type of Organization:	An HIV/AIDS clinic providing comprehensive care for adults and adolescents. Part of Albany Medical Center (AMC), founded as one of the first private medical schools in the US.
Focal Micro-System:	AIDS treatment center
Size:	The ATC serves over 1400 patients with a staff of 70, including specialists in HIV medicine, dentistry, pharmacy, psychiatry and case management. ATC is a central unit within AMC's AIDS Program, the largest provider of HIV-related care in upstate New York.
Location:	Albany, New York (the state capital). The catchment area of AMC, the only academic medical center in the northeast region of the state, encompasses 3 million people across 25 counties. The ATC is located a half mile outside the main AMC campus.
Country:	United States
Awards and Recognitions:	Granted status as a 'Designated AIDS Center' (New York State Dept of Health 1987); a leading site in the federal HIV/AIDS Bureau's first QI learning collaborative (2000); initiated the Center of Excellence in HIV Correctional Health Care, nationally recognized video series for HIV education in incarcerated settings (2002); University HealthSystem Consortium's Customer Service Excellence Award (AMC as a whole, 2001).

KEY CONCEPTS

Social Movement: sustained collective action aimed at bringing about broad-scale, fundamental change in social systems. Social movements, such as for civil rights, gay rights or HIV/AIDS in particular, represent sources of considerable influence on organizations, as well as offering insights into strategies and processes of change within organizations.

Mobilization: the process of marshalling and organizing various resources, including funding, physical assets and, not least, the energy, talents and commitment of people, to achieve common goals.

Given the ATC's principal identity as a clinic serving HIV/AIDS patients, it is not surprising to note the strong effects on the organization of the AIDS movement, one of the most successful American health movements during the past three decades,[6] and which is closely associated with wider movements for gay rights and patient rights.[7] Indeed, recent research within and outside of healthcare has emphasized the influence of social movements on organizations, as well as the utility of understanding the role and potential of movement processes for change within organizations.[8,9]

In reviewing each of the micro-system's organizational strengths, we explore how these dynamics have played out in the case of the ATC. For example, ATC staff exhibit the same hope, caring and idealism that is associated with commitment-based movements whose goals focus on improving society. In particular, they are deeply devoted to improving the lives of people living with HIV and AIDS, and to a philosophy of holistic care that addresses the diverse needs of patients. We also highlight the role of one movement process with distinct relevance to the ATC – 'resource mobilization', the marshalling and organizing of varied forms of financial, human, social and political capital, either from within organizational settings themselves or from the wider environment, to achieve common goals.[10,11] We explicitly examine the proficiency of the ATC and its leaders to mobilize the energy, talents and commitment of their staff, as well as other resources, such as funding streams, specifically towards support of quality initiatives and a proactive approach to improvement. It is in relation to this latter process that the ATC has distinguished itself, even from other HIV/AIDS treatment centers.

The case study then examines two prominent milestones in the development of the ATC's strengths and quality journey: its participation in a national quality improvement program, the HIV Collaborative, and one of its major subsequent improvement initiatives, the ACE campaign. We return in the end to consider lessons from the ATC's quality journey and the implications of a social movement and mobilization perspective for understanding sustained quality improvement in healthcare organizations more generally.

Macro system: Albany Medical Center

Albany Medical Center (AMC) is a large local and regional tertiary care hospital and medical college, with more than 1200 affiliated physicians. It has an upstate New York catchment area of over 200 square miles, spanning 25 counties, encompassing three million people. The medical college, founded in 1839, was one of the first private medical schools in the US. That they are the only academic medical center for the region provides them with unique responsibilities:

> I think we are a sleeping giant among American academic medical centers. We're off the beaten path. We are stand-alone, which is quite unusual. Typically, the academic centers, as you may know, are clustered together in large metropolitan areas, whereas we're in a – I guess the word is remote – a remote geographic area. The delivery of our mission is more difficult because of our position, but that never meant that the people here, inside the institution, and the people outside, who support the institution, were any less determined to make us the first-class deliverer of healthcare . . . (Senior AMC executive)

AMC employs 6700 people, and has an annual revenue of $532 million, including $30 million in grant funding for research. This makes it one of the larger players in the local health economy. AMC hospital, with 650 beds, is the regional transfer center for the critically ill, and provides the hub of area-wide medical teaching activity. There are other hospitals in the region and there is competition for certain services, but AMC differentiates itself from competitors through its educational program and specialized services, some of which have received national quality awards:

> In this region we are the only academic health science center. We have some very fine, larger teaching hospitals, whose residency programs we support from here, but this is the mother ship for everything, whether it is for programs where we send the residents

out to other hospitals, or the fact that we are the regional transfer center for critically ill and injured people. (Senior AMC executive)

The medical center has, for example, the region's only kidney and heart transplantation program and the only children's hospital. The stroke and urology departments received commendation in 2001 from the HCIA-Sachs Institute and US News and World Report, respectively, and the center as a whole was one of three US hospitals to receive a 2001 Customer Service Excellence Award from the University HealthSystem Consortium.

AMC leadership recognizes the uniqueness and the high quality of the HIV services at AMC, especially its main outpatient unit, the AIDS Treatment Center. They attribute much of the success of the ATC to the continuity of its staff and leadership and the additional external funding they are able to acquire:

> No, it's not a surprise that the ATC was selected for this study. I think there is recognition that it is a high-performing group, and they have received a lot of national recognition. I don't think we could do a better job at that. (Senior AMC director)

> First of all, the HIV clinic has had pretty stable membership and has been able to work effectively to drive change through the organization. So, I think that's a key to its success. To be blunt about it, the HIV treatment is very good. They've got significant resources that are extramural that allow them to continue to focus on patients even when things get tight. (Senior AMC physician leader)

Micro system: AIDS Treatment Center (ATC)

The AMC AIDS Program (AMCAP), also known as the Division of HIV Medicine, has been serving patients since 1981. Started at Albany Medical Center hospital, it now has two outpatient clinics, in addition to 25 dedicated beds in the hospital. AMCAP is the largest provider of HIV-related care services in upstate New York State, and in 2003 served approximately 1500 outpatient and 470 inpatient clients. AMCAP has been designated a regional AIDS treatment center by the State of New York, and it participates in the federal government's AIDS Education and Training Center program. AMCAP is also the largest provider of HIV correctional healthcare in the country, financed through a managed care contract with the New York State Department of Correctional Services.

The outpatient AIDS Treatment Center (ATC) is a major component and the main outpatient site for AMCAP. Located a half mile away, it is one of the few AMC medical programs located off the main AMC campus. The ATC provides a full range of HIV-related services, including primary medical care, obstetrics/gynecology, dental care, adherence, nutrition, case management, substance abuse counseling, mental health treatment, and pharmacy. The total staff numbers 70 people, which includes eight physicians, three physician assistants, one nurse practitioner, a dentist, four case managers, a psychiatrist and mental health worker, and five registered nurses. Most ATC physicians are integrally linked to the HIV inpatient services at AMC, caring for HIV patients in the medical center and teaching residents and medical students from the medical college. The ATC also oversees a smaller satellite outpatient clinic with a staff of approximately 10 people in Kingston, New York, an hour's drive away.

Most AMCAP outpatient programs were either initiated by the ATC or are currently led by ATC staff. The ATC also indirectly serves 4000 HIV-infected inmates through its partnership with the Department of Correctional Services and educational programs they conduct for healthcare providers in 20 state correctional facilities. On the national level they have conducted videoconference training for over 800 clinicians working in correctional facilities across 44 states.

ATC resides in a plain three-story cement building on a mixed residential–commercial street. There is no sign to indicate what activities go on inside, which deliberately provides some degree of anonymity for patients. Staff refer to the ATC as '66 Hackett' in reference to the large address sign on the lawn leading up to the building. It also helps distinguish ATC from Albany Medical Center's campus and from the satellite facility in Kingston.

Although affiliation with AMC undoubtedly contributes to the quality of care at the ATC, it is important to note the relative autonomy of the unit. One senior leader in the medical center went so far as to refer to the ATC as an 'orphaned child' of AMC. The ATC, among all of AMC divisions and programs, is unique in its relative independence from the medical center – physically and financially (as mentioned previously), and in terms of information technology, as commented on by a senior ATC administrator:

> Well, we're one of the only free-standing entities within Albany Medical Center itself that has its own file server, has their own information systems staff, manages their own data, protects the security and confidentiality of that data and has really state-of-the-art computer equipment for every single staff member. There aren't a lot of programs that have that. It's not cheap, but it's something we need as a program and something we committed to a long time ago in terms of being able to look at potential technologic solutions. (ATC administrator)

Organizational strengths of the ATC

As described above, the ATC demonstrates a remarkable breadth of organizational strengths. Here we review in detail four of the most salient underlying dimensions whereby ATC excellence has put the center among the ranks of high-performing healthcare providers, as opposed to simply good or very good quality organizations. These include:

1. *Balanced leadership* – leadership in the ATC is shared in a well-balanced partnership between clinical expertise on the one hand and administrative, management and financial expertise on the other. A close examination of the leaders involved illustrates complementary – and not always obvious – processes of effectively mobilizing highly committed people, financial, and other resources towards high-quality care and service improvement.

2. *The commitment and work ethic that pervades the ATC* – for a variety of staff throughout the organization, working at the clinic is not merely a job, but rather a 'calling', more typical of an activist or deep professional mentality than a bureaucratic mentality, which elicits intense passion and effort, so much so that burnout remains a perennial concern.

3. A *patient-centered focus* – this lies at the heart of ATC's mission and imbues all decisions and plans with the question: 'How will this improve the satisfaction and quality of care of our patients?' ATC staff are motivated in particular by a desire to meet the comprehensive needs of HIV/AIDS patients, and they enjoy a regulatory and funding environment that is generally more amenable to such an approach than in other areas of medicine in the US.

4. A *proactive approach to improvement* – the development of a culture and related systems supportive not only of high quality care, but specifically of continuous improvement and improvement methodologies and mindsets. The shift to this type

of approach to improvement at the ATC has its roots in a variety of both voluntary and mandated quality initiatives, while also drawing on the Chronic Care Model (CCM) which promotes a rethinking and reorganization of outpatient care for chronic conditions.[12]

Balanced leadership

Prophets and gurus of healthcare improvement have long harped on the role of leadership in change efforts, issuing a variety of maxims, such as a leader's job is to challenge the status quo and provide a vision for change,[13] a positive 'change concept',[14] and a context and motivation for change;[4] the need in particular for top-level support from senior leadership;[15] and flexibility in the use of different sets of leadership skills – from sharing technical expertise, to supervising, to delegating – at each level of the healthcare system.[1]

Yet lacking in these writings is a perspective on leadership as a process that can shed light on the ways that leadership for improvement occurs in practice and how the elements of leadership come together in actual healthcare settings. The ATC case study demonstrates how leadership can be effectively distributed (*see also* the Reinier de Graaf Groep case, Chapter 5), with individuals contributing complementary roles and skills in mobilizing an organization towards quality.

The senior leadership of the ATC is shared between the clinic administrator and the medical director. The administrator is responsible for identifying and obtaining resources for ATC and manages all non-clinical staff. The medical director sets the tone for clinicians; he is depicted as hardworking, compassionate, committed to patients, approachable, non-threatening, and highly respected. Staff give him a lot of credit for the organization's reputation for high-quality clinical care.

The administrator, who holds a PhD in public administration, describes himself as having two main roles. First, he ensures the financial strength of the organization or, in his words 'resource acquisition':

> In two words, my role is best defined as resource acquisition. I'm responsible for obtaining external support, managing that support for the program as well as internal support, hospital budget, college budget, managing those resources, the space resources, and information resources. In a broad sense, all that resource acquisition is my role. To clarify what that means, I spend a lot of time in grants management. We bring in a lot of grants, 80% of our financing comes from grants. As a result, a multitude of grantors who support us believe that, in fact, I work for them. So, I have a lot of external bosses. Just being able to do all the things that need to be done in terms of that external environment and management consumes a lot of my day. (Clinic administrator)

His success in this role is evident in the approximately $3 million dollars in grants the ATC receives annually, equivalent, as he mentions in the quote above, to about 80% of the clinic's operating budget.

Second, the administrator has management responsibility for all non-medical staff. The departments and related personnel that report to him represent a significant portion of the ATC's human resources, including both direct services such as case management, mental health, substance abuse, and dietary/nutrition, as well as support services such as information systems, quality improvement, grants and accounting. Through this role in particular, he is heavily involved in promoting the vision and goals of the HIV program within the organization, with particular emphasis on improving the quality of services.

For the administrator, these two roles are intertwined in helping to empower and activate staff by providing the opportunities and resources they need to innovate and create:

> Our adherence program is a good example. We got funded three years ago to start this program, designed to help patients take their medication and to develop the life skills they need to do that. And, no one in the world, to the best of my knowledge, knew how to do that. There isn't necessarily one best way, so we had this lump of clay and we had a project officer. One of our nurses took this on and created a program from nothing. Took the clay and molded it into what ended up being a very nice sculpture by the time she was done. (Clinic administrator)

The decentralization of authority alluded to in the above quote has also been attributed in the social movements literature to the mobilization and building of solidarity among individuals.[16] When given authority and responsibility, members give back to the organization in terms of increased commitment.

Another aspect of leadership that involves both his external and internal roles – perhaps comprising a third major function for the administrator – is what he has termed 'cheerleading' on behalf of the organization. Thus, his external role is not merely acquiring financial resources, but serving as a kind of ambassador and public relations manager. He is often the public face of the organization, attending conferences (e.g. the American Foundation for AIDS Research annual meeting), giving presentations on ATC's accomplishments, serving on regional committees (e.g. upstate New York's Persons Living with AIDS Advisory Committee), and meeting with regulators and donors. He makes external constituents aware of the organization, highlights the quality work they are doing, and ensures that funders and potential funders are kept informed of the ATC's programs and activities.

The administrator is the main accountable person to external funders (who, as quoted above, tend to 'believe that . . . I work for them') such as the state and federal grant agencies, as well as upper management within the AMC system, which has oversight of the Division of HIV Medicine and provides financial support, space, and other academic, clinical and laboratory resources. In addition, the administrator acts as a buffer between all these external constituents and the clinic's staff, cushioning them from the varied demands, regulations and bureaucracy of AMC, government agencies, and private funders (*see also* the Royal Devon and Exeter case regarding micro-system leaders' 'protective' role). In this sense, the administrator provides a distinct set of both buffering and bridging functions for the ATC.[17]

The other half of the top management team is the medical director, a physician who has practised at ATC for over nine years. Unassuming and friendly, he inculcates high standards among his clinical team through example and teaching. Attention to detail and quality is one of the attitudes he strives to instill:

> I teach this to the house staff: if you want to know about a test result, you have to see it with your own eyes. You can't believe what somebody else tells you. It's hearsay until you know it. Then to maintain that attention to detail . . . the devil being in the details, and take it to a higher kind of organizational level. I think that's been part of the goal. (Medical director)

At heart, the medical director is a highly skilled clinician who thrives on helping and showing great compassion for patients. This comes through in his description of an encounter with a patient who, for reasons due to his psychological condition and cognitive impairments, presented a number of challenges:

> When he came to us in the hospital he was so demented we couldn't consent him for an HIV test. It was inspiring to see someone who's that ill – and he's simple, he's not an Einstein – and yet he appreciates it at a certain level, all 350 pounds of him. Recently we had a hard time getting his viral load under control. It's like trying to get your blood sugar in the correct range. But we were able to do that. He worked with our adherence program and our adherence nurses. He's here a lot – here he feels special. When he got his viral load result from his nurse that was just very special for him, and likewise special for me. When I saw him he just grabbed me and picked me up – he was so excited. It's so gratifying. I knew it was a special event – you just knew that this was a great thing. (Medical director)

The degree to which the clinical staff value his expertise and guiding example is evidenced through their admiration and respect:

> He works amazingly long hours; he is completely dedicated. When he's on vacation, he calls from wherever he is. If he's on a beach somewhere, he calls to find out how his patients are doing. He's amazing. He sets a very high standard by his own actions. (Nurse practitioner)

The medical director's unique qualities and contributions to the wider system have not gone unnoticed by the medical center, which awarded him AMC's employee of the year in 2000, the first-ever physician to receive this recognition.

Moreover, the clinic administrator and medical director have set the tone for leadership throughout the ATC. Other clinicians and staff in management and supervisory positions receive equally high praise for the same balanced set of leadership qualities, such as being supportive, providing guidance, and expressing openness to new ideas, as described here by a nursing clinician.

> I feel very close with the doctors. The GYN doctor [that supervised me] had an endless amount of patience for new ideas and tons of energy, and commitment. She would go the extra 50 miles, and the same with the other doctors . . . when I have troubles or I have new ideas, or I need help, they are right there, to tell me how to do this. (Nurse specialist)

Staff commitment and work ethic

As mentioned above, there is an 'internal solidarity'[16] among staff, which is fed by and contributes to the satisfaction that people feel from working in the ATC. Staff are energized by knowing that they are helping patients and contributing to the ATC's mission of caring and compassion:

> Yes, there's a camaraderie, there's an understanding that we're all in this together, nobody's here to be a millionaire or earn a handsome income – you're treating patients and you like providing care to these patients, you like the work that you do and you like to be part of the inspiration and hope, as they struggle with this disease. That's very, very important. (Medical specialist)

Many individuals on the staff at the ATC have long tenures – eight or more years of service is not uncommon – with a number having been involved in HIV care since the beginning of the epidemic, when a diagnosis of AIDS almost surely amounted to a death sentence for most patients within a period of months.[18] Staff members also typically have other direct experience with the disease, including current family and friends infected with HIV and, for some, being HIV-positive themselves. Consequently, it may not be surprising that people working in the ATC tend to strongly identify with the goals of the AIDS movement, which center on voice, compassion, treatment, and resources for people with HIV and AIDS.[7] In a sense, through their work within the ATC, staff have been able to transform their personal experiences into collective action, a fundamental process of mobilization noted within social movements.[19]

This commitment to improving the lives of people infected with HIV is described by staff at various levels within the clinic as a 'cause' and a 'calling'. While careers in medicine and the healing professions are often portrayed as such, this characterization appears especially prevalent among those attracted to the field of HIV care:

> The advantages are you end up with a high calibre staff, many of whom are patients, many of whom are not just motivated – this isn't their job – this is a mission, it's their life, it's a cause that they're committed to. (Senior administrator)

> I think with HIV it really has to be more of a calling than a profession. You have to have your heart and your soul in it. Everybody has different reasons to be here, but it is a calling. (Support services provider)

At the ATC this dedication has translated into, as one staff person termed it, a 'very strong work ethic'. A senior manager within the clinic describes the power of focusing the commitment of such highly motivated staff through co-ordinated effort:

> I grew up ten miles from school and four miles to the nearest corner store and I would wake up, look out, and see the horses in the pasture across the street. From a farming perspective, you can take two horses and one horse alone could pull 500 pounds and the other could also pull 500 pounds, but if you get them working together correctly, they could pull 2500 pounds. That's what we've got here. (Senior manager)

A key to ensuring a set of shared commitments and an ability to harness them towards common goals starts with the hiring and training of staff. Recruitment of new clinicians, for example, is highly dependent on whether senior physicians believe candidates share the ATC's philosophy and approach to HIV medicine. Less experienced clinicians are given extensive on-the-job training to acquire not only the necessary skills but also to be enculturated with the clinic's core values and sense of teamwork that distinguishes the ATC even from similar programs in the area:

> I think a lot of it relates to personalities and the type of folks that are drawn to the field of HIV, or maybe we're just lucky. People who don't have that kind of philosophy don't last long in this field. They either don't want to deal with it, or everyone works 300%. There's no slacker here. We have very high standards for ourselves; everyone works late – everybody sticks around – and I would expect a higher rate of turnover due to burn-out. But actually we have higher staff retention than many of the other programs in the area, and I think that's because there's a team feeling; I think it's because we are all committed. (Senior nurse)

Examples of this internally driven work ethic are numerous. A senior administrator stated how he is always surprised at the number of staff he finds on Saturday or Sunday when he comes in to catch up on his own work when the clinic is closed, and the concerns for the wellbeing of staff that it raises for him:

> That atmosphere makes it personal, makes it so that routinely staff think nothing about putting in a 60-hour week. That's just common. If the work needs to be done, there are staff that absolutely commit to doing it. There's a downside to that in that we don't always have a breather, we're fire-fighting a lot. If a staff member has an emerging crisis at home, problems with the family or whatever, this job can be so all consuming that

family stress on top of the stress of being in this environment can cause difficulties. (Senior administrator)

Testimonials of individual staff attest to the toll that this level of effort can take:

> When I get out of here at night, I just pant all the way to my car. I am just so exhausted, and I'm a tough broad. Nothing can take me out, but you go home and you almost decompress. It's the toughest job I've ever had. (Nurse specialist)

Because of the pace of work and the emotional and psychological strain associated with the care of chronically ill people, ATC managers try hard to keep an eye on staff who show signs of burn-out. There is a morale committee that plans parties and other events, including an annual 'roast' of the ATC leadership. The committee also organizes opportunities for bereavement counseling for staff when patients die. Fortunately the frequency of these incidents has declined dramatically in the past six to eight years since the introduction of more effective anti-retroviral therapies. Staff burn-out has likewise been a constant concern within the HIV field in general.[20] One factor that has been suggested as protecting HIV providers against the effects of stress is the level of personal commitment to their work,[21] which may also explain the capacity of staff within the ATC to maintain the intensity of effort they have demonstrated over time.

Patient-centered focus

The workplace that we have been describing within the clinic is one imbued with a strong, commitment-based culture that mobilizes individuals toward collective action. The overriding focus of these commitments and action at the ATC has been to provide the most comprehensive, responsive and highest-quality care possible for each patient.

From its early inception in the 1980s, AIDS care in general in the US has been exceptionally focused on patient perspectives and needs. This is largely attributable to the efforts of HIV patients and activists in the AIDS movement, who, following in the footsteps of the earlier patient rights movement that had emerged in the 1960s,[22] were quick to challenge the traditional doctor–patient relationship, demand patient involvement in treatment decisions, create better-informed patients and caregivers with an almost expert status in HIV biomedicine, and advocate for the range of needs faced by people affected by the disease.[7,23]

One of the strengths of the ATC is the degree to which it has been able to actualize this philosophy of empowerment and comprehensive care in the way services are delivered within a healthcare organization. First, the ATC has a highly developed model of comprehensive care, treatment and support through – as described earlier – a broad range of medical, other clinical and social services. The holistic package of care provided by the clinic, including preventive and supportive services, is viewed not merely as a convenience to patients, but as a critical complement to attaining key objectives of medical treatment and health outcomes:

> If you don't address the patient's mental health, substance abuse, and other issues, you're not addressing the core problem. You are putting on a band-aid that isn't going to solve really long-term issues. (Senior administrator)

This package of services is facilitated by the major source of federal support for HIV care, the Ryan White Comprehensive AIDS Resources Emergency (CARE) Act, which explicitly includes funds for various ancillary and wrap-around services for HIV patients (e.g. mental health and case management). New York State also offers enhanced reimbursement under its Medicaid program to HIV clinics, like the ATC, that are granted status as a 'Designated AIDS Center' (or DAC) in exchange for providing a broader array of services. The ATC is able to supplement this approach even further by means of the substantial grant revenue it attracts. This stream of monies allows the clinic to provide additional services not typically covered by traditional sources of funding, such as its innovative nutrition program, which includes delivery of food and cooked meals, food-shopping assistance, and distribution of food vouchers.

The ATC's model of comprehensive care, however, extends beyond the number and types of services offered to the way in which care is organized and providers relate to one another. While care teams have become increasingly common in American healthcare, the ATC's approach relies on a highly interactive, interdisciplinary team to ensure that the variety of services and treatment provided to each patient are appropriately tailored and co-ordinated:

> The care team members come together. They develop an individualized, very problem-focused treatment plan that recognizes that it's not enough to treat the patient's illness. If we don't also address substance abuse issues, their lack of housing, their lack of mental health support, then when we discharge them from the hospital we're going to see them again soon. Because, the root cause – they came into the hospital with pneumonia – is HIV related. If they get discharged and go back out onto the street and don't have a home the chances of them having recurrent pneumonia are pretty high. So, making sure that the mental health, the substance abuse, those concrete social services, housing, food, etc, all those things that they need to survive get addressed, is a big issue. We come up with the whole plan that everybody's aware of. (Senior administrator)

Another distinctive element of the ATC's patient-centered focus is the importance the clinic places on patient input and involvement in improving care. Input from patients is obtained in several ways. First, clinicians emphasize the need to incorporate patient goals and objectives in their own treatment plans and encourage patients to participate in treatment decisions, a principle of patient self-management shared by the Chronic Care Model described below. At the clinic level, the ATC is aided in its work by a formally constituted consumer advisory board run by patients, which meets six times a year and makes recommendations about improving care. A senior ATC manager also participates in an area-wide committee outside the clinic that actively looks at consumer needs from the regional perspective. These activities are regularly supplemented on an ad hoc basis as staff request patient input for particular programs or initiatives. For example, the food program's project manager held patient focus groups to find out what parts of the program the patients liked, and what aspects they would like to see changed.

Finally, there are a number of staff who are HIV-positive themselves and active patients at the ATC. These individuals occupy a hybrid role, serving as 'two-way windows'[24] able to bridge the patient and provider worlds. Their participation in clinical and management meetings comprises a less formal, yet effective, mechanism for ensuring that the patient perspective is represented in clinic operations and decision-making:

> There are a number of staff who are patients here. They know best – because they wear two hats – what works operationally from a patient perspective and what we can do realistically given whatever limitations are imposed in the environment in terms of resources and regulations. Their input and perspective [are] very valuable. It's the cornerstone of what our quality improvement is based on, getting that active feedback. (Senior administrator)

This does not mean that maintaining a patient-centered focus is without difficulty. Because of the high prevalence of poverty, substance abuse and mental health disorders, the patient population at the ATC can pose a number of challenges. For example, on occasion a patient may act out and become verbally abusive. Staff are generally adept at handling such outbursts, given their experience and knowing individual patients well. Yet working with these patients can require an extraordinary amount of compassion and can test the self-confidence of even the most dedicated providers.

> I guess people [suited to work here] have compassion and understanding and are not so quick to judge. We have to be able to meet the patient where they're at, at that time. If they're not ready to take their medication, we try to be understanding and try to work with them to get them there. (Support services provider)

Helping to counterbalance these experiences are the positive and appreciative responses from patients. Patients seem to sense the difference in quality of care they receive here compared to other clinics. One staff member described an occasion when patients were interviewed by a local newspaper. In describing their care experiences, patients said how they were made to feel welcomed and respected at ATC. One of the patients told a reporter, 'It's the first time in my life I've ever been called "Mister".' A nurse sums it up:

> Patients are out there, in the public, talking to each other and saying, 'Well, I go to Albany Medical Center HIV program and they're really good to me.' (Nurse practitioner)

The end result is a culture with a strong focus on the patient and services organized around providing comprehensive patient-centered care. Even the language used within the clinic reflects this orientation. When talking about their patients, clinicians and staff frequently use words such as 'respect', 'empower', 'compassion', 'understanding', and 'on the patient's terms'.

Corresponding with the emphasis on improvement, this orientation also incorporates a striving for perfection and the highest-quality care for patients, a goal expressed by managers and clinicians alike:

> What we're in business for is providing the highest-quality care we can for the patients we serve. The patients come first. (Senior administrator)

> The most important thing is that the patients have the best care. We wish it were perfect. (Nurse specialist)

Proactive improvement
While high quality of care has long been a priority of the ATC, the strategic use of the paradigms and methods of service improvement in order to achieve that objective has been a more recent emphasis. Leaders within the ATC characterize this shift as going from a 'reactive' to a 'proactive' approach to quality, which has included developing a particular culture, set of skills, and organizational supports for continuous improvement.

This emphasis on quality improvement at the ATC has its roots in the mid-1980s, when the New York State Department of Health created a program to certify select HIV clinics as 'Designated AIDS Centers' (or DACs). Given New York's position as one of two main epicenters of the AIDS epidemic in the US, affecting a disproportionate share of its residents (with 18% of the nation's AIDS cases and only 9% of the total population), the state government took an early lead in dedicating substantial resources and creating policies to encourage the expansion of services for people living with HIV/AIDS. Such political directives have also been shown to positively affect the diffusion of innovative services.[25] As described earlier, the DAC program provided additional resources to the selected clinics while mandating certain service requirements, including a more comprehensive model than traditional primary care due to the fact that many HIV-infected persons have had complex health and social problems.[26] The Albany Medical Center applied, and received the distinction of becoming one of 33 such DACs in 1987. Thus the DAC model was the impetus for both the ATC's holistic package of service and its multi-disciplinary care team:

> We got approved in 1987. The cornerstone of that whole approach was the interdisciplinary care team. So we are required to have a social work counselor, provide mental health services, and provide dental services. Over time we have adopted an approach that requires the various professions to come together in a formal way and develop an integrated treatment plan for each patient. (Senior administrator)

In addition, the New York Department of Health established the AIDS Institute, an agency tasked with helping to monitor and improve the quality of care for HIV patients across the state. As part of its charge, the AIDS Institute developed a national program of quality improvement called HIVQUAL, which utilizes specialized HIV-care software to collect routine clinical data for tracking and improving quality of care. The ATC has taken advantage of HIVQUAL and other AIDS Institute initiatives, but has also participated in a variety of additional quality monitoring efforts, including: the University HealthSystem Consortium national benchmarking program; programs offered by the Island Peer Review Organization (IPRO), an independent state-level healthcare quality review organization; the national Joint Commission for Accreditation of Healthcare Organizations (JCAHO) general accreditation requirements, with which they also must comply; and Albany Medical Center's own quality monitoring and improvement standards.

As we have seen, the current clinic administrator and medical director arrived in the early to mid-1990s and they are viewed as providing visionary clinical and financial leadership – two key elements often considered prerequisites for improving chronic care services[12] – and deserving much of the credit for the current culture, style, and mission of the organization. Yet they characterize the approach to quality in their first four to five years at the clinic, including many of the above programs, as primarily 'reactive':

> I'll give you a little history first. For a very long time we were in what I would call a reactive mode, in terms of quality issues. The institution [AMC] or some regulation or the Health Department would provide more edicts in terms of addressing a concern that they had identified and then we'd react to that. That was our quality program up until about three years ago. (Senior administrator)

During this time senior management at the ATC had grown weary and a bit jaded with this old approach to quality and its typical method of attempting to improve service delivery. When a new idea was identified it would be immediately implemented center-wide, but the expected improvements would often fail to materialize:

> Six years ago what we would do is identify an issue: patients are not coming to their appointments. So we would come up with a plan that would then be introduced system wide. And nine times out of ten it would fail because it was not tested and it was not completely thought out in terms of what it would do. And there wouldn't be any follow up or evaluation. In six months we would find nobody was even following it any more because it didn't work. (Senior administrator)

Repeated past disappointments, as well as financial incentives from the federal HIV/AIDS Bureau (one of the ATC's main funders) to try something new, led to openness to joining a program in 2000 developed by the Institute for Healthcare Improvement (IHI) specifically for HIV/AIDS services, called the HIV Collaborative. Despite initial skepticism, the IHI program seemed to resonate with senior managers and clinicians.

In particular, the IHI-adapted plan-do-study-act (PDSA) methodology for rapid cycle improvement of testing innovations on a small scale and then refining them made sense, was practical and, more importantly, produced results. The ATC's experience with the HIV Collaborative was also directly related to a number of important structural changes, including creating a position for a full-time quality of care co-ordinator and establishing a clinic-wide structure to help manage and implement quality initiatives:

> It resulted in some fairly concrete things that we've been able to do, one of which is dedicating resources specifically for process improvement. We hired a quality co-ordinator, used information systems to provide analysis and evaluation of tests that we do. We also created – and again this is directly out of [the HIV Collaborative] – a core team and a home team that in a small group identifies agenda items and issues, and then in a larger group looks at ways in which these issues can be addressed, things that we could test in terms of change. (Senior administrator)

A senior clinician reiterates the critical contributions that the quality co-ordinator has made to ATC's achievements in recent years:

> [The quality co-ordinator] is the number one factor. She's a person who has taken quality control and run with it. She is not a shy person, but she would never tell you that she is the person that is really making it go, but she is, because she is the one that keeps us coming to the meetings and she is the one who is on the tasks at the meetings and keeps reminding us of things that we have left behind and need to come back to. (Senior physician)

The clinic-wide structure that emerged took shape in the form of a 'core team' and a 'home team'. The core team consists of senior leaders who have strategic responsibility for quality improvement, and includes the administrator, director of operations, and the quality of healthcare co-ordinator. The home team (also known as the process improvement team) includes the core team members, plus those managers representing the clinic's functional areas: clinical care, nursing, adherence, case management, information technology, and clerical, medical records and appointments. Pointing to this structure, staff report a sense of representation and participation in the clinic's improvement agenda and general decision-making process.

In addition, involvement in the HIV Collaborative has changed how the clinic approaches and uses data for quality. Previous programs have mandated the collection and tracking of data, but the IHI approach renewed emphasis on using measurement for continuous, hands-on improvement.[14] ATC specifically relies on measurement in a selective way – where they really want to focus attention, they measure things:

> There are a lot of things that we have worked on where we can't substantiate anything positive through data, but we might still think that they were good changes. For some simple system changes we don't take the time for measurement. For big things we want to focus on, however, we do measure, like with the ACE campaign and PAP, and those types of things. (Manager)

Management has also come to realize that measuring and reporting data is only part of the equation. If data are to be useful and assist with achieving higher-quality outcomes, then communicating and interpreting the numbers is just as important as measuring. This is often the more difficult part of quality improvement, and again the quality co-ordinator has played an especially important role in this regard:

> There are sometimes discussions about how to interpret the numbers. One of my biggest shocks here is that I thought medical people with their scientific training would therefore be able to interpret the numbers I provided, e.g. this percentage, derived from these numbers, lets us conclude X or Y. But in fact, many people couldn't grasp my logic. So sometimes we will have explanations of not only the percentage, but also how we arrived at it, what it means, and why. [The quality co-ordinator] has a much greater grasp of that than she gives herself credit for and is excellent at communicating it to people. She's very, very good at it. I think knowing what those numbers mean and knowing what the targets are, is very beneficial. (Senior manager)

Finally, the ATC emphasizes the education of clinicians and staff, and the constant upgrading of skills and knowledge, as another key ingredient to maintaining continuous improvement in the level of service. The senior leadership makes multiple education and conferencing opportunities available, despite the financial investment this policy presents. As a result, participation in the HIV Collaborative and the changes that ensued have proven a turning point for the ATC to a more proactive approach, including the culture, the techniques and the resources for continuous quality improvement:

> We've always been a quality healthcare provider, but we didn't have the culture, we didn't have the methodology, we didn't have the commitment of a resource person to really help co-ordinate what we do in a planned way. (Senior administrator)

An underlying foundation for such a proactive culture of improvement has been the overall climate of the clinic, most noticeably its flat organizational structure and the considerable autonomy granted to teams and individuals. These features are conducive to types of organizational cultures – such as a group culture which values teamwork and participation, and a developmental culture based on innovation and tolerance for risk-taking – that have been associated with the successful implementation of quality improvement.[27,28,29]

At all levels within the ATC, staff and clinicians make changes to improve service, care and efficiency, and they are able to do this without getting bogged down with unnecessary levels of permission:

> It's sort of like the experiments of the counter culture of the 1960s, where small groups went off and built their own little communes and they had some successes and some failures. [The senior management's] style is they'll give you enough rope. If you choose to hang yourself, then you'll hang yourself. But sometimes you get the right person, you give them enough rope, you give them the opportunities and they can build some tremendous pockets of success. (Senior manager)

As a consequence, the ATC leadership has allowed innovation to thrive, as much by giving creative people the autonomy to attempt new ideas as by instituting specific improvement-related structures and policies:

> There is a lot of change that happens in individual pockets of areas. Like [the adherence manager] who, with her assistant, might figure out a better system of running clinic or

getting patients in rooms quicker or preventing a backup of patients getting their blood drawn. (Manager)

In sum, the ATC has made sustained, continuous improvement an ingrained orientation and habit within the organization. The extent of the clinic's progress becomes especially apparent to members of the ATC who have opportunities to compare their efforts with those of other HIV programs around the country:

> At a national conference in Miami that I recently attended it was once again clear to me that what we're doing here is three to five years ahead of what they're doing in other parts of this country. (Senior administrator)

Participating in the HIV Collaborative

The ATC came to our attention for this series of case studies through its participation in the HIV Collaborative, an 18-month national quality improvement program developed and organized by the IHI. It was one of eight clinics (out of 70 participating) that organizers identified as making substantial progress in adopting the quality improvement techniques advocated by the program. The ATC was also one of the few clinics to show success in increasing the number of HIV patients with suppressed viral load, a key outcome measure in HIV/AIDS care.

The ATC was invited to participate in the HIV Collaborative by one of its main funders, the HIV/AIDS Bureau of the federal Health Resources and Services Administration (HRSA). The HIV Collaborative, like other similar disease-specific programs conducted by the IHI, combines their plan-do-study-act rapid-cycle improvement change methodology with a framework for chronic disease care and management called the Chronic Care Model (CCM). This model recommends system change in six areas in support of chronic illness care: delivery system redesign, patient self-management support, decision support, information support, community linkages, and health system support.[12,30] For example, patient self-management, which fits nicely with the ATC's patient-centered focus, includes the clinician and patient jointly defining the key issues for treatment, making plans and setting goals, and following a disease management approach, which, for HIV, often focuses on adherence to anti-retroviral treatment.[31]

The IHI-sponsored collaboratives typically bring together 20 to 40 healthcare organizations to focus on improving some aspect of healthcare, and have included diverse topics, such as lowering Caesarean-section rates, reducing waiting times in doctors' offices, and improving diabetes care. Each organization sends a team of between two and five clinicians and managers to three or four learning sessions. The learning sessions usually consist of two days of intensive programs of lectures and discussions structured to identify and overcome barriers to quality improvement specific to the types of services and settings targeted by the collaborative. In between learning sessions, teams try out changes, collect and report data to the rest of the participants, attend monthly conference calls for reinforcement and assistance with their changes, and write monthly reports of their progress.

At first, reactions within the ATC to the invitation to the collaborative were ambivalent at best:

> I had been involved in TQM and you name it, it was total quality management, it was quality circles, it was various quality assurance kinds of things, and IHI, at first, I thought was another gimmick . . . I'll be honest and tell you that I went into that with a somewhat jaundiced view. (Senior administrator)

Financial incentives and strong encouragement from HRSA provided the impetus for the ATC to decide to take part in the collaborative:

> I think the reason we participated is because there was an underlying sense that we would come out of it better, but I've got to say money was a big motivator. Our Title IV grant [administrator] said, 'You will participate,' and it didn't seem terribly optional at the time. We have a way of making the best out of things; we'll turn those lemons into lemonade given half the opportunity. (Senior manager)

The collaborative also gave management licence to introduce changes that otherwise might have met with greater resistance if not for the 'organizational cover' that participation provided; i.e. that the clinic was simply trying to comply with the funder's quality improvement program:

> It gave us a little bit of shelter. It allowed us to hide behind the fact that we're mandated to do this. We could say, 'We have to track these numbers and we have to get these data.' We could say, 'It's not me that's saying this has to be done, it's the [federal government]' and we could grumble along with the rest of them saying, 'We don't like this any more than you do but we've got to do it.' (Senior manager)

As described above, the HIV Collaborative was a major milestone in the ATC's shift to a more proactive improvement approach. The strategies and tools learned in the collaborative eventually won over the ATC team, in particular the PDSA change methodology and use of measurement, information systems, and data for improvement:

> . . . what IHI did . . . was it helped us do the PDSA cycles: to start small and try and do a small piece and then replicate it. That's the single biggest thing that we learned . . .

> . . . the other big thing it did was it forced us to configure our database a little bit better and take it to the next step so that we could report out on some of these numbers. (Senior physician leader)

Likewise, the collaborative initiative placed heavy emphasis on involving the ATC's broader clinical and management leadership in the program. This strategy was viewed by key players as a critical precondition for successfully adopting the collaborative's methodologies and implementing improvements within the clinic:

> The other thing that IHI did was getting the leadership involved. Because if you don't have buy-in there, it's easy to just get cynical, as opposed to realizing that there is hope. Improvements can be made and we don't have to resign ourselves to mediocrity. (Senior physician leader)

Many of the HIV clinics in the collaborative chose to work on a relatively large number of small changes to their organization (e.g. new flowsheets, new patient reminder systems, clinician reminder systems for preventive services, etc.). The ATC decided to place most of its effort in one far-reaching, multi-faceted initiative: implementing an annual patient visit, which they called the annual comprehensive exam (ACE).

The ACE campaign

In HIV treatment, a challenge for the care team is to monitor, screen for and take preventive action (if necessary) for any of a number of potential comorbidities, such as tuberculosis, cervical cancer, flu and pneumonia. Most HIV clinics try to incorporate these screenings and preventive health services during acute care or disease monitoring visits. The ACE campaign represented a new approach for the ATC. Rather than place the onus on individual physicians and nurses to check each patient's chart on an ad hoc basis before a visit, the clinic decided to address these screening and preventive services systematically.

Under the new procedure, each patient undergoes a separate ACE exam once a year lasting an hour (double the usual visit length). Half an hour is spent with a nurse or physician assistant assessing and completing all necessary preventive care and education, and the other half hour is spent with the patient's regular primary care clinician monitoring symptoms and reviewing clinical status (e.g. viral load and CD4 counts). Utilizing the methodology of the HIV Collaborative, the new procedure was tested before rolling out across the organization:

> The ACE campaign was created because we had this quality initiative on improving our annual exams. We made lots of changes: we changed the system, we came up with a new system we tested it, and we liked it. It wasn't perfect yet, but it was at a good enough place to actually start it. (Manager)

The framing of collective action – how a new initiative is justified, rationalized or 'spun' to different audiences – is an essential process in initiating and building momentum for movement and change.[32,33] In this regard it is interesting that the ATC framed the roll-out implementation of the initiative as a 'campaign', a term that connotes an activist-oriented, broad-scale effort to win the hearts and minds of staff and mobilize the whole clinic around the goal of providing all patients with an ACE. The campaign involved not only physicians and nurses, but also the medical record manager, receptionists, case managers, and adherence staff – all were encouraged to contribute to improving the coverage of clientele under the new procedure. The secretary, for example, could talk to patients on the phone about the ACE, the chart manager could see who had and had not had one, etc. A member of staff responsible for quality improvement described how the campaign evolved:

> [A senior manager] actually came up with this idea. He said, 'We need to have a campaign and really create a team to work on this.' He and I talked more about it and I brought in [another provider] because she's good at coming up with creative ideas. So we decided to have this competition. We divided into teams, and said the winning team would get a special lunch. And then we decided it would be good if we had some sort of individual incentive. So we made an individual incentive where every month the person who made the most effort towards an ACE could win a prize. (Manager)

To keep attention on the campaign, the clinic offered both team-based incentives (the special catered lunch, pizza parties) and individual prizes (gift certificates from a nearby store) for contributions to the ACE initiative, with clear rules for how teams and individuals could accumulate 'points' towards these awards. Far beyond their monetary value, the intention behind these incentives was to generate a sense of friendly competition and a spirit of inclusion in the campaign:

> It has been a campaign making everyone feel like they have a role in it. We don't just say the doctor just needs to do it, and then blame him or her when the annual exam doesn't get done. The reality of it is there weren't enough hours in a year to schedule this many patients for an annual exam in our current clinic structure. So we had to develop another structure with the chart review and the historical piece. And the figuring out what immunizations are necessary, the PPD, the PCP, the Pap smear, the mammogram, and

on and on. Now that's done ahead of time by the nurse, and so we can still schedule their annual exam and have it still be a 30-minute visit for the provider. (Senior physician leader)

Nurses were generally keen to participate, willingly taking responsibility for half of the hour-long ACE appointment. This has been viewed as a positive expansion of the nurses' roles and further empowerment of the nursing staff within the clinic.

So it's extended nurse roles. But they've loved it because it gives them buy-in and they're not just checking (vital) signs and drawing blood. (Senior physician leader)

In contrast, physicians were less easily convinced of the value of the ACE. Many were concerned the new exams would require a large time commitment and felt that preventive services were already adequately covered through the current system. One nurse described the initial reluctance but eventual acceptance and appreciation of the idea among the physician staff:

... with the ACE ... doctors [said], 'There's no way or time to do these. Why are we doing this? I do this piecemeal over the year, why do I need to do it in one fell swoop?' And now they're just starting to see the results – 'Oh, this is a good idea, I didn't realize how many things I overlooked.' (Senior nurse)

The HIV Collaborative provided the ATC with the capacity to identify and deal with such challenges, as well as an opportunity for introducing changes to their process of care. However, a major question about collaboratives and other healthcare improvements, especially those initiated by or heavily relying on external change agents (e.g. IHI and HRSA), is whether they can be sustained.[34,35]

In the 12-month period prior to our site visits to the ATC, the proportion of patients covered by the ACE initiative (and in the system to get a repeat annually) had risen from 8% to 26%. During the fieldwork for this study, quality improvement meetings observed by the study team included a number of rolling items on the agenda related to the ACE campaign, and managers and clinicians expressed optimism that the program would continue and expand. Slightly over a half year after our fieldwork, the coverage of patients in the ACE campaign had increased to 41%.

Conclusions: movements, mobilization and sustained improvement

This case study has reviewed a number of reasons why the ATC at Albany Medical Center has been able to continually achieve high levels of performance and improvement. In one sense, these reasons boil down to strong leadership, committed staff, a patient-centered focus, and the application of improvement methodologies. While certainly true, this study explores how the ATC got to be so good: what exactly do the clinic's leaders do, how has the clinic attracted, retained, and developed such a committed staff, and how are they able to work together effectively and regularly implement changes to care for their HIV patients when quality improvement often falters in many healthcare organizations? Delving into the quality journey of the ATC at this level has illustrated the utility of a movement and mobilization perspective to sustaining quality and service improvement. This perspective includes the role of social movements in providing impetus, support and resources for high-quality care and improvement (a particular form of 'receptive context'), as well as the potential of movement processes for introducing and implementing change within healthcare organizations.

The AIDS movement in the US has been an especially strong and pervasive influence in the wider environment of the ATC, and of HIV services in general. The AIDS movement is a health social movement which represents 'collective challenges to medical policy and politics, belief systems, research and practice that include an array of formal and informal organizations, supporters, networks of co-operation, and media'.[6] In the US the AIDS movement, through its ability to identify and attract resources, has been instrumental in the development of HIV/AIDS policy and the expansion of service delivery.[36]

A senior administrator in the ATC described the impact of the AIDS movement and its convergence with the modern patient rights movement:

> I think a strong argument could be made that AIDS has, in fact, been the impetus behind the [current] patient rights movement. Because, [AIDS] patients in the late 1980s had no drugs, no long-term solution to the problem, very limited governmental commitment for either prevention or care. There was no 'industry'; there were just a lot of angry patients. [AIDS patients] demonstrated, and they were fairly influential in terms of mobilizing society, and educating society about the true impact that AIDS was having. It absolutely, influenced – and continues to influence – state politics. The state is very responsive to that political pressure. (Senior administrator)

Another senior manager discussed the influence directly on the ATC, both in terms of funding resources and innovation, of what has become an AIDS 'industry' in New York, one of the epicenters of the HIV epidemic in the US:

> There is an AIDS industry that exists in New York City. It truly is an industry. It employs thousands of people. That generally has a lot of positive consequences for what we do because it's influential, it's powerful in terms of lobbying government for funding and for change. And because there is a lot of money thrown at it . . . I think there are some innovative, exciting things that go on there and so we, more from what we get from New York City and what we get from New York State, I think we are on the cutting edge of what we do, who we are. (Senior manager)

In terms of human resources, the field of HIV/AIDS services tends to attract individuals – the kind of professional healthcare activist profiled in this case study – with a strong commitment to serving and empowering people affected by HIV. Akin to the spirit of innovation noted above, the nature of HIV/AIDS care also promotes a familiarity with adaptability and change. As one ATC staff member put it:

> We are continually in a state of change – it is the reality of working in HIV – you have to adapt to new infections, new medications, and new guidelines, often multiple times a year.

In terms of specific opportunities and support for improved services, the ATC was able to take advantage of a number of quality-related programs. It early on became one of New York State's Designated AIDS Centers, dedicated to offering a full range of services to assist patients not only with clinical treatment, but also with mental health, substance abuse, housing, nutrition, and other needs. Likewise, the ATC benefited from other state programs such as HIVQUAL, which recommended more careful tracking of patients through data collection and the use of a patient registry. Its later participation in the HIV Collaborative, a national program sponsored by the IHI and the federal HIV/AIDS Bureau, eventually led to a transformation from a 'reactive' to a more proactive approach to quality improvement. As a result of its involvement in this program, the ATC instituted a number of structural and procedural changes, such as the creation of a new quality co-ordinator position and two improvement-related teams. The teams have substantially changed the way care is delivered, with the prime example being the introduction of the ACE.

Yet, in being able to successfully profit from these resources and opportunities, and maintain high levels of both service excellence and quality improvement, the ATC appears far ahead of many healthcare organizations, perhaps, as a senior administrator estimated above, 'three to five years ahead' of other HIV/AIDS centers. Much of this success can be attributed to the proficiency of the ATC and its leaders in mobilizing people and resources.

Of distinct note, the ATC has cultivated an organizational structure and climate that are purposefully designed to engage and mobilize – rather than stifle – the commitment, effort and creativity of members (internal movement-like dynamics). This issue mirrors a long concern within social movement research about whether and to what degree organizing and giving formal structure to collective action may dampen the idealism, passion and energy of dedicated activists.[37,38] The ATC's flat hierarchy, generous autonomy for teams and individuals, and inclusion of voices from all parts of the organization are notable features helping to encourage bottom-up initiative and ideas for change.

Similarly, the case of the ATC draws attention to the relative advantages of 'loose coupling' in the organization of health systems, reflected most notably in the clinic's relationship to the AMC. Such arrangements can afford the freedom and autonomy for groups to pursue constructive innovation and change, as long as they are accompanied by mechanisms to support vital functions, exchange critical information, and share knowledge and strategies related to improvements.[39,40]

Our study of the ATC also underscores the extent to which organizations – especially the pluralistic forms that predominate in healthcare – are permeable to external influences that may act directly on individual units and micro-systems, rather than necessarily being filtered through higher levels of the organization chart.[41,42] An example is the depth of commitment associated with the AIDS movement that professionals in HIV care and in the ATC, in particular, display. Not all healthcare organizations operate in fields such as HIV services, which are shaped so conspicuously by an identifiable social movement. However, individuals working in many areas of medicine harbour similar commitments to a greater calling, cause or identity (*see*, for example, the San Diego Children's Hospital and Royal Devon and Exeter cases, Chapters 2 and 3), which may serve as reservoirs of sentiment for mobilization.

Finally, the quality journey of the ATC reveals how effective mobilization is a multi-dimensional process that requires combining these commitments and passions with tangible resources (e.g. the 'resource acquisition' function of the clinic administrator), know-how (e.g. improvement methodologies and skills learned in the HIV Collaborative), and a sense of group accomplishment and momentum towards valued goals (e.g. the ACE campaign). Mobilization depends on money and work, as well as trust and moral engagement.[16] Gaining mastery with this process can be a powerful force – as demonstrated by the ATC – for sustaining a trajectory of high performance and continuous improvement in healthcare organizations.

9

A practitioner's codebook for the quality journey

As we collated, read, fed back and shared the organizational stories we had been told (as summarized in Chapters 2 to 8), we began to realize that despite the huge variety of solutions and strategies that had been – and were continuing – to be implemented in the organizations we visited, there were common elements or themes emerging and repeating themselves. Through our familiarization with the stories it became increasingly clear – and intriguing – to us that these high-performing healthcare organizations had all encountered similar kinds of challenges when seeking to develop their improvement systems and processes.

Although not anticipated at the outset of this research, the idea of a set of common challenges with different solutions across several contexts is far from original. This finding is referred to across the social sciences as the 'universal but variable' thesis, which states that there are only 'a limited number of basic human problems to which all people at all times and in all places must find a solution',[1] but the number of possible solutions to them is almost unlimited – hence the co-existence of similarities (common problems) *and* differences (varied solutions) between all human systems, social or organizational.[1,2] Such variations, in our case between healthcare QI processes, stem from the infinite number of ways in which people have sought to resolve these life or, as in our case, quality challenges or problems.

The remainder of this book takes this broad 'universal but variable' thesis as its organizer. With this in mind, our tasks in the next two chapters are to:

❐ identify for practitioners what the common core challenges and practical solutions are (or may be) for QI efforts in healthcare organizations generally (Chapter 9)
❐ explore in more detail the similarities and differences between our case study sites in terms of their varied efforts to solve each of these challenges (Chapter 10).

In the context of healthcare QI processes, and drawing on our real-life cases, we represent this thesis here as six common challenges that are problems to which any organization will need to find solutions that will work for them in their particular context, and that if they do not do so will ultimately lead to disappointment and failure in the quality arena. Although these six challenges are broadly similar for all healthcare organizations, the possible solutions (or, more pertinently, as we shall show in Chapter 10, the possible *combinations* of solutions) are assumed to be practically innumerable.

Furthermore, what works for one organization may not work for another: San Diego Children's Hospital (Chapter 2) does not require a Cedars-Sinai (Chapter 4) or a Royal Devon and Exeter (Chapter 3) approach. Hence, the broad advice to any healthcare organization seeking to learn from the stories outlined in Chapters 2 to 8 is to:

a. be aware that one needs to take up each and every one of these six organizational challenges (as did our case study sites), given that they are imperatives or 'must do's', not luxuries or add-ons to a QI effort
b. find answers to each that fit locally and are contextually appropriate (find the right key for the right lock)
c. build them into your ongoing organizational and service improvement processes.

Our overarching thesis is simply that 'successful' organizations (in terms of quality and performance generally) will be doing (a), (b) and (c), even if only implicitly. Conversely, we propose that low performers in terms of healthcare quality will be failing on one, some or all of these fronts, although this remains to be tested empirically.

The purposes of this chapter are therefore to help healthcare managers, practitioners and researchers to:

- understand these six common challenges that every healthcare organization will need to face up to if it is to successfully implement, spread and sustain quality and service improvement processes
- establish the extent to which their own organization has risen to and been able to meet these challenges
- leverage a model and a language that allows the complex and difficult developmental issues associated with these challenges to be thought about and debated, and effort and attention to be focused on where the 'gaps' lie and where QI interventions need to be targeted.

The six common challenges

The organizational stories recounted in Chapters 2 to 8 saw all of our organizations struggling to attend to and manage the same set of core challenges, and doing so by adopting and employing a wide range of different methods and approaches.

For example, the main theme of the Royal Devon and Exeter case revolved around organizational identity and pride, concepts closely tied to *cultural processes* within organizations. Yet cultural challenges and solutions were prominent across virtually all the cases, from a similar culture of excellence at Cedars-Sinai, to the culture of mindfulness discussed in the San Diego Children's Hospital chapter, and the development of group-oriented cultures at Peterborough. Similarly, the predominating theme of a distributed leadership system in the Reinier de Graff Groep case, and of intelligent socio-technical systems design in the Luther Midelfort case, each imply *structural processes* within organizations. The Peterborough case, with its emphasis on empowerment, drew attention to *political processes* within organizations. This theme of empowerment was also present at the Albany AIDS Treatment Center, while the issue of engaging clinicians in quality efforts, which involves deep political challenges particular to healthcare organizations, was a consistent theme across all of the cases. Likewise, the Cedars-Sinai case highlighted the need to link organizational *learning* to improvement, as did San Diego and Royal Devon and Exeter, in the form of strong mentoring by micro-system leaders, and Luther Midelfort, which dedicated 'slack' resources to support QI training and 'knowledge harvesting' from other organizations.

The Albany case was unique in its emphasis on mobilizing processes that tap into the commitments and passions of individuals at an *emotional* level. However, other cases, each in their own way, also addressed emotional processes inherent in the quality journey in the form of generating collective momentum for the quality agenda (*see*, for example, the Peterborough case) and seeking to 'move' people by inspirational leadership (for example, the San Diego case).

Finally, there were numerous references to the design and use of both *physical and technological* infrastructure throughout the narratives, including such issues as the placement of facilities and organizational units (e.g. Royal Devon and Exeter, Luther Midelfort), different roles for information technology in the improvement process (Cedars-Sinai, Peterborough), and the aesthetics of the built environment (*see*, especially, the San Diego case).

Previous studies of the quality journeys of healthcare organizations (e.g. Øvretveit and Aslaksen[3]) have mirrored our case-based approach but have not sought to explicitly draw out such commonalities and differences across the organizations under study. With this in mind, and driven by a desire to rise above the idiosyncrasies of each case and at the same time leave our readers with something practical, we revisited the organizational narratives and were able to pull out the six universal challenges, which in turn became the organizer for the specific sub-themes or elements that we identified in our repeated readings of the cases and which now provide the spine of the quality codebook that follows.

We have already stated the six challenges in our opening chapter:

1. **structural** – the whole challenge around structuring, planning and co-ordinating quality efforts
2. **political** – the challenge of addressing the politics and negotiating the buy-in, conflict and relationships of change surrounding any QI effort
3. **cultural** – the challenge of giving 'quality' a shared, collective meaning, value and significance within the organization
4. **educational** – the challenge of creating and nurturing a learning process that supports continuous improvement
5. **emotional** – the challenge of inspiring, energizing, and mobilizing people for the QI effort
6. **physical and technological** – the challenge of designing physical systems and technological infrastructures that support improvement and quality of care.

As already stated, every organization in our research has, to varying degrees, found different ways of meeting these challenges, reinforcing the point that there is no one best way of reaching one's goal. Because local conditions and contexts vary so much, particular solutions also need to vary, and therefore need to be locally cultivated, home-grown and situation-specific. In this sense it is better to assume that 'solutions' travel poorly and cannot simply be copied or co-opted from elsewhere. Furthermore, most or all of the case studies describe key interactions and pressures with parties or influences external to their organization, hence the need to factor in the effect of the wider institutional and social environment. Without this 'contextualist'[4,5] and 'institutionalist'[6–9] framework, any attempt at making sense of the stories would risk overlooking or misattributing critical sources of organizational behavior and change.

It is not always a case of there being a difficult or hostile environment to manage.

External conditions can be enabling too, echoing the related notions of 'structural conduciveness'[10] and 'opportunity structures'[11] in social movement theory, and 'receptive context' in organizational theory.[12] For example, the US Institute of Medicine reports *To Err is Human*[13] and *Crossing the Quality Chasm*[14] both gave a terrific boost to Cedar-Sinai's internal improvement efforts (Chapter 4), as did the IHI Pursuing Perfection initiative in RD&E and Reinier de Graaf (Chapters 3 and 5). The explicit inclusion of external contextual factors in our framework stems from the importance these were given in the cases as sources of knowledge, as well as influences and impetus in reinforcing (or detracting from) the development of an organization's quality agenda and journey. In many of the cases the internal–external divide was also an important locus of boundary-spanning activities (as described, for example, in the Luther Midelfort case study in Chapter 6). One of the particular strengths of the case study approach is its ability to show *how* these internal–external dynamics play out around QI in healthcare.

A 'color-codebook' for quality and service improvement

The six challenges described above are depicted by the large circles in Figure 9.1 (*see* color plate section), along with the major categories of contextual influences (from within and outside the organization), as shown at the top of the figure.

For ease of use as a diagnostic tool and heuristic (aid to thinking), we have translated the six common challenges into a color-coded schema, allocating a different color to each of the core challenges. We have found the color code to be a simple and readily accessible way for people to think and talk about complex issues in the change/ improvement domain. There is nothing particularly new or original in this idea, since our use of colors as a visual metaphor is merely an adaptation and extension of Vermaak and de Caluwé's 'color-code for change'.[15]

In our view, the color code they developed for organizational development efforts can apply equally to quality and improvement efforts (themselves a form of organizational development). In our own color code, the blue, yellow and green remain broadly the same in concept as in Vermaak and de Caluwé's scheme (namely, concerned with structure, politics and learning respectively). Based on our data, however, red has been changed from a human resources to a cultural perspective, defined as the need to create strong collective ideas and values around QI such that the meaning and identification with quality efforts are system-wide and part of the working ethos of the organization. We have also amended white, based on two of the current authors' related social movements work,[16] to indicate the 'white heat' and energy of a truly mobilized organization (everyone behind the quality 'cause'), and have introduced the new color, pink, to represent the 'flesh' of organizational systems and infrastructures for improvement. Finally, we have also added in codes for the wider 'inner' (organizational) and 'outer' (external) context using the (admittedly less suggestive) colors of grey and black, respectively, to draw attention to the influence of environmental conditions on successful QI efforts (as discussed above).

Each of the six main 'process' colors was chosen to evoke the essence or fundamental nature of the challenge with which it is associated, as follows.

Blue

Blue (*structural* challenges) represents the cold, hard steel of structural and strategic support for the QI effort, acting like the metal hoops around the barrel to pull the various quality activities together. This first challenge encompasses – among many other issues, as listed in the codebook at the end of this chapter – the establishment of quality systems, structures and roles, data and monitoring systems, and QI training programs, as well as the issue of strategic leadership for QI. This is illustrated by the following quotation from one of our case study organizations:

> ... going into next year, we have five strategic goals in this organization and one of them is about quality and safety. That's going to be on everybody's plate next year and that's a long way from a decade ago when we were looking at finances as number one. So, it's sort of setting the institutional priorities for quality and safety, and then asking what's going to happen in any particular neighbourhood in the institution.

Examples of 'blue' solutions from our case study organizations would include the development and organization-wide implementation of integrated care pathways at San Diego Children's (Chapter 2), the work of the central transformation team at Peterborough (Chapter 7) and the elaborate QI structure (or 'wiring diagram') that has evolved at Cedars-Sinai (Chapter 4).

Yellow

Yellow (challenges relating to the *power and politics* of organization) represents the frictional 'heat' of politics and the search for common ground between stakeholders, and sufficient appeal to their 'what's in it for me', to get them lining up behind the quality endeavour. In this regard, Kelman suggests that:

> ... rather than saying that 'people resist change' ... it is more appropriate to see initiation of a change process as setting in motion a political struggle inside the organization.[17]

Or as Stensaker and Langley put it, 'power and politics ... are simply an integral part of organizational reality necessarily affecting all associated with organizational change'.[18] We would extend this to QI efforts, which are after all one type of change. Or, as one of our interviewees at RD&E (Chapter 3) suggested:

> We've got to open the doors and we've actually got to listen – we may not agree but if somebody wants something, think of what you want to do and then see if you can hang it on their hook and then you can move forward. But let's start learning how to play politics – because if we don't all we do is damage our service.

This second challenge includes issues of clinical engagement, staff and patient empowerment, and partnership working with external stakeholders, with Bill's parties with key primary care stakeholders, as described in the Peterborough case study (Chapter 7), being a good example of a solution to the latter.

Red

Red (*cultural* challenges relating to creating a shared mindset or ethos around quality) stands for the blood or viscera of the organization: 'the way we do things around here', 'the pattern of basic assumptions', the organization as a social construction; in short, the culture of the organization.[19] Culture is important to all aspects of the QI process, but particularly to the sustainability ('making it stick') aspect, 'anchoring' and 'fixing' the change – as it needs to do – in new 'habits of thinking'[20] and new patterns of behavior:

> In large-scale change efforts, we use the power of culture to help make a transformation stick ... For our purposes here it means the norms of behavior and the shared values in a group of people. It's a set of common feelings about what is of value and how we should

act. A good test of whether something is embedded in a culture is if our peers, without really thinking, find ways to nudge us back to group norms when we go astray. The keys are *peers* – that is, a group activity – and *not really thinking*, which means behavior with roots deeper than rational thought.[21]

We have seen red at work in so many of our case study organizations, making quality more than just another project or goal, but a deeply embedded ideal, even mission, that is collectively valued and supported; not something that is enforced top down, but reinforced in peer-to-peer interactions and everyday, taken-for-granted behavior. Examples include the way quality was embedded in both the professional and corporate cultures of RD&E (Chapter 3), and the philosophies underlying the physician compacts at Luther Midelfort (Chapter 6) and Cedars-Sinai (Chapter 4).

Similarly, Weick introduced the idea that sustainability in an organization is essentially a social accomplishment, incorporated in the binding commitments that people make to each other in relation to a particular enacted change or innovation.[24] As the following quotation from one of our interviewees at Cedars-Sinai (Chapter 4) suggests, healthcare organizations that have successfully embedded QI in their culture may 'feel' very different from those that have not:

> When I look back at some of the other hospitals I worked at . . . [they] were hospitals that were to some degree really proactive in their quality programs, or were interested . . . but their priorities were different. They say they have their structures, they have the corporate quality person and then they also have to ensure that everything is in place, but they weren't building the culture, they were building the structure for it but it wasn't really embodiment or belief in that philosophy.

Green

Green represents *growth and learning*. This fourth universal challenge is all about how one begins to accumulate and pass on the knowledge and lessons about quality from generation to generation: in the jargon, how does one build a learning organization around one's QI and service improvement endeavours? Perhaps the clearest example of this from our case studies was the formal knowledge management system that had been established at Cedars-Sinai (Chapter 4). This overlaps to some extent with the blue structural challenge described above (around co-ordinating the QI effort) and we shall come to the interactions between the six challenges in Chapter 10. For the moment, this specific challenge asks: what will test people, what will develop them and what will stretch them to higher things (the notion of continuous improvement)? Importantly, like red, overcoming this challenge can be seen as a key stage towards sustainability (something of the holy grail of healthcare improvement). As Oliver Wendell Holmes the younger said, 'Man's mind, once stretched by a new idea, never regains its original dimensions.'

Learning about new approaches to QI, albeit one small part of the learning and development process, featured strongly in all of our case study sites:

> All of us have come back from different meetings, have seen things, have reviewed things, or we see things in the literature, and we think, 'Boy, this will be a great idea,' and we put together a team and say, 'Here's something we've seen, let's explore it, let's examine it, and let's figure out how to make it fit our organization.'

Other green issues – beyond learning about formal QI approaches – include knowledge harvesting (witness the specific boundary-spanning role created for this purpose at Luther Midelfort, in Chapter 6), experimentation and piloting, and leaders who take on a mentorship role to encourage reflective practice and personal development (as we saw in the micro-systems in our San Diego Children's and Peterborough case studies, *see* Chapters 2 and 7 respectively).

White

White stands for the white heat of *emotion and mobilization*, the energy that is needed behind a quality and service improvement effort to get it going and then to keep it going. This is Kelman's notion of unleashing the passion and energy for change and improvement.[17] Similarly, the stories we were told were not about improvement programs or targets, but simply about exciting people and making quality something that had to be done:

> We started rolling these concepts out ... engaging people in the decision-making process ... We found a huge number of people at the frontline who said, 'Yes, that's what we should do.' It resonated with them, they were prepared to adopt it, they were very excited about it, they saw the connection with what we had explicitly said was our mission and they felt it was very important.

White is what changes an improvement 'effort' into a 'burning wish', or even a 'cause', and a quality program into a 'movement for improvement', terms that were actually used by some of our case study sites (in particular, Albany in Chapter 8) to describe that special something in change and improvement processes where they acquire a life of their own, and an unstoppable forward momentum.[22]

Pink

Finally, pink is symbolic of the *flesh* of the organization, the physical and technical infrastructure that is needed to regularize quality and deliver it on a routine, everyday basis: 'tangible improvements to the estate and environment which just means that it is a different hospital to visit now than it was 10 years ago'.

This was not something we had anticipated would end up with its own color, nor is there any mention of it in Vermaak and Caluwé's original color-code for change. However, it became clear very early on how important a role physical environment (both functionally and aesthetically) and technical infrastructure (including IT systems) play in an organization's improvement journey, and how necessary it therefore is to have this challenge represented in the codebook.

Different failures of QI efforts

Before detailing these six challenges we invite readers to speculate on the flipside to all this: the implications of *not* responding to any one of these listed challenges. The main point here is to recognize that different kinds of failure are associated with each of the six challenges. Which is to say, improvement efforts do not just fail or succeed; they can fail or underachieve in many different ways. Hence, we wish to propose that if there is no effective:

- ❐ structural process (blue), the result will be *fragmentation* and a general lack of synergy and joined-upness between the different parts of the organization doing QI (reminiscent of the 'Six West problem' described in Chapter 1)
- ❐ political process (yellow), the result will be *disillusionment*, because QI is just not happening on the ground and because individuals and groups are blocking and resisting change; the failure scenario here is that the change process has become stymied or gridlocked as the result of the 'impossible politics' being played out in the organization, and people simply give up trying

❏ cultural process (red), the result will be *evaporation*, because the change has not properly anchored or become rooted in habitual everyday thinking and behavioral routines; this is highly reminiscent of program- or project-based approaches to QI, where the drive for quality lasts only as long as the flavour of the current program or project

❏ educational process (green), the result will be *amnesia or frustration*, as lessons and knowledge are forgotten or fail to accumulate (as in the notion of sedimentary learning), and improvement capabilities and skills fail to keep abreast of growing aspirations

❏ emotional process (white), the result will be *disinterest or fade-out*, as the change effort runs out of energy and forward movement; improvement theorists and practitioners like to talk about the accumulation of small steps or increments leading to final 'lift off' and transformation (think of a long-jumper running down the track to the board), but without the white, the effort is more likely to end up running into the sand than taking off

❏ physical, technological and systems design process (pink), the result will be *exhaustion*, as people run around trying to do it all by hand or word of mouth, not having the luxury of a system or standardized set of routines to take the weight of necessary everyday activities.

As noted above, participants in our case study organizations talked about the many and various solutions they had applied to these challenges at various points and stages on their quality journeys, and it is our contention that these solutions either helped them in a positive sense to meet the six core challenges, or in a negative sense to avoid the pitfalls associated with them that we have just described.

The codebook

Based on systematic review and coding of the cases, multiple illustrations of the different types of challenges and solutions were extracted from the individual case study narratives and assigned to the different colors. This is how the color codebook was born (*see* pages 177-85 below). In total, the codebook includes 56 such solutions spread across the six challenges, all derived ground-up from the cases themselves.

The codebook defines each of these solutions in turn, and Annex 1 illustrates how each may contribute to sustained quality and service improvement in the healthcare setting by drawing on quotations from the study participants (a sort of thesaurus or lexicon for the codebook). This 'quality thesaurus' needed to be included, first to support the codebook with real, empirical illustrations from the cases and to help readers with the definitions; but second because we considered it important to retain the words used by the participants themselves to define the various challenges and solutions, not to impose our own. Of course no single organization can be expected – or needs – to implement each and every one of the 56 'solutions'. Rather, the list of solutions is presented here to illustrate the whole range of responses made by high-performing healthcare organizations in our sample to the six common challenges we have identified.

Using the color codebook

We believe the codebook on pages 177-85 can serve a number of useful purposes, but let us begin by saying what it cannot do. It can tell organization members what the various challenges are and can illustrate the range of solutions, but, as we have insisted all along, it cannot give them the 'correct' solution or answer – people still have to find these for themselves. Local context, whether it be cultural, structural or economic, is so unique and different as to require a properly tailored QI solution or set of solutions, and this can only mean that the QI system or process has to be home-grown, inside-out and bottom up, not appropriated or imported from elsewhere.

Wilkins made exactly the same point in relation to organizational culture when he observed, 'You cannot buy a distinctive organizational culture and you cannot copy it from someone else. You must grow it.'[23] The fact that our quality organizations did exactly this – that their process of selecting and constructing the solution was intelligent and effective – is the main point we want our readers to take away, even though there may be some initial disappointment that (unlike many of the best-selling business book authors) we cannot offer any universal plug-in or off-the-shelf solutions.

So, the codebook cannot be used prescriptively to come up with the right solution. Nor, for that matter, can it be used predictively to model the ideal theoretical solution. These limitations apart, we believe that it can help organizations to carry out an intelligent search for a solution by:

- ❒ providing a checklist of the areas and topics any QI effort will need to cover (a map of the terrain, including its main barriers and obstacles)
- ❒ giving improvement activists a way of charting where they and their organization are on their improvement journey, and a method for identifying any 'gaps' in their own QI activities that will need to be addressed (a self-administered diagnostic tool)
- ❒ allowing implicit assumptions about the theory and practice of QI to surface, and to be thought about, perhaps for the first time (a reflective model)
- ❒ providing people with a framework and language for talking about and debating the issues (a dialogical tool).

The codebook is mainly for practitioners, but QI theorists might also be able to use the tool to develop and then go out and test some of the sub-topics in the form of hypotheses – something we were not in a position to do at the start of our journey.

Leadership

At this point a few words about leadership and where it fits in to the overall scheme of things may be in order. We have so many wonderful examples of different kinds of leadership in our case studies, ranging from the distributed collective leadership system at Reinier de Graaf (Chapter 5), to the charismatic leadership of single individuals described at San Diego Children's Hospital (Chapter 2); the knowledge leadership at Cedars-Sinai (Chapter 4) and San Diego; as well as various forms of leadership at the micro-level, such as the mentoring leadership within the Asthma Clinic at San Diego and the Radiology Department at Peterborough (Chapter 7), the leadership-by-example and mobilization leadership of the medical director and administrator at Albany (Chapter 8), and the division of leadership between technical and political tasks in the Emergency Department at Cedars-Sinai.

Readers will notice that these different forms of leadership are provided as solutions throughout the six challenges contained in the codebook rather than leadership being represented as a challenge in its own right. While initially tempted to give leadership its own category – not least to underline its crucial importance in QI efforts – we finally decided against this on the grounds that leadership is not a challenge that can be separated from the other challenges but is integral to them. Blue (structuring) and pink (infrastructure), for example, call for leadership skills in design,[24] whether this be organizational, software or facilities design; whereas yellow (politics) requires a conciliative, brokering form of leadership that is capable of 'uniting the various parties in thought'.[19] Different again, green (learning) requires leaders like the head of the Asthma Clinic at San Diego who, according to his staff, was mentor and teacher rolled into one. Red and white leaders also bring special and very different skills in engaging and mobilizing staff, and turning individual improvement enthusiasts into a community for improvement. In short, leadership, whether defined as a person or a process, is the means for delivering success on these challenges, not an abstract or independent challenge in its own right.

How to apply the codebook

A general word of warning about the use of the color codebook: the idea of a color code is attractive, but the 'doing' of effective QI is not the same as painting by numbers. In order to understand the interactions, timing and unfolding of these solutions in actual organizational settings and in real time, we strongly recommend that readers read this codebook in conjunction with both the companion case studies from which it was produced (Chapters 2 to 8), and with Chapter 10 in this book, which explores how the dynamic *interactions* between these solutions actively shaped the quality journeys in our case study organizations. Its proper place – and strength – therefore, is as a guide book to accompany fellow travelers on their quality journeys rather than a detailed do-it-yourself guide to home improvement. Its limitation is that, as with any book, it contains only the still photographs of the journey and no moving pictures at all. However, it is to these, the dynamics of QI processes, that we turn our attention in Chapter 10.

Achieving and Sustaining Healthcare Quality

A COLOR CODEBOOK FOR QUALITY AND SERVICE IMPROVEMENT PRACTICE

Organizational challenges and solutions

A checklist
- ❐ The structural challenge
- ❐ The political challenge
- ❐ The cultural challenge
- ❐ The educational challenge
- ❐ The emotional challenge
- ❐ The physical and technological challenge

Assess your own organization against the six universal challenges by checking (individually or as a team) how close you think it is to achieving each of the specific solutions within each challenge (in terms of either 'a long way to go', 'some way there' or 'already there').

Reviewing your overall responses across the six challenges can help identify current gaps and opportunities and help facilitate discussions on the necessary direction of travel of the organization's future QI efforts. (For example, does your organization have 'a long way to go' on most or all of the structural solutions? Is it 'already there' in terms of the majority of the political solutions?)

Annex 1 at the back of this book provides quotations from the case studies to further define and illustrate the various elements and solutions.

The structural challenge

Structuring, planning and co-ordinating the quality and service improvement effort, and embedding it within the organizational fabric.

SOLUTION	DEFINITION	'WHERE ARE WE?'		
		A long way to go	Some way there	Already there
Quality strategy and plan	A formal strategy for quality and service improvement (Q & SI), and a plan for implementation	☐	☐	☐
Strategic leadership	Strong and decisive executive leadership, providing a clear, strategic direction and a disciplined and detailed focus around Q & SI matters	☐	☐	☐
Whole-systems organizational design	A coordinated Q & SI effort that involves joined up whole-systems design and cross-functional improvement initiatives (as opposed to discreet local projects)	☐	☐	☐
Devolved authority system	A 'flat' organizational structure that minimizes hierarchy and provides opportunity and encouragement for bottom-up improvement and change initiatives	☐	☐	☐
Quality leadership positions	Formal roles and responsibilities in relation to Q & SI are shown on the organizational chart, which also shows a senior person at the top who is leading on quality	☐	☐	☐
Multi-level leadership structure for quality	A dispersed, multi-level leadership structure that sees leadership in Q & SI being exercised simultaneously at the micro-system, intermediate/middle-management, directorate, medical board and corporate levels of the organization	☐	☐	☐
Quality facilitation team or group	A dedicated 'core' improvement/ change team comprising improvement specialists and a wide range of Q & SI skills in areas such as process mapping, continuous quality improvement (CQI), organizational development (OD), team building and facilitation	☐	☐	☐
QI training programs	Formal education and training opportunities for staff development in the Q & SI area	☐	☐	☐
Enabling administrative role	Central HQ departments, managers and staff that function more as a performance and quality service to frontline units in Q & SI matters than a central, directing authority	☐	☐	☐

SOLUTION	DEFINITION	'WHERE ARE WE?'		
		A long way to go	Some way there	Already there
Boundary-spanner roles	Hybrid dual, bridging, liaison, interlocutor or boundary-spanning roles, such as clinical leader/manager, which allow for lateral contact and communication between different groups, and the linking of resources, people and ideas around the Q & SI effort	❏	❏	❏
Communities of practice	Cross-organizational and occupational networks, groups, and fora that come together to debate, share knowledge and take forward the Q & SI agenda	❏	❏	❏
Results-oriented planning	Formally constituted procedures for planning and monitoring improvement projects with clear timelines and robust project management mechanisms	❏	❏	❏
Quality governance system	An organization-wide infrastructure of Q & SI meetings and groups for co-ordinating and spreading improvement throughout the system	❏	❏	❏
Organizational slack for quality	Deliberate provision of slack resources or headroom in the organization (be it money, time, airline tickets or space) that enables staff periodically to stand back from everyday operations and think and work on service development issues	❏	❏	❏
Data and monitoring systems	Formal data collection and information processing systems for constant monitoring, measuring, benchmarking of organizational and clinical performance (e.g. dashboards, clinical information, etc.)	❏	❏	❏

The political challenge

Negotiating the politics of change associated with implanting and sustaining the improvement process, including securing stakeholder buy-in and engagement, dealing with conflict and opposition, building change relationships, and agreeing and committing to a common agenda for improvement.

SOLUTION	DEFINITION	'WHERE ARE WE?'		
		A long way to go	Some way there	Already there
Politically credible leadership	Senior leaders with the authority and skill to broker and manage the 'politics of engagement' associated with improvement work, including dealing with resistance, and selling the case for engaging in Q & SI activities	☐	☐	☐
Clinical engagement	Strong and active clinician engagement in, and ownership of, the Q & SI process	☐	☐	☐
Peer-to-peer relationships	Strong peer-to-peer lines of communication and influence, from clinician to clinician, manager to manager, that enable QI innovations to spread rapidly and effectively down through the organization	☐	☐	☐
Clinical–managerial partnering	An agreed clinician and management compact (formal or informal) binding them to work together on the Q & SI agenda	☐	☐	☐
Staff empowerment	Empowering staff to be able to influence and exercise real control over their local service environment	☐	☐	☐
Patient empowerment	Empowering patients to be able to influence and participate in improvement work	☐	☐	☐
External partnering	Strong and close partnership and mutual interaction between internal staff and relevant external stakeholders in the improvement process	☐	☐	☐

The cultural challenge

Building shared understanding, commitment and community around the improvement process.

SOLUTION	DEFINITION	'WHERE ARE WE?'		
		A long way to go	Some way there	Already there
Culture of excellence	A culture that places a premium on excellence in delivering quality care to patients (reflected in the mission, values, language, systems and symbols)	❑	❑	❑
Values / symbolic leadership	Leaders who are committed to developing a culture in which quality is the key and overriding concern, and who actively role model this commitment in their own everyday language and behaviors	❑	❑	❑
Patient-centered ethic	A strong patient/customer care ethic that infuses every part of the service, large or small	❑	❑	❑
Culture of mindfulness	A culture of mindfulness that keeps staff constantly vigilant and alert as to their personal and group standards and practices – being awake to quality and safety concerns, and avoiding automatic or standard cookbook practice	❑	❑	❑
Group/ collaborative culture	A strong 'we group' culture that promotes teamwork and co-operation between staff, placing a premium on human values like respect, integrity, trust, pride, honesty, inclusion and openness	❑	❑	❑
Scientific culture	A scientific culture that values data, measurement and evidence in both medical and managerial practice, while being strongly task- and results-driven	❑	❑	❑
Culture of learning	A culture of innovation and learning that values risk-taking and experimentation, and constantly encourages people to do more and differently, and to develop and share new knowledge, skills and expertise	❑	❑	❑
Formal culture	A culture that emphasizes the need for formalized disciplines and enabling structures to ensure efficiency, effectiveness, and personal accountability	❑	❑	❑
Culture of empowerment	A culture that genuinely nurtures and supports empowerment and 'self-leadership' at all levels of the organization, and that demonstrates this commitment in its reward systems and everyday practices	❑	❑	❑

SOLUTION	DEFINITION	'WHERE ARE WE?'		
		A long way to go	Some way there	Already there
Cosmopolitan culture	An outward-facing organizational culture that is sensitive to the dangers of isolation, arrogance and ethnocentric mentalities and behaviors, and is prepared to learn from others	❏	❏	❏
Long-term culture	A culture that supports the longer-term perspective on Q & SI (the long haul rather than the quick sprint), and is alert to the dangers of fads and short-term quick fixes	❏	❏	❏
Organizational identity	A strong sense of organization pride and history, identity, legacy and tradition	❏	❏	❏
Recruitment and retainment	Recruiting and rewarding people whose personal values closely align to the quality values of the organization	❏	❏	❏
Acculturation	Socialization, induction and training processes that help people tune-in and acculturate to the core Q & SI values of the organization	❏	❏	❏

The educational challenge

Embedding and nurturing a continuous learning process in relation to quality and service improvement issues, including both formal and informal mentoring, instruction, education and training, and the acquisition of relevant knowledge, skills and expertise.

SOLUTION	DEFINITION	'WHERE ARE WE?'		
		A long way to go	**Some way there**	**Already there**
Pedagogic leadership	Influential organizational leaders who champion reflective practice, and encourage staff and colleagues to engage in continuous learning and development in relation to quality and service improvement (Q & SI) issues	❑	❑	❑
Organizational change knowledge	The acquisition and application of existing knowledge and an evidence base relating to Q & SI, and organizational development and change management knowledge	❑	❑	❑
Quality improvement knowledge	The acquisition and application of knowledge relating to specific Q & SI methods and techniques (e.g. PDSA, process mapping), and clinical care/ improvement models (clinical pathways, chronic care model, etc.) in their work.	❑	❑	❑
Knowledge harvesting	Formal or informal activities to search for and bring back (i.e. harvest) new Q & SI methods, concepts and ideas from conferences and other sources outside of one's own organization or group	❑	❑	❑
Experimentation and piloting	Developing, piloting and systematically testing (and learning from) the application of new Q & SI methods and approaches	❑	❑	❑
Evidence-based learning	Learning and developing new understanding from review and analysis of routine evidence and data (e.g. clinical auditing, benchmarking, and other activities to evaluate and measure the impact/benefits of Q & SI applications)	❑	❑	❑
Experience-based learning	Learning and developing new understanding from the involvement of patients and caregivers in the design of their own care, including the ability to listen and learn directly from the 'voice of experience'	❑	❑	❑

The emotional challenge

Energizing, mobilizing and inspiring staff and other stakeholders to want to join in the improvement effort by their own volition and sustain its momentum through individual and collective motivation, enthusiasm and movement.

SOLUTION	DEFINITION	'WHERE ARE WE?'		
		A long way to go	Some way there	Already there
Mobilizing leadership	Inspirational leaders who see Q & SI as much a mission or movement as a project, and who have sufficient skill in scripting/framing ideas for various audiences and sufficient standing within the organization to be able to mobilize large numbers and a wide cross-section of staff to join their 'improvement movement'	❑	❑	❑
Clinical and other change champions	Clinical champions and similarly influential others in the organization who are able to energize, mobilize, and engage fellow professionals and co-workers in the Q & SI effort	❑	❑	❑
Collective momentum	Building powerful momentum around the Q & SI effort such that it ultimately takes on a life of its own, spreading and feeding off its own energies, and no longer needing to be driven from above	❑	❑	❑
Professional and social affiliations	Local quality activists mobilizing and driving the improvement effort through their informal networks of professional and social affiliations	❑	❑	❑
Quality as a mission/calling	Staff are energized and self-motivated around Q & SI, knowing they are helping people and contributing to the humanitarian goals of the organization – more than a job, it's a mission and a calling	❑	❑	❑
Emotional involvement	Staff are emotionally involved and invested in the improvement effort – it has become a matter of the heart as well as the head	❑	❑	❑
Improvement campaigns	Mounting improvement campaigns to speed up and carry the improvement work forward	❑	❑	❑

The physical and technological challenge

The design and use of a physical, informational and technological infrastructure that improves service quality and the experience of care.

SOLUTION	DEFINITION	'WHERE ARE WE?'		
		A long way to go	Some way there	Already there
Functional design	Functional design of architecture and the built environment to support and encourage Q & SI (i.e. does the job it is supposed to do, safely and effectively, and improves the usability of the service)	☐	☐	☐
Aesthetic design	Aesthetic design of architecture and the built environment supporting and encouraging Q & SI (i.e. improves the patient's and carers' experience of care)	☐	☐	☐
Technology/ design leadership	A leadership that is aware of the positive effects of the built environment (both functionality and aesthetics) and/or of clinical and information technology on the patient experience, and incorporates these design elements into service improvement efforts	☐	☐	☐
Location of infrastructure and technology	Location of physical infrastructure and technological systems (e.g. free-standing vs. integrated facilities, proximity to other organizational units, separate vs. integrated IT systems, etc.)	☐	☐	☐
Supportive information technology	Design and implementation of IT and communications systems that support and encourage Q & SI efforts	☐	☐	☐
Supportive medical technology	Design and implementation of medical equipment and clinical technologies to support and encourage Q & SI efforts	☐	☐	☐

Towards a process model of organizing for quality

The need for something more

The codebook in the previous chapter outlines the six universal challenges that all healthcare organizations involved in QI will face at some point, and the practical solutions that were devised and applied by the particular group of high-performing organizations in our study to meet these challenges. The codebook's focus on the organizational and human dimension of the QI effort – challenges and solutions – is deliberate, first because so far they have received scant attention in healthcare research and practice relative to the clinical and technical dimensions, and second because of the inescapable fact that every aspect of quality is delivered by people working in organizations. In our view this makes it impossible to ignore these missing dimensions any longer.

In our first chapter we also stressed the need for quality research to move from a focus on factors to one on processes. So far, however, this notion has been only faintly developed in our color-coded framework. Indeed, critics would be justified in pointing out that the codebook in Chapter 9, although extracted from the rich descriptions of organizational processes in the case narratives, still represents challenges and solutions as single elements, and in that sense offers little more than the typical menu of key success factors we ourselves criticized, with barely a glimmer of a process in sight. However, we hope this will now begin to change as we try to bring our model to life.

But first let us be clear where we are starting from and attempting to reach. Meyer *et al.* is a fairly typical example of the traditional approach to researching QI in the healthcare context that we feel now needs to be challenged and extended. This research study identified and described the *key factors* that contributed to the success of four high-performing hospitals in the US.[1] In passing, the factors listed were: developing the right culture, attracting and retaining the right people, devising and updating the right in-house processes, and giving staff the right tools to do the job. The authors presented '18 action steps for hospitals', but as the likes of Whelan-Berry *et al.* have rightly argued, such steps have rarely been conceptualized or synthesized into any kind of process model.[2]

The important thing to be said here is that change and improvement models – even those that go further than 'factors' to describe stages and steps (referred to by OD writers as 'recipe' or 'n-step models') – actually tell us little about process, because process is not so much the sequence or steps themselves as what happens between them. Typically – and disappointingly – n-step models will say little about the dynamics of how one step leads to, influences or transitions into another. Indeed, it is almost as if there is nothing beyond or between the stepping stones, and the reassuringly straight and logical line they follow: 'first do A, then do B' and so on (think of a dance choreography, hopscotch or road directions from the internet), always progressing, and always clear and well signposted.

Recipe- or stage-based 'planned change' models like these abound in both the quality and healthcare fields (lean, PDSA, pathways, etc.), and one could be forgiven for thinking that they are the only models on offer. But what if the change and improvement process they purport to describe (linear, sequential, etc.) is not really like this at all? Perhaps such representations are more the kind of simple, uncomplicated and manageable process we would *like* to see rather than the complex, messy and circular one that it *actually is*?

The problem is that such linear models have largely untested assumptions standing in place of facts, and a paucity of empirical research concerning the organizational processes in question. An additional source of concern is that for most of us the conventional models and assumptions do not accord with our *experience* of the change process, which, whether in work or social life, tends much more towards the complex, messier or foggier end of things. The really discomforting thought is that if the assumptions about the processes in question are indeed flawed, then the change and QI interventions and methods themselves will also be flawed: we may be *doing* change and improvement wrongly.

Some change writers are in no doubt that for this reason we should be challenging the n-step or recipe models and the theories and practice that go with them, and finding out what change processes are really like.[3] We also share the view that there is an urgent need to go further in order to acquire a deeper and more empirically informed comprehension of the fundamentals of change processes. As Morgan[4] put it more than two decades ago (and the need he identified is still there): 'We need to try and understand how the discrete events that make up our experience of change are generated by a logic unfolded in the process of change itself.' More recently, organization researchers have stated that the time has come to stop talking about process and actually go out and study it.[5] Quality and healthcare studies might wish to consider doing likewise.

Moving from factors and steps to processes

The reason we need to resist the temptation to merely (and endlessly) list and categorize key variables is that the key to quality – if there is one – is not to be found in the factors as such, but in the processes that connect them.

The starting point is to recognize that we cannot approach human factors in the same way as we would technical or clinical factors – as independent and dependent variables in closed cause-effect relationships with each other. As previously stated, organization researchers have repeatedly drawn attention to the weaknesses and limitations of the variables paradigm and the particular type of scientific language associated with it.[6] Thus, while nice if only it were true, there is rarely a single or even dominant set of factors that explain why only 55% of patients receive their recommended care,[7] or why some national healthcare systems do significantly better or worse than the average on particular quality and performance measures.

Rather, studying organizations as systems and processes requires:

❐ holistic case studies of the kind we have been carrying out (still rare), which at least open up the possibility of our being able to see how system dynamics emerge and play out (especially, as our cases have shown, between the different levels of the system)

❐ a way (e.g. complexity or systems theory[8]) to explore the patterns of relationships, interconnections and interactions among the organization's or system's parts, ideally over time

❐ a particular sensitivity to the positive and negative feedback loops that link factors and processes together, what we described metaphorically in Chapter 1 as the positive thermals that can – sometimes slowly, sometimes quite suddenly – take an improvement effort skywards (the notion of synergy[9,10] or lift-off) or the negative downdraughts that can take it crashing to the ground.

Motivated by these objectives, the particular 'process' questions that we now want to go on to address via our case studies include:

❐ were the various quality solutions identified in the codebook related or joined together in some way?

❐ what was the process whereby these different parts of the 'quality engine' burst into life – or not?

❐ were there different kinds of relationships and interactions between certain colors or shades (i.e. elements and sub-elements) that led to different kinds of dynamics and outcomes?

❐ were the colors (e.g. structure and culture) even connected at all, and if so, which ones were most strongly associated or bonded to which? In short, what quality *processes* were at work in the organizations we studied?

Building on the work of a small number of others who are interested in this perspective,[2,11–13] and using formal network mapping as we describe below, we developed an approach that offers an imperfect, but still rare and privileged, glimpse into the machinery that drives successful QI processes – a machinery whose workings differed markedly from organization to organization, making each one of them, and their stories, so unique.

A quotation from Pettigrew *et al.* defined the task at hand and the required paradigm shift necessary for the next stage of our analysis:

> Focusing on interaction moves away from the variables paradigm toward a form of holistic explanation. The intellectual task is to examine how and why constellations of forces shape the character of change processes rather than 'fixed entities with variable qualities'.[11]

Following a number of process theorists, and Weick in particular (1969 through to 2001), we aim in the remainder of this chapter to show how the improvement processes identified in our sites were interconnected and symbiotic, and 'part of an unfolding process . . . a conjunction of open-ended interactions occurring in time'.[5] Kelman uses the phrase 'change feeding on itself' to characterize system effects.[14] Masuch similarly demonstrated how certain sets of organizational processes form cycles or closed loops, which can be virtuous (upward improvement spirals) or vicious (downward/ degrading),[15] both of these being present in an organization at one and the same time. Perlow *et al.*, on the other hand, in an ethnographic study of work groups across three national contexts,[16] use the term 'mutually reinforcing relationship', illustrating once again the same basic idea of a virtuous cycle or positive feedback loop. Our overall argument here is that it is in the patterns and dynamics of these connections or relationships that the fate of any healthcare improvement system will lie.

Visualizing quality improvement processes in healthcare organizations

As Langley suggests:

> . . . both narratives and visual maps can serve as intermediary databases for the . . . formulation of hypotheses and propositions. Since narratives are closer to the raw data than visual maps, they may also precede their development.[17]

Following Langley's advice to the letter, we have presented our narratives and now it's time for the visual maps.

For this we turned to the method of social network analysis,[18–20] or at least a variant that examines patterns of relationships among social and organizational *processes*,[21–22] in contrast to relationships among people or organizations, *per se*. The network analysis and visual mapping strategy we adopted aims to detect patterns in order to make sense and facilitate comparison of the organizing processes documented in the case narratives. According to Miles and Huberman[23] (as cited by Langley[24]), graphical forms have several advantages over narrative approaches, such as the one adopted to present each of our seven cases earlier in this book: they allow the presentation of large quantities of information in relatively little space, and they can be useful tools for the development and verification of theoretical ideas. Visual graphical representations are particularly attractive for analyzing process data because they allow the simultaneous representation of a large number of dimensions. It is for all these reasons that we also decided to pursue a network and visual mapping strategy for the process analysis of our cases.

The first step was to systematically identify and code the validated case narratives for any stated connections between two process elements or solutions. A simple example of an interaction between two solutions *within* the same color (see the Codebook) would be the way in which (a) awards or recognition for QI work and (b) pride and identity in the workplace reinforce each other (these are both red – solutions to the cultural challenge). More interestingly, perhaps, examples of interactions *between* colors would include (a) the way in which people playing boundary-spanning roles (blue) connect with the outside world and bring back learning (green); (b) how taking believers and non-believers to external conferences and QI fora (green) can help deal with some of the political issues around getting people on board (yellow) and mobilized/engaged (white); (c) using official (blue) reports like *To Err is Human* to disengage people from old patterns of behavior and mobilize (white); and (d) using a physician leadership program (green) to mobilize and engage clinicians (white/yellow) and deal with some of the cultural challenges of developing peer camaraderie and building a wider community of practice (red).

All of the examples cited so far are of positive loops, but there are also negative loops. Refer back, for example, to the potential problems of information overload resulting from the quality infrastructure at Cedars-Sinai (blue has a negative impact on green), which can also put busy physicians off (negative impact on white/yellow) – what one interviewee called the 'double-edged sword' of that particular QI infrastructure.

Before we present the results of our mapping of all these interconnected processes from a selection of our case study organizations, here, as an example of our coding method, is a very brief extract from the final narrative of the Cedars-Sinai hospital in Los Angeles (Chapter 4). This extract concerns a physician who took a particular role in the QI effort. The square brackets indicate where we were able to see and note connections between the solutions (see Annex 2 for the solutions or sub-processes that the alpha-numerical codes used in this example represent).

> In this spirit, the hospital decided to hire this physician to lend clinical background and credibility to the quality effort [S.10 to P.1].
>
> So he . . . went around looking at evidence-based stuff, and began to bring to the institution a whole discipline around analyzing process, flow diagrams, cradle diagrams, privatization approaches . . . and we began to infuse the organization with that approach. We linked up then with the national demonstration project later becoming the Institute for Healthcare Improvement, [he] became faculty in the IHI, as you probably know, and kept us connected with a network of people who had a growing similar interest around these kinds of things. [S.10 to ED.4]. (Senior medical administrator)

So, if we just take the first interaction shown here (code S.10 to P.1), this link reveals how a specific individual occupying a boundary-spanning role between physicians and managers (a blue structural challenge) came to provide credible leadership to the QI effort (a yellow political challenge). From the extract we also learn that in this role he was able to bring ideas and suggestions back to the organization from the wider QI network in US healthcare (that is the blue S.10 to green ED.4 link shown on the final line). In the narrative the extract then goes on to suggest that such roles were becoming more common because of managed care trends in the US, an example of the influence of outer context, which needs to be mapped in addition to the interactions between the colors themselves.

Having coded the case study narratives in this way, we then input these data into network analysis and graphing programs to produce network statistics and visual process mappings of the network of connections (also termed 'ties' or 'links') among process elements for each case.* The raw results of this procedure are illustrated for the Cedars-Sinai case in Figure 10.1 (see color plate section) using short descriptive identifiers of the process elements in place of the alpha-numerical codes above.† The

---

* UCINet 6 for Windows (Borgatti *et al.*, 2002)[25] was used to transform the data for network analysis and provide statistics on network characteristics. The visual graphs for the detailed sub-process mapping of Cedars-Sinai (Figure 10.1) was produced using NetDraw 1.0 (Borgatti, 2002),[26] and the high-level process mappings (Figures 10.2 to 10.5) were produced using the Pajek 1.08 network analysis software program (de Nooy *et al.*, 2005).[27]

† The thickness of lines in Figure 10.1 is proportional to the number of times a relationship was identified between two solutions or sub-processes, often considered to signify the strength of ties between two nodes. Note also the one 'isolate' in the upper left corner of the graph, 'OrgSize'; this was a contextual feature that was mentioned in the case narrative, but not in relation to any of the other process or context themes in the codebook.

key to the colors is shown on the bottom right of the figure, and Annex 2 provides a list of the sub-processes and the shorthand labels used.

Figure 10.1 is essentially the story of Cedars-Sinai's journey to sustained QI in graphical form, based on the codebook and the six generic challenges. If nothing else, this first map – fairly typical of those for the other sites – confirms that improvement processes are dense and complex, and difficult to disentangle and to make any sense of (which is worrying, because if you want to design interventions to improve things then first you have to understand how this system works!). The map also confirms that organizing for quality in healthcare does indeed comprise a complex system; in other words, it is the interactions between many elements and processes that produce outcomes, not single factors or simple cause-and-effect relationships. If we then cast our eye over the colors themselves, we see lots of blue (structure) and red (culture), with some yellow (politics) and green (learning), providing some insight into the key factors and processes at work.

Although we were not sure what, if anything, these early raw snaps were showing or capable of showing us, our interest was stimulated on a number of levels. First, they were allowing us to see the QI process in all its glory, arguably for the first time – our very own DNA of quality! Second, they offered at least the prospect of quick and dirty comparisons to be made between the sites without having to wade through page after page of narrative data. Third, even in these early rushes there was confirmation of our hunches about how complex and dynamic the QI process actually is and how limited the traditional 'Chinese menu' of key success factors is in dealing with this. Here indeed was a volatile system with different atoms knocking into each other and creating lots of heat and energy.

However, before moving on we needed to take stock and ask what maps like this are for, and what we were trying to accomplish. The problem was deciding what constituted a useful model in this context (for this was clearly not a theory), 'useful' being something that would assist and deepen our own sensemaking and analysis of the QI process.[28] Models are both representations (maps of the reality) and idealizations (simplifications of that reality). The main issue for any model is how complex or simple one wants or needs it to be: if too simple it can end up misrepresenting or distorting the reality it purports to describe – an oversimplification; if too complex it can be too much like real life, thereby undermining the very point of a model which, by leaving details out, aims to make the reality more accessible, comprehensible and manageable (as, say, a map does in order to get you from A to B). Clearly all the signs were that our first design model[29] was too complex, and that the second design would need to leave out some of the detail if we were to stand any chance of understanding, explaining or making sense of the QI process at both a deeper and more general level.

The conclusion we arrived at was that we could not have our cake and eat it; that in our second design we had to find a way of reducing the complexity – in Langley's[17] terms, go to a higher level of abstraction – in order for any patterns and shapes buried within the multiple links between elements and challenges to emerge and come more sharply into view. We did this by aggregating all the processes up to the six generic challenges to illustrate the relative emphasis on the various process challenges. The following sections present and discuss the resulting higher-level process maps from four of our seven case study organizations – Cedars-Sinai, Peterborough, Royal Devon and Exeter, and Albany.

Apart from reasons of space (which prevented inclusion of all seven), the maps of these four sites were selected because they provide the greatest range and contrast among our case studies in terms of map profile and shape. In the aggregate maps that follow, each of the six universal challenges is color-coded as before, as are the inner and outer contextual factors. These higher-level maps allowed us to go up one level and take a step back from the detail, but of course we were still able to refer to the detailed sub-process maps (as illustrated in Figure 10.1) and the original case narratives if we wanted to inspect any of the organizations more closely.

Cedars-Sinai

The first example of this higher-level model (Figure 10.2, *see* color plate section) is derived from our case study of Cedars-Sinai in Los Angeles (Chapter 4). On the following pages we analyze and explain this particular map in greater detail than in the later examples in order to familiarize and orient the reader to these representations and some of the ways they can be read and interpreted.

The size of the circles in Figure 10.2 indicate the proportion of all process ties in the narrative of Cedars-Sinai's quality journey that included a solution or element related to a particular challenge color (i.e. the bigger the circles, the relatively greater frequency a particular color was implicated in the Cedars-Sinai story).* Immediately, a pattern comes into view that was not evident in the more detailed version (Figure 10.1). We see that Cedars-Sinai appears relatively strong on the structural (blue) and cultural (red) aspects, and less strong on learning (green) and political (yellow). Emotional (white) and physical and technological (pink) processes appear to be of much less importance (i.e they are not central to the story). Contextual factors (both inner and outer) do not seem to have played a central role in sustaining Cedars-Sinai's journey to quality either (a small circle indicates that context was checked only a few times as being connected to other elements of the story).

The table at the bottom of Figure 10.2 shows:
- ❏ the total number of times processes within each of the challenges was coded as connected to another process ('Total sub-process ties')
- ❏ what proportion of that total related to a tie between two processes within the same challenge ('W/in process'; e.g. red to red)
- ❏ what proportion were ties originating from another of the challenges ('IN-ties'; e.g. blue to red)
- ❏ what proportion were ties emanating from that challenge ('OUT-ties'; e.g. red to blue).

The final column in the table lists the 'Most central sub-processes'. These were the individual sub-processes that had the highest number of ties to other sub-processes in the detailed map displayed in Figure 10.1, a measure referred to in network analysis as 'degree centrality' (we used a centrality score higher than one standard deviation above the mean as our guideline for identifying these central sub-processes). So, in the case of Cedars-Sinai, 11 sub-processes stood out from the rest: communities of practice, quality governance systems, distributed leadership, boundary-spanner roles, data and monitoring systems, group culture, values/symbolic leadership, culture of learning, organizational identity, QI training, and knowledge harvesting. Our interpretation would be that they have had a special role to play in Cedars' QI journey and success, as have blue (structure), red (culture) and green (learning) generally, of which these particular sub-processes are part.

---

* Using the relative frequency of sub-process ties for each challenge (as opposed to the straight number of sub-process ties shown in the first column of the table beneath the map in Figure 10.2) allows comparison of the size of the circles across case mappings (e.g. with Figures 10.3–10.5).

Moving on, not only does the map allow us to pinpoint where to begin look for the success; it also enables us to draw some tentative conclusions about what made a particular site different from the other case study sites. For example, when readers begin to compare this picture with the others, they will see that there is no other like it in terms of the strong dual emphasis on structure (blue) and culture (red). Depending on whether we want to include learning (green) as well, which is the third largest node, we can say, again tentatively, that Cedars' success was based either on the axis of structure and culture (the notion of an organic, living form), or the triangle of structural, cultural and learning processes (the notion of a well-formed, communitarian, learning organization). We say 'tentatively' because it is always best to read the map alongside the case study narrative itself, to see whether the two accord, which here they most certainly do.

As in the detailed map in Figure 10.1, the thickness of the lines between the colored circles in Figure 10.2 is also proportional to the sum of the ties between each of the colors (the more ties, the thicker the line). The thickest line in this process map actually relates to structural processes reinforcing other structural processes (i.e. the arrow looping back to the blue circle), which accounts for 31% of the total of 100 structural ties. By cross-referring back to Figure 10.1, we can see that examples of these self-reinforcing structural (blue) ties include Cedars-Sinai having a 'QI facil team' (a dedicated QI facilitation/change team), which links into 'Enabling admin' (a supportive/enabling oriented role of central administration) and 'DistLdrs' (a multi-level leadership structure for quality), which in turn feeds into – and is fed by – 'QStrategy' (an explicit organizational strategy for quality').

So what early insights into sustained quality and service improvement can be gained from this analysis of the Cedars-Sinai case study using the codebook and the colors as a heuristic (aid to thinking)? First, the high visibility of the quality infrastructure (blue) at Cedars has a significant cultural impact (red) in terms of valuing and according high priority to quality and safety. The infrastructure is also the process through which various interests are worked and tensions managed (see the thickish line between blue and yellow), so the infrastructure acts not only as a co-ordinating mechanism for the improvement effort but also as a political system.

The thick arrow connecting blue and green shows that the infrastructure is also a knowledge management process, a specific example of this being the sub-PICs (blue) that carry out tests of change from which learning results (green). Another thick two-way arrow in Figure 10.2 between blue and red shows that structural and cultural processes are closely entwined and mutually reinforcing. For example, data and monitoring systems (blue) can promote collective consensus around quality (red), and the culture of collegiality and inclusion (red) promotes multi-level quality structures (blue) – a good illustration of the kind of virtuous cycle described earlier.

Second, as we have seen, Cedars-Sinai has a lot of blue (structured quality), but it also has quite a lot of green (learning-related issues). An effective learning process – in this case based on well-developed exploration and exploitation sub-processes – is one that enables an organization to be capable of double-loop learning, not endlessly repeating old recipes and routines (single loop). As the narrative of Cedars-Sinai revealed, this organization was also successful in its 'retrospective sensemaking' – learning from the past in order to set a course for the future, including being aware of the dangers of getting trapped in thinking routines, or of not responding to a changing environment.

We already know from the narrative that an effective selection process ('search, filter, make sense') had enabled the organization to choose between the many options, including the type and scale of change, when to adapt and when to transform, as well as the overall change methodology and approach. Successful healthcare organizations have to be able to learn the right lessons. Selection (a combination of blue and green – systematic organized learning) is what makes the learning process active and intelligent, as opposed to blind fashion or fad following. Adler *et al.* call this the 'knowing-doing' gap and suggest that any organization's 'improvement capability' is closely related to its 'learning capability'.[30]

Third, it is interesting, although perhaps not surprising, how a learning process (green) can become a culture-building process (red), indicated by the moderately thick arrows in both directions between the two. As mentioned above, educational processes (with 54 total sub-process ties) are one of the most central after structural and cultural, and contribute two of the most central sub-processes in the case (QI training and knowledge harvesting). Educational (green) processes are also strongly associated with two of the most central sub-processes listed under other colors (i.e. communities of practice under blue, which are by definition learning-centered; and culture of learning under red). This suggests that learning at Cedars-Sinai is also relatively dispersed throughout a variety of strategies.

On reflection, we might begin to ask where the value lies in a map like this. In some respects we must accept that it tells us little more than what we know already from the story itself; namely, that structural, cultural and learning processes were, and probably continue to be, key in Cedars' success in the QI field. On the other hand, it also tells us that it is not these processes working independently but together in a virtuous, positively reinforcing way that has undoubtedly given the Cedars' QI system its special magic in QI excellence.

This point has important implications for the QI intervention itself. From a traditional factors perspective, practitioners might be tempted to attribute Cedars' success to its quality infrastructure (which would be right in part), and as a consequence try to replicate this in their own organizations. However, we know from Cedars' own admission that it can be (quote) 'a double-edged sword'. The proper term for this is 'polyvalent' or 'multivalent': almost anything, including complexly wired infrastructures like this one, can be bad *or* good, positive *or* negative, functional *or* dysfunctional. The 'thing' in question has no inherent properties as such that can make it one or other of these things: it all depends on the context. Without proper attention to this context an organization may end up with a quality infrastructure identical to the one at Cedars but one that is rigid, overly bureaucratic and ultimately paralyzing for the organization.

What made Cedars special was not so much that it had a quality infrastructure, but that it had succeeded in linking it in such a positive, synergistic way to its wider cultural, learning and political processes, thereby enhancing and enriching both itself and them. In short, it was its system effects rather than the factor itself that had made the infrastructure (and its process) successful as a community-building process (culture), a knowledge management process (learning), and an interest-harmonizing process (politics). Conversely, it was their presence within that infrastructure that had prevented it from ossifying or turning into a bureaucratic nightmare. A good example is the way that green, the learning organization that Cedars clearly was, had itself enabled the QI team to see that its hard-wired infrastructure was, or could be, a double-edged sword, and therefore that one needed to be aware and constantly mindful of this and ensure that any excesses or dysfunctions in this area were detected early and corrected. Arguably, this mindfulness towards structure (also reminiscent of San Diego Children's, *see* Chapter 2) was crucial in keeping the structure fresh and in check.

In our view, Cedars had succeeded in creating a classic virtuous circle, and this can be clearly seen in Figure 10.2 as the black lines and loops connecting the structural, cultural, educational and political processes. The message for QI practitioners must therefore be: focus on building a QI *system* (although not necessarily the same as this one), looking not so much at the individual challenges as the connections between them, and the opportunities these hold. Obviously, to build a system such as this requires systems thinking – one of the central theses of this book.

Kanter[31] expresses this well as the ability to 'see the whole as opposed to parts and challenge the established patterns rather than walling off a piece of experience'. Beckhard and Pritchard[32] do the same thing, usefully addressing their comments to the change effort:

> Systems thinking involves viewing the 'world' as a whole composed of many parts that interact with each other in a dynamic way . . . Thinking in systems terms means being aware of the web of inter-relationships that exist between the parts . . . and being aware of the parts themselves . . . Systems thinking also implies concern for and attention to 'connections'. In a fundamental change effort the parts are all connected in a dynamic manner.

Peter Senge's somewhat more dramatic description of this systems perspective[33] is also worth including because it links this discussion back to our earlier comments about the need to find the 'thermals' and positive feedback loops within systems if one's QI effort is going to 'fly':

> A cloud masses, the sky darkens, leaves twist upwards and we know that it will rain. We also know that after the storm, the runoff will feed into groundwater miles away, and the sky will clear by tomorrow. All these events are different in time and space, yet they are all connected within the same 'pattern'. Each has an influence on the rest, an influence that is usually hidden from view. You can only understand the system of a rainstorm by contemplating the whole, not any individual part of the pattern. Business and other human endeavours are also systems.

Unfortunately, erudite though all these writers are, none of them (as with many systems writers) give much information about what the 'whole' or the 'patterns' are, or how to identify them, and to this extent offer little practical guidance to QI leaders and students of QI processes. Our network maps, on the other hand, do at least do that, making visible both the QI system and the patterns and challenges within it, and providing some clear co-ordinates for targeting the OD and QI intervention.

Peterborough

The process map for Peterborough (Figure 10.3, *see* color plate section) is similar (although not identical) to that for Cedars-Sinai – a point of note in itself given the different countries and entirely different contexts within which the two healthcare systems operate. (We come back to this context point later when we question whether writers may have been guilty of overestimating the importance of external contextual dynamics relative to internal systems dynamics). Interestingly, the two maps are similar with respect to the relatively marginal role that physical and technical (pink) and mobilizing (white) processes appear to have played in their overall QI efforts, which is only partly true in the other organizational maps.

As with Cedars-Sinai, there is the same strong quartet of blue, red, yellow and green, and the same strong axis between the structural and cultural (blue/red), but with more emphasis this time on the politics of change (yellow), and to a lesser extent on organizational learning (green). The direction of the arrows in the Peterborough map suggest (more strongly than Cedars) that sustained QI here starts with structure (72% of the structural processes are driving other processes), which shapes the cultural, political and educational processes within the organization (73%, 63% and 50% respectively of these are being driven by processes emanating from other challenges).

In this regard, the roles played by the central QI facilitation team and other central administrative support services seem to be key elements in the structure for quality at Peterborough (as described in Chapter 7), driving many different parts of the QI process. Though smaller in scale to Cedars, the Peterborough QI infrastructure may have ended up more central as the driver of quality processes because it does not have the same strong culture (what Cedars staff described as the Judaic immigrant heritage) acting on and keeping a check and balance on it. This would be consistent with the 'simultaneous loose–tight principle' found in organization research (usefully discussed in a QI context by Watson and Korukonda[34]), which states that the stronger or tighter the organization's core culture or values (described at Cedars as its 'excellence ethic'), the looser it can afford to be in its norms and formal reporting structures.

Just returning to Cedars for a moment, it is possible that it was its culture rather than its structure that provided the necessary mainstay of co-ordination and consensus for its QI efforts (not, as most believe, the structure), whereas at Peterborough its structure did this, with culture being more of an outcome or residue – an important difference.

The other central sub-processes shown in the table reflect the meta-narrative of empowerment, as described in the summary of the Peterborough case study in Chapter 7, demonstrating the consistency between map and narrative. Outer context, inner context, physical and technological and emotional processes all play a relatively minor role (again), although contextual processes do appear to be having some impact on the cultural challenge particularly.

In comparing the Peterborough and Cedars-Sinai process maps, we would make a number of observations. First, the size of the nodes clearly illustrates the relative emphasis on the various process challenges within each case: for example, the (green) educational node is bigger for Cedars-Sinai while the (yellow) political node is bigger for Peterborough. This variation is not unexpected given that we have seen already how the Cedars-Sinai case narrative found organizational learning (green) to be a central focus, whereas in Peterborough the emphasis was more on brokering relationships, engaging people in the improvement effort and empowering them (yellow).

What we found most striking – the second point of comparison between Cedars and Peterborough, already touched on – was that the structural and cultural circles were the largest process domains in both cases. It would appear, at least from the first two of our sites, that no matter what the specific organizational strategy for sustaining QI, the structural and cultural elements are central. This is nicely illustrated by the 'iron triangle' – the thick lines back and forth among a triad of processes – of the political, structural and cultural in the Peterborough map and educational, cultural and structural in the Cedars-Sinai map. This point is also illustrated by the types of sub-processes that are identified as most central to supporting the main strategic theme of each case.

Organizational structure and culture have been extensively studied, but separately and rarely together, and so we still know little about the nature of the relationship or the interactions between them. Our thesis is that this relationship is crucial to the dynamics of the wider QI system, and therefore if any early focus of attention were required it should probably begin here. One of the present authors (Bate) and colleagues previously developed this thesis in the wider OD context, but in the light of the present work we would now suggest extending it further into QI.

> The evolution of an organization's structure is integrally related to the evolution of its culture – and vice versa. Structure and culture co-evolve: each shapes and is in turn shaped by the other. The emerging role for organization design and organization development (OD) specialists – and for organizational leaders – is to attend to the dynamics of simultaneous structural and cultural change. For this, a 'both-and' model of change and change management is required: one that can realize the synchronicity and complementarity between cultural and structural processes within an organization.[35]

Third, here, as in traditional social network analysis, it is often informative to look at what is missing or ends up more peripheral, as well as that which is central on the map to which the eye is naturally drawn. This led to a few surprises, not least with regard to some processes that did not feature heavily (if at all). First, context, whether inner organizational features such as size and performance, or influences from the external environment, appears to have played a relatively minor role in sustaining the quality journeys of these two organizations. This would suggest that although contextual influences or events may provide an important initial impetus to an organization's quality journey (e.g. the advent of managed care cost pressures for Cedars, and to some extent political mandates from the NHS to improve service in the case of Peterborough), whether the quality journey is sustained may depend more on how the organization responds and acts (or does not act) to these stimuli.

Similarly, in these two case narratives physical and technological factors did not appear central to sustaining QI. This is not to say that factors such as IT and clinical technology were unimportant, only that they were seen as rather less central to sustaining quality and QI processes than some of the other factors within these two particular organizations. This is a reversal of the way they are usually portrayed in the improvement literature, where technology (reflected in the pink challenge) is always the fall-back panacea to the ills of healthcare, as to a lesser extent is the enhancement of the physical healing environment. The pink circle is slightly more pronounced in the Cedars process graph (a case narrative that included a great deal on IT), but it remains much smaller relative to the five other challenges, with the sole exception of the emotional challenge at Peterborough.*

Although not being definitive, our findings put a large question mark over what can be expected solely from IT in terms of impact on healthcare quality, efficiency and performance, a point echoed by Chaudhry *et al.* following a systematic review of the evidence.[36] Such a finding also echoes the argument often heard today about the importance of human and organizational factors to the successful implementation of IT systems (the socio- part of the socio-technical system).[37–39] One can have the greatest

---

* This is not an artefact of the coding: the pink challenge has only one less sub-process code than, for example, the political challenge, and theoretically each sub-process code is equally likely to have been mentioned. Moreover, the case narratives were reviewed by the site participants, and if we had grossly understated the role of technology in sustaining improvement (separate from how to use it, which a number of sub-processes in the other categories deal with), we would have most likely heard about it during the case validation process.

technology in the world, but if no one knows how to use it (learning), it is not perceived as important or useful (cultural), it doesn't fit into existing work systems and routines (structural), or it rubs against substantial vested interests and inertial resistance to change (political and emotional), then this technology will probably not add much benefit in terms of levels of service or QI activity.

We now consider three further aggregated process maps much more briefly.

Royal Devon and Exeter

Even at first sight we can see that the map from the RD&E case study (Figure 10.4, *see* color plate section) looks markedly different from those for Cedars-Sinai and Peterborough. This map is dominated by the cultural (red) challenge and by the self-reinforcing nature of many of the cultural sub-processes within it (the thickest arrow loops back into the red circle). We would interpret such dominance as a reflection of the very strong identity we found within the macro- and micro-systems of this organization (*see* Chapter 3), identity being very much a cultural issue. In contrast to our other cases, there were only two central sub-processes and these were (not surprisingly) organizational identity and group culture.

As with the preceding two cases, the structural (blue) and cultural (red) axis remains prominent, as does the two-way symbiotic relationship between them. The political challenge (yellow) is of greater importance than the educational (green), emotional (white) or physical and technological (pink) challenges. Inner contextual processes appear to be driving some of the cultural processes, but again there appears to be little part played by outer context in the RD&E story of sustaining improvement, despite the initial shock to the institution of the very public breast cancer screening scandal early in the Trust's quality journey.

This map confirms that – as seen through the eyes of the participants themselves – strong professional and corporate identification affects quality of care, the most obvious reason being the heightened levels of energy and commitment people bring to their jobs and the quality challenge because of this strong inner sense of professional self and unswerving loyalty to the organization and their profession.[40] As described in Chapter 3, the journey to quality of the orthopedics department was infused with a strong sense of commitment and tradition, intense awareness of its international reputation for clinical excellence and innovation (originating in the 1950s), and staff strongly identifying with the department (and its high standards).

Meanwhile, the strong emerging corporate identity of the macro-system as enacted by a new senior management team – partly born of a serious crisis that had led to patient deaths in another micro-system within the organization – had helped to reinforce the orthopedic department's own long-established local commitment and professional identity, while enhancing its contribution to the image and identity of the hospital as a whole. This case study suggests that identity represents a powerful interior motive to quality to the extent that is self-regulating and immanent, and therefore does not require external regulation or policing. High standards of quality come from within the community and are implicit in the compact the citizen has with that community; history is the referent, not any external protocol or measure.

Whereas the literature on TQM and CQI tends to present quality as a scientific technique, method or discipline, an identity focus reminds us that it is as much – if not more – a question of value orientation and outlook. One glance at RD&E's map is sufficient to show that, while still a QI system, there is no doubt where the main power and heat for that system are coming from: the red of culture, organizational and professional. And so back to loose–tight: perhaps this particular hospital did not need a hard-wired infrastructure like the one at Cedars (blue), given that the professional and organizational cultures operating within it were largely self-regulating and self-policing. The salutary implication for QI interventions is that we should perhaps be spending more time developing professional and corporate commitment than directly trying to improve quality, particularly bearing in mind that programs or projects quickly run out of energy, whereas being professional is a lifelong vocation and the very fuel of giving service.

Albany

The Albany map (Figure 10.5, *see* color plate section), the last of our examples, is interesting for several reasons. First, in the Albany map emphases are much more spread around all the major challenges than in the other cases, reflecting a point made in the case study narrative that Albany was strongly balanced across many organizational dimensions. Second, the emotional process (white) is much more prominent than in any of the other case maps, reflecting the strong mobilizing theme in the case narrative. Third, the outer context is also much more prominent than in other cases (mostly revolving around professional/cultural social movements; for example, see also the centrality of the external partnering sub-theme under political process).

In fact we have not seen two of the structural (blue) sub-processes that occur in the Albany story much, if at all, in any of the other cases presented; the first of these sub-processes is task-centered leadership, which was important in this case study narrative to the social movement perspective with regard to the ability to organize, not just inspire. The second sub-process is organizational slack, although this is also significant in the case study of Luther Midelfort (*see* Chapter 6), the map of which is not included here.

Finally, there are many fewer interactions among sub-themes within processes (i.e. there are smaller loops going back into each circle in the Albany process map), suggesting a greater emphasis on connecting processes between the six challenges than in our other cases.

A final reflection: different paths up the mountain . . . but some paths are more well-trodden than others

We hope that through the maps in this chapter we have been able to offer the outlines of a different method for conducting cross-case analyses with complex data sets, and, as Eisenhardt[41] puts it in relation to this kind of research, increasing the 'likelihood of creative reframing' of our subject. Erring on the side of caution we would probably prefer 'confirmatory' to 'creative'. The maps have corroborated most of what the longer case studies already told us, presenting the highlights in different but not necessarily new ways. This is not to detract from their value. Long narratives have the virtue of depth and richness, but they are, as most qualitative researchers know well, dense and difficult to handle in a comparative context. The maps, on the other hand, are graphic, pared down to the essential details, all on one page, and one can click between them, comparing and contrasting at one's leisure.

We also hope that, sufficiently freed up from all the detail, we have been able to demonstrate more clearly the universal but variable nature of QI systems with which we began Chapter 9; that is, the same recurring common challenges but the infinite number of variations and permutations of attempted process solutions. Hopefully readers will now have a better appreciation of why the texture of each site's story of its journey to quality felt so different when they read it, but also how common was their quest and general orientation.

As the network maps above and Figure 10.6 (*see* color plate section) show, every site in our research has, to varying degrees, placed emphasis on different solutions to the universal challenges, demonstrating the old adage that there are many paths up the mountain and many starting places, and no one best way of reaching one's goal. The color-coded lists of the most central sub-processes in Figure 10.6 give a quick comparison of the favored – and very different – paths for each of the sites, this also being reflected in the maps. Essentially, they found their own way up the mountain, recognizing that blindly following others was not what the ascent to quality required.

That being said, there were more similarities than we had expected, examples of some paths being more well-trodden than others or trodden over by teams of climbers from more than one site (although never following precisely the same path). So while the white and pink paths remained almost deserted routes, the blue (structure) and red (culture) paths were well-trodden and clearly marked, as to only a slightly lesser extent were green (learning) and yellow (politics). Without over-privileging some processes at the cost of the wider systems view, it does therefore appear that some processes may be more important than others in helping teams reach and stay at the top – as all of these did.

It is important to say this. After all, we have focused on only the small élite that have actually made it to the top, barely sparing a thought for those who have not – those who got lost on the mountain or, worse still, fell off, or those who found themselves going round and round the mountain or spiralling downwards; or yet again those who, finding themselves not up to the challenge, settled for the lesser but still pleasant view from the slopes.

So if there are lessons to be learned from those that did make it, they would probably be, don't try to do everything:

❐ focus on getting the basic structures in place (blue)
❐ take time to build camaraderie and strong team work (red, culture)
❐ deal with conflicts and tensions (yellow, politics)
❐ learn from your mistakes (green, learning)
❐ feel and share the passion for getting to the top (white, mobilization)
❐ avoid being distracted too early by high-tech solutions (pink)
❐ above all, don't look down (manage the context).

11

Journey's end: epilogue and final reflections

All journeys have secret destinations of which the traveler is unaware.
(MARTIN BUBER, 1878–1965)

So, where has our long-haul journey to discover some of the secrets of high-performing, high-quality organizations within the healthcare domain ultimately led us?

The first thing we should say is that as in most largely uncharted journeys, we have found ourselves visiting places and discovering things on the way that we simply could not have anticipated when we embarked. In this sense our own journey has been very similar to that of the stories of QI we heard from the organizations we studied: emergent and unpredictable, and full of twists and turns. Indeed, the journey metaphor is one that is commonly applied to stories of organizational change, both in healthcare[1,2] and in other sectors,[3–5] and we think we are now beginning to understand why.

In this vein, for example, Pettigrew[5] (cited and summarized by Bate[2]) develops the engaging metaphor of 'journeys as wagon trains', comparing the organizational change journey to the traditional story of the nineteenth-century US wagon train heading westward from the relative safety of the eastern seaboard to California (ironically a destination for us, too, in the case of two of our studies, San Diego Children's and Cedars-Sinai). Pettigrew's aim is to draw attention to the hazards and uncertainties lying in wait in the punishing contextual terrain that has to be crossed, the waxing and waning of hope and despair, and above all the dramas and politics that get played out between the mixed bag of settlers during their long haul towards the land of milk and honey: the enthusiasts, career opportunists and malcontents, resource providers, scouts, and the innocent and not-so-innocent bystanders who observe this band of travelers but mostly choose not to participate in the journey themselves.

As the journey proceeds there is a sense of emotional relief as landmarks are reached. But there are ups and downs of energy as obstacles are rounded and blind canyons and other deadlocks encountered. For some (the lost and bewildered) there is journey's end, but not where anticipated. For the fortunate there is the prospect of a new life in California now that this particular stage in life's long journey has come to a successful conclusion. For the less fortunate there is failure and disappointment.

During our own particular, and similarly eventful and (mostly) westward, travels, the focus has been on seeking to explain both the how and why of achieving sustained QI in healthcare organizations, despite the hazards and uncertainties portrayed above. We already know from the large body of existing research that there is striking variation between (and even within) organizations in terms of how they implement, spread and sustain QI. The ambition of our research was to preserve a commitment to the description of what happened in the form of holistic, full-length narrative accounts of these seven organizational journeys to quality (Chapters 2 to 8), while seeking to offer interpretations and explanations of how and why these variations had come about. To these ends, the codebook presented in Chapter 9 of this book reveals how QI happened, and hopefully our conceptual analysis in Chapter 10 helps readers to understand why these organizations have been successful in their QI efforts over a sustained period of time.

Limitations of our research

There are three limitations of our research that we must acknowledge and address head-on. Each was a result of necessary trade-offs in the research design.

First, and obviously, we cherry-picked our organizational case studies. We deliberately set out to find successful (and early) adopters of QI and did not include the majority of middle or late adopters. However, such selection bias can be justified on various grounds, and typically is found among those who are interested less in statistical significance and are more intrigued by what Weick terms a 'bountiful supply of socially interpreted everyday life', and therefore represents an argument for 'detail, for thoroughness, for prototypical narratives, and an argument against formulations that strip out most of what matters.'[6]

Second, although there was (inevitably) variation *within* the organizations we studied, we were not able to explore those variations and, for instance, compare high-versus low-performing micro-systems.

Finally, we explored only a limited number of organizations, nine in total, of which seven are represented in this book, so that even among high-performing healthcare organizations we have clearly not captured the full range of experiences (from a qualitative research perspective) and certainly not a representative distribution of experience (from a quantitative perspective).

We therefore realized from the outset that our findings would be less than definitive. However, our own measure of success of the research, and the driver for this journey, is whether it provides new avenues and hypotheses (particularly around organizational processes) for research and new directions and topics for attention and reflection (rather than continuing certainties) for practitioners.

Although our research is more concerned with hypothesis-building than hypothesis-testing, and has all of the limitations described above, the focus on what we have termed organizational and human processes and the in-depth nature of the fieldwork across multiple sites have yielded an array of rich and instructive insights, which we believe open up new perspectives on QI in healthcare settings for practitioners and researchers alike. So what are these insights that we have gleaned from our travels and would wish to offer, firstly to practitioners and then to fellow researchers?

Implications for practitioners

QI needs a particular kind of change model and a particular kind of leadership

In conducting this research, we explicitly did not set out to seek 'the development of a model that predicts and explains a comprehensive organizational change process'.[7] We simply did not believe this would be possible given the known complexity and non-linear qualities of organizational change. One unsurprising finding, therefore, is that there was no single best way to achieve service excellence. Huge variety was the order of the day, with each organization having found its own unique path up the mountain:

> Some travel into the mountains accompanied by experienced guides who know the best and least dangerous routes by which they arrive at their destination. Still others, inexperienced and untrusting, attempt to make their own routes. Few of these are successful, but occasionally some, by sheer will and luck and grace, do make it. Once there they become more aware than any of the others that there's no single or fixed number of routes. There are as many routes as there are individual souls.[8]

There was, however, a good deal more to it than just 'will, luck and grace'. These organizations seemed to know (i.e. had learnt or discovered) what the challenges were and had proceeded to demonstrate consummate skill in simultaneously managing and dealing with them. The interesting finding was that although the solutions – routes – may differ, the six broad change challenges they faced were the same, whether in the US or Europe. Furthermore, two general processes stood out from our analysis as being the most central across all the maps of sustained QI journeys we presented in Chapter 10: the importance of an enabling structure (blue: form) and an enabling culture (red: shared meanings; what Detert et al.[9] very appropriately refer to as the 'cultural backbone' of QI efforts). These processes acted as a kind of axis around which all of the other processes orbited. Both need each other: structure without underpinning shared meanings will be disconnected and empty; culture without form and structure will be unfocused and undirected.

Above all the conclusion has to be that sustained QI is dynamic, processual and emergent, and therefore requires a more flexible opportunistic mindset than the rigid planning mindset normally recommended in the change and improvement literatures. Mirroring Pettigrew,[5] Kanter et al.[10] describe what improvement travelers can expect to encounter, and why the detailed planning model is unsuited to such a quest:

> While the literature often portrays an organization's quest for change like a brisk march along a well-marked path, those in the middle of change are more likely to describe their journey as a laborious crawl towards an elusive, flickering goal, with many wrong turns and missed opportunities along the way. Only rarely does an organization know exactly where it's going, or how it should get there.

Weick also throws his weight behind these views, describing very clearly what the broad approach to organizing, including organizing for quality, the title of our book, needs to be – probably best summed up as lightening up and trying to relax into the rhythms of the journey!

> . . . organizing is never very tidy or foresightful, despite the necessity of its practitioners to make it appear otherwise. Efforts to maintain the illusion that organizations are rational and orderly in the interest of legitimacy are costly and futile. They consume enormous energy and undermine self-acceptance when managers hold themselves to standards of prescience that are unattainable. To appreciate organizations and their

> environments as flows interrupted by constraints of one's own making, is to take oneself a little less seriously . . . and to have a little less hubris and a little more fun . . .[11]

His punchline – probably the punchline for this whole book – being:

> In the last analysis, organizing is about fallible people who keep going.

We urge practitioners, therefore, to begin to see QI as an exploration, not totally loose or open-ended, but based on broad stratagems that can be improvised and adapted to whatever conditions, events and situations present themselves. This calls for good preparation (skills, mental strength, resources, fitness for purpose) and not just good planning.

Waterman[12] refers to this as 'informed opportunism', with equal emphasis placed on both words. The task for leaders, he says, is to set a direction for the QI effort, not detailed strategy:

> They are the best of strategists precisely because they are suspicious of forecasts and open to surprise. They know the value of being prepared, and they also know that some of the most important strategic decisions they make are inherently unpredictable. They think strategic planning is great – as long as no-one takes the planning too seriously. They often see more value in the process of planning than in the plan itself.

The leaders of such expeditions also need to recognize that the visionary, 'Great Leader' form of leadership backed up by management fiat may not be as effective as they might have hoped or expected given the particular kind of terrain and journey they are on (think of Napoleon's Russian campaign).

Certainly the leaders we have met on our travels have generally preferred a quiet collaborative style of leadership to the visible and visionary, charismatic, directive kind of leadership often portrayed on TV shows and in the airport business literature; much more low key, yet still an interesting combination of courage (gutsy, bold, determined, persistent) and humility.[13] In this vein, Collins warns that 'companies built around a cult of personality seldom last' and our view is that this is also true of QI programs.[14]

Leaders must seek to develop their own local solutions and continually respond to outside pressures

As others have argued, 'Leaders can adopt ideas that have worked elsewhere, but they need to create their own one-of-a-kind change model through experimentation, learning, blueprint creation, and, most of all, a strong focus on results.'[15,16] So first, the bad news: organizations cannot 'buy' a high-performing, quality culture off the shelf, and they cannot copy it from someone else. There are no universal solutions. But then the good news: we know what the key ingredients or elements are (there are universal challenges), and we now have a way of reading, up, down and across the whole range of options as the first step towards constructing workable solutions and effective interventions.

The codebook described in Chapter 9 offers how-to insights into 56 different ways (solutions) to address and navigate the six universal challenges, based on the paths up the mountain that successful organizations have already taken. In this way, the code-book provides a simple model that allows complex issues to be appropriately identified and debated, and effort and attention to be focused when improvement interventions need to be made. Moreover, if managing quality is indeed about making the right strategic choices, then now at least we have a fuller range of alternatives from which such choices can be made.

But leaders need also to understand, if only partially and incompletely, how these organizational processes interact (and can be successfully managed) over time. The exemplar process maps in Chapter 10 are one way, as is reading the case narratives themselves (Chapters 2 to 8) with the framework (Chapter 9) as a guide. The latter approach will help illustrate how such journeys played out over time in our case study organizations, and provide insight into how managers and practitioners can customize and adapt the lessons from these journeys for their own healthcare organizations.

Hence, the local leadership task is to develop a greater awareness of where the gaps, weaknesses and blind spots lie and start to construct an approach, or repertoire of approaches, that is appropriate to their own time and place. Even if practitioners do not have the time or resources to do this kind of detailed network mapping, the images they take away with them from this book will hopefully help them to 'think connections', to 'think whole systems' and to 'think process rather than variables'.

There is also a good deal of value in organizations putting together case study narratives of their own as their story unfolds to assist in reflection and ongoing sensemaking. Such sensemaking is crucial when so much of the terrain in question is unknown and unsignposted, and where travelers have to be constantly struggling ('scratching around', to quote Weick below) to find out where they are or should be trying to get to. Sensemaking is not the same as decision-making; it is about trying to figure things out through *interpretation of one's ongoing experiences* (which is not the same as collecting data); and it is the quality of this sensemaking process – individual and collective – that will determine ultimate levels of success in meeting each of the six core QI challenges.

> It is the job of the sensemaker to convert a world of experience into an intelligible world. That person's job is not to look for the one true picture that corresponds to a pre-existing, preformed reality . . . Instead the picture of sensemaking that is suggested is 'that there is nobody here but us scratching around trying to make our experience and our world as comprehensible to ourselves in the best way that we can . . . there are only maps that we construct to make sense of the welter of our experience, and only us to judge whether these maps are worthwhile for us or not'.[17] (as cited by Weick[11]).

Even when they have done all these things this may still not be enough, however, for as we saw in our very first case study (San Diego Children's, Chapter 2), no matter how embedded quality may appear to be in an organization's culture, events can still conspire against even the most persistent and skilled advocates for QI in healthcare. Not all contextual events are hostile, however. Indeed, despite the differential nature of policy and competitive environments across countries – such as the predominance of private market forces in the US and public mandates in the UK – environmental shocks or jolts from each appear to have provided a similar impetus to the quality journey of the organizations we studied. The Albany case study (Chapter 8) also illustrates that external support from the wider healthcare and social context can sometimes have even greater influence than the upper levels of the organizational chart.

Pay attention to human and organizational processes (as well as clinical and technical)

As we previewed in Chapter 1 (*see* Figure 1.1), the journeys to quality described in Chapters 2 to 8 clearly demonstrate that quality and QI is a human and organizational, not just a technical or mechanical systems, phenomenon, and that if we are to truly understand why there is a 45% defect rate in healthcare[18] and how to reduce or eliminate it, then we have to look to the myriad of human and organizational causes.

In this regard, the hard left-brain technical and operating systems factors have received by far the greatest attention in quality research. However, what this research has revealed is how important the softer right-brain organizational, cultural and human factors are to improvement efforts – issues such as identity, aesthetics, politics, leadership, value systems, organizational slack and learning, none of which have received anything like the same amount of attention. We argue that future research, policy and practice need to address the sociology of improvement in equal measure to the science and technique of improvement, or at least expand the discipline of improvement to include these critical organizational and human processes. Practitioners, especially, would be well advised to follow the wonderful example set by Luther Midelfort hospital (*see* Chapter 6) in achieving a perfected balance between the socio and the technical, as indeed they also would that of San Diego Children's Hospital (*see* Chapter 2). Modern 'lean' practitioners should also take note, as did Luther, that lean without the socio may improve system performance and efficiency but not necessarily service quality.

Implications for researchers

The need for longitudinal organizational case studies: the pace and sequencing of QI efforts

The use of cross-case analysis such as that presented in Chapter 10 increases the likelihood of generating novel theory:

> ... attempts to reconcile evidence across cases, types of data, and different investigators, and between cases and literature increases the likelihood of creative reframing into a new theoretical vision.[19]

One hypothesis resulting from the longitudinal case studies presented here is that, although these successful organizations have dealt with the six common challenges at one point or another regardless of where they started their journeys, there are some challenges that are more important than others at certain points in a quality journey. Further research is needed to confirm and delve deeper into these issues of the pace and sequencing of a change effort.[20] There also still remains a need for similar case studies of organizations that have attempted quality journeys but with less success, having got lost, found themselves going in circles, fallen off the path, or settled for a lesser goal along the way (to use a metaphor from Chapter 10).

The need for multi-level process models of QI

The codebook presented in Chapter 9 allows us as researchers to begin to explore the interactions between the macro- and micro-systems within each of the organizations we studied, thereby responding to the challenge set by Whelan-Berry *et al*:

> ... the existing organizational change literature does not fully describe the relationships between the change process at the organizational level and the change processes at the inherent individual and group levels ... [There is need for more] research that considers change initiatives across levels of analysis and related transition points in the process.[7]

The cases, and our analyses, point strongly to the need (and illustrate ways) to distinguish between the roles of the macro- and micro-systems within healthcare organizations in implementing and sustaining QI, and enable practitioners to attend to the relationships and interactions between these levels. Both macro- and micro-system levels of organizational systems have different, as well as overlapping, contributions to make in sustaining QI processes in healthcare (e.g. *see* Table 2.1 in Chapter 2).

However, most of the literature remains heavily focused on leader actions and pays little attention to change processes on organizational front lines. Mohr and Batalden, who in studying the characteristics of effective clinical micro-systems are an exception to the rule, suggest that senior leaders of the micro-system should look for ways in which the macro-organization connects to and facilitates the work of the micro-system[21] (*see* also Nelson *et al.*[22]).

Further empirical work is needed to clarify the relative contributions of the macro- and micro-system contributions to the overall QI effort. As Dawson and Buchanan remark, 'corporate narratives are typically constructed as rational-linear events, [but] this masks an array of competing narratives each of which has a story to tell about change'.[23] It is at this point that House *et al.*'s[24] notion of the meso-paradigm (which had an important influence on our thinking) leads naturally on to questions of how to investigate and analyze the interactions among levels, and what questions researchers need to ask. Another useful conceptualization which may assist future research is that of 'front' (formal expectations of change agents and senior managers) and 'back-stage' change efforts (social processes taking place in organizations).[25]

Use novel approaches to identify and analyze organizational processes and their interactions

We have attempted here to use novel approaches to identify organizational processes and their interactions,[26] and have presented three ways of making sense of the process data we have collected: the color code heuristic (Chapter 9), the (detailed and aggregated) process maps (Chapter 10) and the narratives themselves (Chapters 2 to 8). Using Thorngate's[27] (adapted by Weick[28]) three-dimensional categorization of models in terms of accuracy, generality and simplicity, we have come to view each of our attempts at making sense of the data we collected as follows: the colors heuristic is general and simple, but not accurate; the aggregated process maps have moderate accuracy, simplicity and generality; and the case study narratives are high on accuracy but low on simplicity and generality. Our approach is just one of many possible, but we would encourage building on the network techniques we have used, as well as applying other approaches that add new, constructive ways of looking at this type of in-depth, longitudinal case study data, especially those able to more fully tease out the sequencing of processes over time.

New theoretical insights for QI in healthcare

Finally, our initial objective before we set off was to introduce and demonstrate the application of organizational theories that have remained relatively untapped in health-care QI research and practice up to this point. In this collection these theories embrace concepts such as mindfulness (Chapter 2), organizational and professional identity (Chapter 3), organizational learning and bricolage (Chapter 4), multi-level leadership (Chapter 5), socio-technical systems (Chapter 6), empowerment (Chapter 7) and mobilization (Chapter 8). These concepts emerged from our re-readings of the stories we were told but represent only the beginning of efforts to bring new thinking to bear on what, at times, appears to be a stilted and narrow view of QI in healthcare. The 'leadership of quality' theme in particular would reward further study.

The final observation we would offer is that like most explorations, our own and those of the organizations we studied do not necessarily have a neat beginning and end. The organizations studied here have not reached a final end point in their quality journey. As conventional wisdom in the quality movement holds, quality is a continuous process, not an end, and we know from some of the cases how fragile and short-lived success can be. The healthcare organizations we studied have been working at the quality challenge for between 10 and 20 years, and each of them expressed how far they have yet to go in fully rooting quality and QI throughout their respective organizations. Nonetheless, we hope that by sharing their stories so far they may help those who wish to follow in their footsteps. Initially, all that it requires is the willingness – and the courage – to take the first step. As Theodor Seuss Geisel (Dr Seuss) put it: 'Today is your day! Your mountain is waiting. So . . . get on your way.'

ANNEX 1: Achieving and sustaining healthcare quality: a codebook for quality and service improvement

Definitions and examples
- The structural challenge
- The political challenge
- The cultural challenge
- The educational challenge
- The emotional challenge
- The physical and technological challenge

Quotations are taken verbatim from the interview transcripts in order to illustrate, in the participants' own words, the nature of each of the organizational challenges.

The structural challenge
Structuring, planning and co-ordinating the quality and service improvement effort, and embedding it within the organizational fabric.

Quality strategy and plan: a formal strategy for Q & SI, and a plan for implementation

'Quality Council is senior leadership coming together to talk about quality initiatives . . . they are kind of the oversight for some of the main priorities that they feel the organization should look at.'

Strategic leadership: strong and decisive executive leadership providing a clear, strategic direction and a disciplined focus around Q & SI matters

'Increasingly, the organization became much more self-governing. Almost like a ship that was steaming ahead operationally. The chief executive didn't drive it operationally – he drove the strategic agenda and set the context.'

'I've got to say that this is one of the few hospitals that I've worked at, or even in my career of consulting, that I have felt is probably on the cutting edge of their quality department . . . usually in most hospitals, I come in and I have to be the one carrying data or quality and forcing people to look at it. But here it's not a forcing nature *per se*, it's really trying to keep up with [the QI director] and the Quality Council and what they want to look at, and there are definitely things going on that are really impressive.'

Whole-systems organizational design: a co-ordinated Q & SI effort that involves joined-up whole-systems design and cross-functional improvement initiatives (as opposed to discreet, one-off projects)

'What we are doing is laying on top of our traditional organizational chart this process management structure which is a much more horizontal approach . . . we are not throwing out the vertical relationships; we are too big not to have those kinds of relationships – and we are not adding any new people – but what is starting to happen is that people are spending part of their day in the vertical world on the organizational chart and part of their time looking horizontally.'

'We take a much broader based framework. It's not just satisfaction we are pushing, it's not just a clinical outcome, but it really is systemic improvement. You end up with improvements within each of the areas, like slowly making water rise, and so what happens is that you start to improve in all areas because there isn't a singular focus; it's not like one day it's going to be finance and one day it's this, and one day it's this. You're making improvements across the board, which pushes the level up into all . . . Everybody rises up, no matter where you are. So if you're here you go up to here, but if you're here you go up to there. If you don't do that you end up with a choppiness factor . . . you don't end up with these pockets, so it just seems much more seamless.'

Devolved authority system: a flat organizational structure that minimizes hierarchy and provides opportunity and encouragement for bottom-up improvement and change initiatives

'The first thing I always say . . . is "it's this relationship thing". I have heard of Trusts where people dare not go see somebody higher up without an appointment. There is a very open structure here. It's not particularly flat, but it is pretty flat, and that I think would mean the open relationships, the respect for each other's area of work, and the mutual support. I think those things make us stand out and which allow us to do the things we do.'

'. . .if you're hierarchical, you all have to maintain your place in the hierarchy, so you have to put other people down in order to maintain your place and I think if you're in a culture where people tend to put other people down, then you end up with divisiveness, you end up with sub-groups, you end up with little cliques where people say they never such-and-such and we always have to such-and-such, and that has been progressively eroded over the years I've been here.'

Quality leadership positions: formal roles and responsibilities in relation to Q & SI are shown on the organizational chart, which also shows a senior person at the top who is leading on quality

'One of the things we have done really right here is to create my post [of service development manager]. Just having project managers put into particular places to achieve particular things at the levels which they've been employed – with all due respect to them – they don't have that organizational development, that organizational management expertise, to actually see what the links are and how you can work through the organization to actually make the big changes.'

'[The quality co-ordinator] is the number one factor. She's a person who has taken quality control and run with it. She is not a shy person, but she would never tell you that she is the person that is really making it go, but she is, because she is the one that keeps us coming to the meetings and she is the one who is on the tasks at the meetings and keeps reminding us of things that we have left behind and need to come back to.'

Multi-level leadership structure for quality: a dispersed, multi-level leadership structure that sees leadership in Q & SI being exercised simultaneously at the micro-system, intermediate/middle-management, directorate, medical board and corporate levels of the organization

> 'Quality is something that needs to be seen as important at all levels of the organization. The employees who are working in their own micro-system in the organization, they all have ideas about their work, how they can do it better, smarter, how can they reduce red tape but in a lot of situations, they cannot make it happen and to make it happen the higher management levels in the organization must be open for this kind of improvement.'

> 'Leadership at every level of the organization. Success doesn't rest in my hands but in everyone else's. Everybody is a leader.'

Quality facilitation team or group: a dedicated core improvement/change team comprising improvement specialists and a wide range of Q & SI skills in areas like process mapping, CQI, OD, team building and facilitation

> 'So we had the heritage of that finite [Business Process Re-engineering] program that lasted three or four years and there was a residual smaller group which carried on – the Modernizing Healthcare Team – who continued to be there as a change management resource within the organization.'

QI training programs: formal education and training opportunities for staff development in the Q & SI area

> 'We've trained about 120 of the medical and hospital leaders to date on our "quality in service improvement course", and that's been over maybe an 18-month period or so. That's all senior leadership, all middle management, and then physician leadership as well – medical directors and chiefs of staff . . . The education is going to drive, I think, much of what we do in performance improvement.'

> 'We trained a lot of the people in the institution and there was a formal training process, about the basics of analyzing quality, process, discipline, diagrams all kinds of things, because we wanted everybody in the institution to have a working vocabulary around these kinds of things.'

Enabling administrative role: central HQ departments, managers and staff that function more as a service to frontline units in Q & SI matters than a central, directing authority

> 'What we have got I think, increasingly, is people out there who know that the modernization team can help them – not do it for them but help them. I am more comfortable with that as it is more robust, embedded in the organization – it's not invested in a few people going out and selling a message because I don't think it works it that way.'

> 'In a lot of organizations quality resources are the people who try to push the improvement projects out there. Here the Quality Resources department is a resource; they are not responsible for improvement – they are responsible in part for measurement – but what happens is that *everyone* is responsible for measurement.'

> 'The role of the Quality Department is not to initiate and manage projects, but to offer support and information to ongoing projects.'

Boundary-spanner roles: hybrid, dual, bridging, liaison, interlocutor or boundary-spanning roles, such as clinical leader/manager, which allow for lateral contact and communication between different groups, and the linking of resources, people and ideas around the Q & SI effort

'They're the jam in the sandwich. If you think about the role that [the directorate manager] undertakes, and all the directors undertake, they have top team and the clinical teams and they have to create some kind of mutual language, so that when we talk targets, there's an interpretation that takes place about what that individual patient needs. I think that's the critical factor and if their translator isn't working then nobody's translator is working.'

'In two words, my role is best defined as resource acquisition. I'm responsible for obtaining external support, managing that support for the program as well as internal support, hospital budget, college budget, managing those resources, the space resources and information resources. In a broad sense, all that resource acquisition is my role.'

'The dilemma is that some people believe you can manage a unit professionally and not have any clinical knowledge and that a good manager will be able to manage that, but I'm still convinced that a hybrid manager – someone with a clinical background going into management, management skills – is the sort of person that is going to take people forward into modernization. And I think we've started to prove that. A lot of my colleagues are the same sort of person.'

Communities of practice: cross-organizational and occupational networks, groups and fora that come together regularly to debate, share knowledge and take forward the Q & SI agenda

'It's docs who . . . are trying to educate ourselves as to what skills may be required for leadership. So we had monthly lecture series [covering] business skills, performance improvement, risk management, [etc] . . . We create a community, and so when we try to change things, as far as philosophies and how you do it, you have to get the right people on board . . .'

'We have [a] physician group meeting twice a month . . . it's a closed community of physicians; we can really preach the gospel when it's necessary on certain quality items and revisit those at the physician group meeting.'

'It's basically creating the collegiality.'

Results-oriented planning: formally constituted procedures for planning and monitoring improvement projects, with clear timelines and robust project management mechanisms

'We identify an issue, a concern, a problem; we develop a planned improvement. We implement it through a plan-do-study-act kind of cycle and if it succeeds we try and implement it on a bigger scale. It's at that point that all staff get communications either in a full staff meeting, a clinical staff meeting or perhaps more commonly, the email.'

Quality governance system: an organization-wide infrastructure of Q & SI meetings and groups for co-ordinating and spreading improvement throughout the system

'The important thing is, the real important thing is, to have a wiring diagram. And a wiring diagram that works for your culture in your setting and that recognizes where the institution is in its quality journey and pushes that as far as it can.'

'. . . in the mid-80s we had something called the medical advisory committee . . . [which] looked at peer review issues, looked at issues in terms of governance and medical staff affairs and relations between the voluntary staff and the Medical Center, and what evolved by the

90s was the performance improvement committees which actually began to focus on quality initiatives . . . actual performance improvement.'

Organizational slack for quality: deliberate provision of slack resources or headroom in the organization (be it money, time, airline tickets or space) that enables staff to stand back from everyday operations and think and work on service development issues

'In the early 1990s the CEO and the medical director recognized slack time is required to work on ideas and innovations. I was that slack time, or part of it, that was created. My job was specifically to go there and change things. They didn't specifically give me a road map on what to change. They said go out and change things. One of the arenas that was, I think, pointed to was the arena of medication safety, but otherwise there was no restriction on what I could or I couldn't work on. In fact, looking back at it, whether it was by design or by chance, it's difficult to tell, but the concept that slack time was necessary and you gave it to someone to work on things, ends up being a way that this organization actually learned about how to do improvement.'

'You have got to give people time and room to do the thinking. Then they can do the critical evaluation. Just coming in and telling them, "Why aren't you doing this?" almost punitively is not a sensible approach. We have to create time and room for the workforce as a whole – we're in danger of making them like hamsters in the wheel, just peddling harder.'

Data and monitoring systems: formal data collection and information processing systems for constant monitoring, measuring, benchmarking of organizational and clinical performance (e.g. dashboards, clinical information, etc.)

'We began taking information analyzed internally and presenting it to medical staff committees and administrative areas, because we felt that if people actually had information, they would be able to use it and make rational decisions, and if we can do that compared against the literature, that means we would have some real opportunities for improvement and that was one of the major turning points.'

'I think more and more . . . one of the advantages of having the dashboards is there is an obligation to measure the foundation and look at the data when [they] come out, and by putting a cover memo on a dashboard, we're pinpointing what the issues are and the observations.'

'The "being exceptional" part of our mission statement has been reinforced consistently through our strategic and financial planning process and our performance improvement reports and our goal settings. We sit there and say that our goal is "exceptional", which means something other than average. So we actually have adopted a policy on how to set goals. If you are below the 25th percentile on any particular metric, then your first objective is to get to that point, and whether it takes one, two or three years, that's where you're at. If you're at the 25th percentile, then set your goal for the 10th percentile, and if you're at the top 10th percentile in your performance, then you should strive to become the absolute benchmark, the absolute best performer on that particular metric.'

The political challenge

Negotiating the politics of change associated with implanting and sustaining the improvement process, including securing stakeholder buy-in and engagement, dealing with conflict and opposition, building change relationships, and agreeing on a common agenda for improvement.

Politically credible leadership: leaders with the authority and skill to broker and manage the politics of engagement associated with improvement work, including dealing with resistance, and selling the case for engaging in Q & SI activities

'On some issues they [micro-system clinicians] will be completely cynical – [the chief executive and medical director] are very skilled at managing that. They are completely on her side – they may have their temper tantrums but they're allowed to voice that and it is valued. [The chief executive] is very skilled at saying, "We take on board what you're saying, however, if we play it this way or that way . . ." She is very skilled at showing them the cunning of playing the game a different way to the advantage of the organization.'

'When we started, we had to convince a sceptical clinical audience and, again, I remember the first presentation we gave to the consultant executive body, one of the senior surgeons turned round saying, "Well, what you're saying is we've been working in a naff way for years . . ." We had to persuade and change and demonstrate, above all else demonstrate, that (a) we can do it, and (b) it's worth doing and that the people doing it know what they're talking about. I've had to develop credibility for the team and protect it and protect its reputation and you can't afford a mistake because that costs you a couple of years. There were a whole lot of factors but the culture has changed . . . Yeah, it's because we try and do it, and the other consultants watching in other specialities, see what's going on. That encourages change.'

'If you ski in France, it becomes apparent very quickly that the French can't queue. At 6 foot three I have the ability by extending my arms to stop the French from getting past me. All they do is succeed in projecting me further forward. That's what you do; you've got to get in the way of all that stuff.'

Clinical engagement: strong and active clinician engagement in – and ownership of – the Q & SI process

'One pathway we did early on wasn't very successful and the reason . . . was because we didn't take the time to get our doctors on board, to make them really understand all the ins and outs of it. The pathway is the end result, but the real change happens – culture change happens – in the process, because . . . if you're in a pathway group then you take this back to your area and you share it and you talk about it and you bring back your ideas. So you're building "buy in". There's a story, I think Dr [x] tells it, about a tree house, build your own versus someone builds it for you. Dad built the kid a tree house and the kid wouldn't go in.'

'Once they take ownership, they're amazing!! You know you can put it in there and it will go. But it's getting them to take ownership because once they take ownership they make it a success.'

'Until the doctors believe that this is their issue, their problem, it isn't going to get better . . . [There's an] expression, 'No one in the history of the world has ever washed a rental car,' which I love because that is exactly true.'

Peer-to-peer relationships: strong peer-to-peer lines of communication and influence, from clinician to clinician, manager to manager, that enable innovation to spread rapidly and effectively down through the organization

'How Dr X approached it is one very effective way to engage, it's very much on a peer-to-peer basis. I don't think that I could walk into a room of general surgeons and get them to agree on how to all do an appendectomy the same way like Dr X or another peer could.'

Clinical–managerial partnering: an agreed clinician and management compact (formal or informal) binding them to work together on the Q & SI agenda

> 'And we've invented and reinvented and reinvented ourselves so that by the end of the second year ... one of the doctors said, "Wait a minute, where's the administration?" ... So we had a little mini-retreat, it was a day retreat, we met with the administration, and basically we said, what are your expectations and what are our expectations? ... We developed a compact.'

> 'If we want to truly improve the quality of care and what we are doing, you need to move much more to a compact concept that encourages more things such as inter-dependence, delegated authority, ownership of issues ...'

> 'One of the successes about QI is good leadership, and that means good leadership in terms of management and in terms of clinicians and also that partnership, because both management and clinicians if they don't work together concrete up the whole process. Consultants can be downright stubborn, so can managers. If you look at areas in the Trust where things have worked out well it is where there is that good managerial and clinical partnership and that is an unstoppable force.'

Staff empowerment: empowering staff to be able to influence and exercise real control over their local service environment

> 'Certainly the Trust environment. Having seen other hospital Trusts, the way they work, the direct systems and the way of the management, allowing the managers to work, not independently but they have a certain amount of freedom has certainly contributed a lot to innovation through this Trust, I'm sure. People are being given the support and the chance to make mistakes.'

> 'Quality improvement processes are sometimes initiated by the cluster and department managers, and not necessarily the board of directors or the Quality Department. The Quality Department does not even have to be aware of these initiatives and only gets involved if the managers approach the department for support.'

Patient empowerment: empowering patients to be able to influence and participate in improvement work

> 'There are a number of staff who are patients here. They know best – because they wear two hats – what works operationally from a patient perspective and what we can do realistically given whatever limitations are imposed in the environment in terms of resources and regulations. Their input and perspective [are] very valuable. It's the cornerstone of what our quality improvement is based on, getting that active feedback.'

> 'We have to be able to meet the patient where they're at, at that time. If they're not ready to take their medication we try to be understanding and try to work with them to get them there. Or if they're not ready to stop drinking, we meet them at that point.'

External partnering: strong and close partnership and mutual interaction between internal staff and relevant external stakeholders in the improvement process.

> 'We got incredible support from PCTs [primary care trusts] ... suddenly there was an air of trust and the feeling that we really could work closer together on everything and we could get a better result all round. I think that changed some of the dynamics within our own top team and we started getting more confident about boundaries or not having boundaries around our organization.'

The cultural challenge

Building shared understanding, commitment and community around the improvement process.

Culture of excellence: a culture that places a premium on 'excellence' in delivering quality care to patients (reflected in the mission, values, language, systems and symbols)

'We are not just training for the local 10km race here; we are training for the Olympics. That is the kind of performance that we are talking about and what would it take to do that . . . this whole concept of organizational transformation is a very, very big piece and part of the approach that we have taken now.'

'No matter how good we are, it's not good enough. We should always try to be better; improvement is part of the job.'

'No, we didn't have the intent to have a homogeneous culture across the system . . . On the other hand, there was no reason why two hospitals couldn't share a common desire to be better in everything that they did.'

Values/symbolic leadership: leaders who are committed to developing a culture in which quality is the key and overriding concern, and who actively role model this commitment in their own everyday language and behaviors

'We weren't distinguished and [the CEO] decided that she wasn't going to accept that. Her legacy was not going to be "I presided over a status quo organization", and she felt that we needed to do something more and better and distinguish ourselves for the sake of our values and our vision and our mission . . .'

'And sometimes you tell stories. In the thinking of older physicians, the VA [Department of Veterans Affairs Health Administration] is a pit . . . but today the VA is one of the safest places in the world, and so when you start telling stories about what's happened in the VA, that is helpful as well, in the sense that if the VA can change then we can change.'

'And I will say, though, that [the physician co-chairs and assistant director] . . . they do go out of their way in terms of social things, to acknowledge the staff, to reward the staff . . . For instance, every other pay period, every employee gets a little coupon in their paycheck for $3.50 off at the cafeteria. They throw the Christmas parties, they generally throw a summer party, they have bought T-shirts for the staff with logos on it, they have a position award. Every month they give a position award to an employee who has made a significant contribution to the department and that goes to whether it's a transporter or a security officer or a nurse. I mean, it's absolutely equal across the board.'

Patient-centered ethic: a strong patient/customer care 'ethic' that infuses every part of the service, large or small

'. . . in the end it always goes back to just actually making a real difference in patient care. Where it's making a difference in patient care, people will engage with it, whatever their reservations are about the process.'

'This is our core value. You have to understand what our core values are. Our core value is the patient is the one who counts. You've got to see it from their perspective.'

'[The organization] has more of a perception of being "hi-touch" rather than "hi-tech", where the care – the compassion element – is more so than the hi-tech.'

'A desire to make a difference to people's lives.'

Culture of mindfulness: a culture that keeps staff constantly vigilant and alert as to their personal and group standards and practices – being awake to quality and safety concerns, and avoiding automatic or standard cookbook practice

'Nurses are very willing to tell doctors about smaller things . . . and so patients actually get better care because the nurses are more willing to say, "Mr Smith just looks funny to me – I don't really know what it is." And the doctor is now aware of it and looking, and it's surprising how often in day-to-day things those are very early signs of something is wrong. The nurse is experienced – she just can't put her finger on it. If you can't have that kind of thing it often slips beyond your screen or your horizon.'

'People keep up with the literature. They also challenge the pathway. They put the references down at the bottom and so you can go back to the literature, and say, "Maybe that's what it says in your pathway but I don't believe it", or you know, "This paper is flawed and I don't know whether I am going to do it this way", or "This is a great paper and I hadn't seen it and this is the way I'm gonna practice." So I hope that is why pathways work here, because people think about it.'

Group/collaborative culture: a strong 'we group' culture that promotes teamwork and co-operation between staff, placing a premium on human values like respect, integrity, trust, pride, honesty, inclusion and openness

'Trust and commitment to each other: that really is the lifeblood of it. You know what, for me as a nurse it's really important to know I'm working with F or I'm working with R, and I've worked with that nurse before and I trust her, so if something's going on with my patient, I know I can say, help, and that person's going to be able to come and we're going to work as a team and bail me out. I can trust her judgement skills and her assessment skills . . . her level of quality of care.'

'It's the common values and beliefs and then there's something about the way they work, the way they understand each other. Isn't it about beliefs and values and isn't that where real quality comes from? You can't teach people that.'

'I grew up ten miles from school and four miles to the nearest corner store and I would wake up, look out, and see the horses in the pasture across the street. From a farming perspective, you can take two horses and one horse alone could pull 500 pounds and the other could also pull 500 pounds, but if you get them working together correctly, they could pull 2500 pounds. That's what we've got here.'

Scientific culture: a culture that values data, measurement, and evidence in both medical and managerial practice, at the same time as being strongly task- and results-driven

'We realized it goes back to knowing what's important, measuring it and setting goals and holding ourselves accountable for achieving those goals. So we created some new processes of performance improvement reports which became milestones to the whole thing – the constant sense of reassessing what we're doing, never allowing a process to go so long without a formal checkpoint in it . . . So everything we do now has a regular checkpoint built into it.'

'I came in with the science of it. I documented variation in this organization, I documented variation between providers for asthma, I documented variation in individual providers over time. [We found] you don't treat asthma the same way two days in a row. Is that the way it should be? And so we documented variation, we documented not following national guidelines and everybody has problems with national guidelines and so there was that. And then I tried to bring in the idea of systems thinking and how complex medicine is and how a doctor trying to do it alone aint going to work.'

Culture of learning: a culture that values risk-taking and experimentation, and constantly encourages people to 'do more, and differently', and to develop and share new knowledge, skills and expertise

'There was a sort of acceptance of the status quo where people would say, "We're 95% compliant so that was ok" . . . We would always seem to be in reactive mode and never proactively looking to improve. The question was what could we do to break this status quo mentality?'

'Our adherence program is a good example. We got funded three years ago to start this program, designed to help patients take their medication and to develop the life skills they need to do that. And, no one in the world, to the best of my knowledge, knew how to do that. There isn't necessarily one best way, so we had this lump of clay and we had a project officer. One of our nurses took this on and created a program from nothing. Took the clay and molded it into what ended up being a very nice sculpture by the time she was done.'

Formal culture: a culture that emphasizes the need for formalized disciplines and enabling structures to ensure efficiency, effectiveness, and personal accountability

'QI 91 was our first effort to take the disparate pieces of quality improvement work that was going on in the organization, and wrap it under a label and an umbrella and give it an organizational identity. And just making it an organizational initiative as opposed to a collection of different programs. That was the first effort at trying to bring it together in some cohesive way. To be able to say to the organization, this is what we're trying to do.'

'One was the creation of a health services research division in our department of medicine here. I'm going to say . . . mid to late 80s, somewhere in that time frame, I think, was an important event that occurred. And so there, you have a situation of the evolution of the core historical mission of the institution as an academic medical center changing with the times of the environment around it, health services research became a legitimate discipline.'

Culture of empowerment: a culture that genuinely nurtures and supports empowerment and self-leadership at all levels of the organization, and that demonstrates this commitment in its reward systems and everyday practices

'Cultivate a culture in which every person is a leader.'

'I've worked at a lot of hospitals but I've never stayed as long as I have here. The reputation of the Trust is that we have can-do culture. You feel empowered to get on and change things yourself . . .'

'It's sort of like the experiments of the counter culture of the 1960s where small groups went off and built their own little communes and they had some successes and some failures. [The senior management's] style is they'll give you enough rope. If you choose to hang yourself, then you'll hang yourself. But sometimes you get the right person, you give them enough rope, you give them the opportunities and they can build some tremendous pockets of success.'

Cosmopolitan culture: an outward-facing organizational culture that is sensitive to the dangers of isolation, arrogance and ethnocentric mentalities and behaviors

'It was about trying to bring the management out and saying, "Yes, you've done a good job internally but unless people out there know what you are doing . . ." The objective for each of the execs was, "You will get yourself actively involved in one project regionally and if you get yourself on something nationally, then that is what you do – your agenda is partly outside as well as inside."'

'A real thirst to go out and get good practice, and stealing shamelessly!'

'In fact everything we do system wide we usually picked up someplace else and brought it into our organization, whether it's risk management or employee benefits or anything else we're doing. But prior to the cultural change, we weren't very open to bringing in things from the outside.'

Long-term culture: a culture that supports the longer-term perspective on Q & SI, the long haul rather than the quick sprint, and is alert to the dangers of fads and short-term quick-fixes

'It's perseverance, hard work, toil and tears, rather than mystery that achieve results.'

'Number one, we said this is going to take a long time to do this, and secondly we made it a 10-year commitment. So immediately people realized we weren't going to be changing approaches every year or two. And so, as we learnt about new things, we resisted the temptation to bring those in and, more, let's understand what those different approaches do and where their strengths are . . . so people aren't saying well gee, this year it's Sigma and what's it going to be next year. It's like no, it's CQI with improvements and enhancements.'

Organizational identity: a strong sense of organization pride and history, identity, legacy and tradition

'I think it's a sense of pride and a sense of history. And I know that sounds crazy – I don't live in the past, I'm not that kind of person, but actually it does make a difference if there is a history to a place or a team of people. It's like when we came across here it was trying to make them understand that it's not the building that makes the place, it's the people that are in it, and I truly believe that . . . I think those people are the people that care about what they do very much and they have a sense of pride in what they do.'

'I am responsible for the legacy of the early Franciscan Sisters of Mary. To do anything less than best, I could not sleep at night because I'd be letting my congregation down.'

Recruitment and retainment: recruiting and rewarding people whose personal values closely align to those of the organization

'One of the ways that the medical leadership, though, has encouraged us is by the quality of the people they hired. They brought some physicians on duty on staff here who have that true collegial belief, some of the younger staff.'

Acculturation: socialization, induction and training processes that help people tune-in and acculturate to the core Q & SI values of the organization

'History I think has a large part to play in it; going back to the Ark really. At least four of the current consultants were registrars, so they've had that cultural thing sort of drilled into them as well.'

'Quality is defined by the six Pursuing Perfection dimensions. In the induction course for new employees these dimensions are tabled and discussed, with people split into small teams to discuss them. This is a good way to get them familiar with the Pursuing Perfection idea, and when the new people start working they instantly recognize these dimensions in their daily practice.'

The educational challenge

Establishing and nurturing a continuous learning process around quality and service improvement issues including both formal and informal mentoring, instruction, education and training, and acquisition of relevant knowledge, skills, expertise.

Pedagogic leadership: influential organizational leaders who champion reflective practice, and encourage staff and colleagues to engage in continuous learning and development around quality and service improvement (Q & SI) issues

'Dr X is one of the best teachers I have ever worked with. If we could all learn to think like him we'd be real smart . . . A lot of the "art" part of it in medicine just comes from watching people like him and seeing how they think about it. I mean with a really good doctor it's fun just to watch them think, and see what they come up with, and hope one day you'll be able to think in the same way. I mean he teaches even when he's not teaching! It comes from loving what you do.'

Organizational change knowledge: the acquisition and application of existing knowledge and evidence base relating to Q & SI, and organizational development and change management

'We have a whole series of middle management development courses . . . it's all part of our CQI curriculum.'

'There was a lot of rotation of members of the Transforming Healthcare Delivery (THD) team back into the organization. We would "grow our own" within the organization which has certainly happened in terms of attitudes having changed fairly dramatically, particularly clinician attitudes. A lot of that was created by the early work of the THD. It's been a case of the organization self-perpetuating, self-generating that.'

Quality improvement knowledge: the acquisition and application of knowledge relating to specific Q & SI methods and techniques (e.g. PDSA, process mapping), and clinical care/improvement models (clinical pathways, chronic care model, etc) in their work.

'But I think what IHI [the Institute for Healthcare Improvement] did for us was it helped us do the PDSA cycles: to start small and try and do a small piece and then replicate it. That's the single biggest thing that we learned, as opposed to tackling some enormous thing.'

'It provided a good start for the quality improvement process in the hospital. Many of the people involved in developing Juran's method are now part of IHI, which promotes a more mature quality management approach.'

'We don't do a kind of a systematic sheep dip approach . . . but for example, when we had a clinical governance workshop a few months ago, we had the Transformation Team there just simply talking about some of the basic processes in change management, and then running some groups and workshops. I didn't quite know how that would go down because we had quite a few consultants, medical staff, and a real mixture – and actually, it went down very well.'

Knowledge harvesting: formal or informal activities to search for and bring back (i.e. harvest) new Q & SI methods, concepts and ideas from conferences and other sources outside of one's own organization or group

'So he . . . and [a non-clinical consultant from the medical staff task force project who previously had been brought in-house] . . . became a team, and they went around looking at evidence based stuff, and they began to bring to the institution a whole discipline around analyzing process, flow diagrams, cradle diagrams, privatization approaches . . . and we began to infuse the organization with that approach.'

'I'm lucky that I can get to travel, get exposed to the latest thinking and have a sense of what's going on, and I can come back and sort of repackage it and talk to the medical executive committee and others in the organization. Although I still see patients in clinic, my position affords me an independent view of quality and safety from the perspective of the patient. My only agenda is quality and safety.'

'Baldridge has given us a framework, focus and discipline . . . a new lens through which to see and evaluate our entire organization. How could we have missed the things that are excruciatingly obvious to others?'

Experimentation and piloting: developing, piloting and testing (and learning from) the application of new Q & SI methods and approaches

'We did it in a classic way. Started with one general practice, tried them out, tried it, and then tried it with about four or five general practices, and eventually its carried on working quite well. It was with the understanding that to do something you don't actually have to have a complete grand process there; you could try it in a very small way.'

'The breakthrough series accelerated and focused our CQI work and helped us achieve more rapid results.'

Evidence-based learning: learning and developing new understanding from review and analysis of routine evidence and data (e.g. clinical auditing, benchmarking, and other activities to evaluate and measure the impact/ benefits of Q & SI applications)

'We discussed the concept of "we do good work, let's document it and let's marry our goals with what the core measures are". So . . . we developed this book for each of our core measures, and the first area is acute coronary syndrome, in which the acute myocardial infarction is a core measure. The core measures that are recognized are nitroglycerin therapy, aspirin therapy. We tagged on some stuff that we studied and basically we go through it and we just review where we are. This is for all the core measures. So you have all the things that we've documented. This is how we do, as a department, over time. This was our baseline but with targeted clinical feedback, we've been able to do improve all of our core measures . . . Then we have each physician. So the physician knows where he performs.'

'[Physicians] will look at data and say, "Ok, I'm performing here and physician A is up here, what's the differences?" If you can focus not punitively but in an educational format what are those differences, and, "Hey, did you know we've got 47 different types of instrumentation here, is there a big difference?" They appreciate the dialogue and it's been very helpful.'

Experience-based learning: learning and developing new understanding from the involvement of patients and caregivers in the design of their own care, including the ability to listen and learn directly from the 'voice of experience'

'[T]his is very important to remember, this is a patient center, because there's lots of places that have put together system maps and that in itself isn't terribly unusual, but the questions came from as a patient experiences their care . . . because the whole issue [is] about patient centered-ness. I'm not sure that happens just by putting some patients on an advisory group or putting patients on a committee. I think it has to fundamentally strike how you view, how you deliver care, how you organize yourselves. So where this comes from is to say, from a patient's viewpoint, how do they experience their care . . . it's an incredibly simple model. This is just trying to recognize that there's lots of things that patients experience in their care . . .'

'We've also been consulting patients about what they think of us for years. I personally for the last six years have been asking 100 patients every year to tell me what they think of me as a person; this is before patient involvement was even thought of.'

The emotional challenge

Energizing, mobilizing, and inspiring staff and other stakeholders to want to join in the improvement effort by their own volition and sustain its momentum through individual and collective motivation, enthusiasm and movement.

Inspirational leadership: inspirational leaders who see Q & SI as much a mission or movement as a project, and who have sufficient skill in scripting/framing ideas for various audiences and sufficient standing within the organization to be able to mobilize large numbers and a wide cross-section of staff to join their improvement movement

> 'Perfect care is something we never reach, but like the North Star, it serves as a beacon to guide us . . . Every day [we] should strive to be even better than before. Our physicians, our nurses, and our staff seek to attain it; our families deserve it.'

> 'But if you find a political leader who really has vision around this, we can move mountains.'

> 'The 13 words of our mission that inspire me are ". . . to reveal the healing presence of God when I deliver best quality care".'

Clinical and other change champions: clinical champions and similarly influential others in the organization who are able to energize, mobilize, and engage fellow professionals and co-workers in the Q & SI effort

> 'He works amazingly long hours; he is completely dedicated. When he's on vacation, he calls from wherever he is. If he's on a beach somewhere, he calls to find out how his patients are doing. He's amazing. He sets a very high standard by his own actions.'

> 'We basically said, "Find physician champions", and that was the key thing . . . someone who was more of a risk taker . . . who was intellectually curious about and open to change, had credibility, and had a connection with a relatively large number of patients at a relatively high amount of resource utilization. So, it was going to create a ripple effect.'

> 'We didn't worry about the nay-sayers. We adopted the real champions of the concept and we worked with them, and gradually there was a big enough group that became the way we did things around here.'

Collective momentum: building powerful momentum around the Q & SI effort such that it ultimately takes on a life of its own, spreading and feeding off its own energies, no longer needing to be driven from above

> 'Yeah, there's a camaraderie, there's an understanding that we're all in this together, nobody's

here to be a millionaire or earn a handsome income – you're treating patients and you like providing care to these patients, you like the work that you do and you like to be part of the inspiration and hope, as they struggle with this disease. That's very, very important.'

'The transformation project would have open days and put notices up in fact sheets and try and get the word around. It's a bit like the fly wheel – it takes some time to get the momentum going but once you get it spinning it gets a bit easier, which is probably the culture changing.'

Professional and social affiliations: local quality activists mobilizing and driving the improvement effort through their informal networks of professional and social affiliations

'It's basically creating the collegiality and a group of individuals who are committed; and I don't think we pressure each other, but . . . there is a certain amount of camaraderie that we drive each other, that when you're in a meeting, it's the same group, we're all motivated, we drive each other, and we go up and down in cycles.'

'[Surgeon B] understands quality improvement and the value of it and he also has informal influence over all the surgeons and can speak to them in a way they understand . . . the dialogue gets started.'

Quality as a mission/calling: staff are energized and self-motivated around Q & SI, knowing they are helping people and contributing to the humanitarian goals of the organization – more than a job, it's a mission and a calling

'That atmosphere makes it personal, makes it so that routinely staff think nothing about putting in a 60-hour week. That's just common. If the work needs to be done, there are staff that absolutely commit to doing it.'

'I think with HIV it really has to be more of a calling than a profession. You have to have your heart and your soul in it. Everybody has different reasons to be here but it is a calling.'

Emotional involvement: staff are emotionally involved and invested in the improvement effort – it has become a matter of the heart as well as the head

'It's almost like you've got there against all the odds – there's a bit of a survivor spirit about it which feeds into the way people feel about the organization. People feel quite passionate about it in a way that isn't always the case . . .'

Improvement campaigns: campaigns to speed up and carry the improvement work forward

'[A senior manager] actually came up with this idea. He said, "We need to have a campaign and really create a team to work on this." He and I talked more about it and I brought in [another provider] because she's good at coming up with creative ideas. So we decided to have this competition. We divided into teams, and said the winning team would get a special lunch. And then we decided it would be good if we had some sort of individual incentive. So we made an individual incentive where every month the person who made the most effort towards an ACE could win a prize.'

The physical and technological challenge

Design and use of a physical, informational and technological infrastructure that improves service quality and the experience of care.

Functional design: functional design of architecture and the built environment to support and encourage Q & SI (i.e. does the job it is supposed to do, safely and effectively, and improves the usability of the service)

'These administrative doors actually tend to cut the end of the dungeon, the emergency fluorescent hell we call home. So we don't get bombarded with the clinical stuff, because there's no way I can do anything administrative and be on the floor . . . But since all of us are either emergency nurses or emergency physicians, we unfortunately find ourselves devolving into administrative planning that is more chaotic than it should be. But I usually calm them, and say, "Hey, we're not in a clinical area. Let's just step back" . . . Fortunately, we're just far enough away where we can have access if there's a problem . . .'

'. . . if it's a typical Monday, half of our patients will be in hallway spots on gurneys . . . the aesthetics may be better, but once you get put in the hallway, the aesthetics are gone. You lose the battle.'

Aesthetic design: design of architecture and the built environment supporting and encouraging Q & SI (i.e. improves the patients' and carers' experience of care)

'There are very practical examples of optimal design. The new stuff that is coming out on noise is incredible. The things on anger and violence in the workplace are amazing, and the correlation between the studies we've done about the calming nature scenes versus abstract paintings in art is remarkable.'

'One of the administrators who no longer works here made a comment and said, "It's beautiful . . . Let's see how long it stays this way with your clientele." The reality is our clientele is not that bad. But to the extent that we do get some of these extreme people, people react to their environment. We've never had one graffiti and this is going on seven years. We've never had one person carve into the wood . . . If you treat people with dignity, they're going to act more dignified.'

'Orthopedics isn't the only one that has it's own front door, it has the best front door coming in. We've done that deliberately, because we've rationalized from five sites down onto this site, and most of the departments that came from separate hospitals have their own entrance, and that's critically important in terms of identity and not being swallowed up. That's very important, because they've got their own front doors, people recognize the need to make sure they don't cut themselves off. I think if we hadn't put their own front doors in, they may feel they have to establish their own identity and the barriers become more fixed.'

Technology/design leadership: a leadership that is aware of the positive effects of the built environment (both functionality and aesthetics) and/or of clinical and information technology on the patient experience, and incorporates these design elements into service improvement efforts

'I think how a lot of this came together was serendipity in that we started out very much on a left brain cognitive path and then, independently of this path, the real transformational experience was when we treated this as a "sick building", when the architect said, "We want to ask you each to give 30 seconds thought to this one question – what do you want this new facility to feel like?" Well, we hadn't thought about that, we'd thought about the functions, how many beds, how many treatment rooms, not what it was supposed to feel like. So, we all filled in this stuff, and came out with things like how playful, how comforting, and inspiring the [hospital] architectural environment should be.'

Location of infrastructure and technology: location of physical infrastructure and technological systems (e.g. free-standing vs. integrated facilities, proximity to other organizational units, separate vs. integrated IT systems, etc.)

'. . . the identity that is still separate, and I think it works fantastically well because it is at the end of the building and we've got our own theatres and our own wards, and I still think that's very good. It's good that we are a separate unit.'

'Well, we're one of the only free-standing entities within [the organization] itself that has its own file server, has their own information systems staff, manages their own data, protects the security and confidentiality of that data and has really state-of-the-art computer equipment for every single staff member. There aren't a lot of programs that have that. It's not cheap, but it's something we need as a program and something we committed to a long time ago in terms of being able to look at potential technologic solutions.'

'It's really nice [to have the computer terminals in the patient rooms]. Some of the nurses have to be in with patients one to one. They can be in there and . . . stay in there so they can do the documentation while they're still with the patient.'

Supportive information technology: design and implementation of IT and communications systems that support and encourage Q & SI efforts

'Perhaps one of the differences between [organization] and elsewhere, two differences possibly, one is that I have always tried to bring in a culture not just of data processing, which often happens – [people] just churn out a spreadsheet. The model that we have got here however is different to that. We've gone down a functional route in that I have experts who develop programs and who understand a service area. So there will be people who know about outpatients or people who know about admissions and people who know about waiting lists. And what we've done with them is trained them up, made them available to understand the area of their subject. What that means is that people can come to them and actually talk to them and engage to them as real people. What we have are skills-based services; for example, we have someone who is outpatient based and that will cover all of the services. That has proved extremely beneficial.'

'I can tell you the trolley weights in Accident & Emergency; I can tell you our waiting lists position, when patients are coming in, real time, which has been developed internally . . . so really good information systems.'

'One is, we're trying to enhance our use of technology to enhance our delivery of care with CPOE [computerized physician order entry] and the use of data mining of data bases to help us identify opportunities for improvement. So that's at the hard technology end.'

Supportive medical technology: design and implementation of medical equipment and clinical technologies to support and encourage Q & SI efforts

'. . . the initiation of thrombolytics . . . had been around for five or ten years, but to really have them integrated into daily practice . . . came . . . in the early or mid 1990s. When we looked at our process, we found things right away like keeping the drugs at the bedside and . . . having a pathway to early data, early EKG. So we've made tremendous gains in that by looking at the system. Then, of course, just as we perfected it, they took away thrombolytics, But, having said that, since we went through and tweaked the system to make thrombolytics available, to re-direct and put it into the PTCA track was a fairly easy process for us.'

Context

Features and dynamics of the environment of organizations that are receptive or non-receptive, enabling or disabling of improvement and the organizational supports and processes needed to sustain it. Examples drawn directly from the experiences of our case study organizations included both inner and outer contextual factors.

Inner context

Organization size and scale
- ❏ large or small player relative to like or competing organizations
- ❏ number of staff and patient episodes
- ❏ scope of services and research activities
- ❏ teaching hospital / tertiary center or not.

Organization structure
- ❏ public/private ownership
- ❏ for-profit/non-profit legal/tax status
- ❏ integrated or stand-alone / degree of autonomy
- ❏ degree of clinical specialization
- ❏ degree of organizational stability (e.g. continuity in leadership, structure, etc.)
- ❏ affiliations (system membership, research and education affiliations)
- ❏ mergers and reorganizations.

Organization performance
- ❏ financial situation (e.g. revenue, turnover, profit and loss, bankruptcy, receivership)
- ❏ clinical performance (e.g. quality of care process, such as adherence to clinical guidelines / standards of care, health outcomes such as mortality, readmissions)
- ❏ patient and customer satisfaction (e.g. patient survey ratings, patient/customer complaints).

Illustrating just a few of these inner contextual factors are some quotations from participants.

'In this region we are the only academic health science center. We have some very fine larger teaching hospitals, whose residency programs we support from here, but this is the mother ship for everything, whether it is for the residents in programs where we send the residents out to other hospitals, or the fact that we are the regional transfer center for critically ill and injured people.'

'The second arm of the success is the stability in this. I don't think that is fortuitous, however, because what we've tried to do is a virtuous circle to push our service as being at the forefront all the way along the line. "It'll do" isn't an approach that we take, certainly in the time that I've been doing this. It's very much pushing the boundaries, which means that we've been fortunate to engage, retain people who have got an interest in and are quite skilled, and we have retained their interest by a number of things, one is by giving them the flexibility, so that they are not stagnating. Based on promotions and staff development I have been able to retain key people because of that.'

'. . . it was a conscious decision to integrate; it wasn't a passive decision . . . things [like integration] don't help in an organization unless you create some sort of slack [resources] and I think integration really did that for us . . . It frees up a tremendous amount of energy in an organization . . . That's a very liberating effect on our position and it really frees you up from having to worry about it . . . So I think what happened as we freed up our energies, the timing was, I think, right, that filled that up in many ways with the commitment to quality and I think a lot of the quality efforts, because if we had been busy doing lots of other things, I'm not sure you would have literally have found time in the day to be able to do much other things you really wanted to do.'

'It finally went public two days after the first Labour government came in after 18 years and [the Secretary of State for Health] was on his feet in the House of Commons . . . the whole screening program had to be reviewed. The quality standards we had in place were rubbish, absolutely rubbish. Taking an organization through that trauma, a new chief executive suspending two consultants, making it public, managing a review: the organization had to pull together.'

Outer context
Political and regulatory environments
❒ accreditation and certification bodies (e.g. Joint Commission for Accreditation of Healthcare Organizations (JCAHO) in the US)
❒ government health- and healthcare-related authorities (e.g. Department of Health and Human Services, Centers for Medicare and Medicaid Servies, National Institutes of Health in the US; Royal Colleges in UK)
❒ external performance measures, such as National Service Frameworks and the Healthcare Commission in the UK, and JCAHO core measures, HIVQUAL, and the Healthcare Effectiveness Data and Information Set (HEDIS) in the US
❒ medical and healthcare policies (e.g. managed care in the US)
❒ formal status and recognition: Foundation Trust (UK) and other absolute and comparable ratings and rankings (including mortality statistics, and national staff and patient surveys)
❒ local community authorities and other organizational stakeholders (links to).

Market and resource environments
❒ competitive environment (e.g. degree of competition, stable/dynamic, certain/uncertain)
❒ degree of service specialization/differentiation
❒ local vs. tertiary balance
❒ demand factors (e.g. customer–patient socio-economic demographics, including education, income, class, race/ethnicity, case mix for different medical/health conditions, population/market size)
❒ supply factors (e.g. funding and reimbursements, such as limitations or new sources provided by health insurance plans or government programs; labour market supply, such as availability/shortages of qualified staff, nurses, general or specialty physicians).

Social, cultural and professional environments
❒ social and ideological movements, such as consumer rights, gay rights, human rights, anti-poverty
❒ health-related social and ideological movements, such as patient rights, alternative/complementary health, HIV-AIDS
❒ quality improvement professions, associations and industry organizations (e.g. IHI, Juran Institute)

❑ medical and related professions associations and industry organizations (e.g. American Medical Association)
❑ national awards for quality and customer care (e.g. Baldridge (US), Health Services Journal (UK) Awards, reputation and level of national recognition)

Technological environments
❑ advances in and availability of clinical therapies (e.g. anti-retroviral therapies, chronic disease management)
❑ advances in and availability of medical equipment (e.g. MRI, ultrasound)
❑ advances in and availability of information and communication technologies (e.g. electronic record-keeping, computerized physician ordering systems, computerized pharmacy dispensing, pagers/cell phones, internet applications).

'It gave us a little bit of shelter. It allowed us to hide behind the fact that we're mandated to do this. We could say, "We have to track these numbers and we have to get this data." We could say, "It's not me that's saying this has to be done, it's the [federal government]" and we could grumble along with the rest of them saying, "We don't like this any more than you do but we've got to do it."'

'There is an AIDS industry that exists in New York City. It truly is an industry. It employs thousands of people. That, generally has a lot of positive consequences for what we do because it's influential, it's powerful in terms of lobbying government for funding and for change. And because there is a lot of money thrown at it . . . I think there are some innovative, exciting things that go on there and so we, more from what we get from New York City and what we get from New York State, I think we are on the cutting edge of what we do, who we are.'

'Some of the patients are really rough. Some days you go home and you think, "Am I the one to do this?" And their lives are so fragile. The world expects them to be able to cope and by the time they were five they were stripped of everything that was ever going to help them do that. There are days when you go home thinking, "I'm so limited and whatever they need I don't have." You can't help that.'

'I think the IOM [Institute of Medicine] report was another place where there was great public credibility about that and suddenly people were talking about safety and harm and that was different . . . IOM is powerful, because I brought it back and I canned it into a PowerPoint presentation and we went around and showed the PowerPoint presentation and we didn't get stuck in the details . . . Thousands of people a year were dying and there might be something we could do about it.'

ANNEX 2: Codes, labels and shorthand descriptions

SUB-PROCESS CODE	COLOR	ABBREVIATED LABEL	DESCRIPTION
Structural process			
S.1	Blue	QStrategy	Explicit organizational strategy for quality
S.2	Blue	TaskLship	Structure/task-centered leadership
S.3	Blue	WholeSysDesign	Whole-systems organizational design
S.4	Blue	Devolved Auth	Decentralized authority system
S.5	Blue	QLdrs	Explicit leadership positions for quality
S.6	Blue	DistrLdrs	Multi-level leadership structure for quality
S.7	Blue	QI Facil Team	Dedicated QI facilitation/change team
S.8	Blue	QITraining Programs	Formal QI training programs
S.9	Blue	Enabling Admin	Supportive/enabling-oriented roles of central administration
S.10	Blue	Bndry Spans	Boundary-spanner roles
S.11	Blue	Comm-of-Practice	Communities of practice and development of other cross-organization/occupation forums or groups
S.12	Blue	Plan Process	Results-oriented planning process for monitoring objectives/timelines
S.13	Blue	QGovern	Explicit governance system for quality
S.14	Blue	QSlackRes	Slack resources for quality
S.15	Blue	DataSys	Data and monitoring systems, data-based management process
Political Process			
P.1	Yellow	CredLship	Politically credible leadership
P.2	Yellow	ClinEngage	Clinician engagement
P.3	Yellow	Peer-to-Peer	Peer-to-peer connections
P.4	Yellow	Clin-Mgt Prtnr	Clinical–managerial partnership
P.5	Yellow	Staff Empwr	Empowering staff
P.6	Yellow	Patient Empwr	Empowering patients
P.7	Yellow	Ext Prtnr	Partnership with external stakeholders
Cultural Process			
C.1	Red	CExcell	Culture of excellence
C.2	Red	Values Lship	Values/symbolic leadership
C.3	Red	Patient-centeredC	Patient/consumer-centric culture
C.4	Red	MindfulC	Culture of mindfulness
C.5	Red	GroupC	Group culture

SUB-PROCESS CODE	COLOR	ABBREVIATED LABEL	DESCRIPTION
C.6	Red	ScienceC	Scientific, rationally oriented culture
C.7	Red	LearnC	Culture of learning
C.8	Red	FormalC	Formal culture
C.9	Red	EmpwrC	Culture of empowerment
C.10	Red	CosmopC	Cosmopolitan culture
C.11	Red	LTermC	Long-term culture
C.12	Red	Org Identity	Organizational identity/self-image
C.13	Red	Recruit Retain	Recruiting/retaining staff with organization's values
C.14	Red	Accultration	Acculturating and socializing staff to organization's values
Educational Process			
ED.1	Green	Pedag Lship	Pedagogic leadership
ED.2	Green	OrgChng Training	Training in organizational change
ED.3	Green	QI Training	Training in QI techniques
ED.4	Green	KHarvest	Knowledge-harvesting activities
ED.5	Green	Experim	Experimentation and pilots
ED.6	Green	Evid-based Learning	Evidence-based learning (evidence/data)
ED.7	Green	Exp-based Learning	Experience-based learning (stakeholder input)
Emotional Process			
EM.1	White	InspLship	Inspirational leadership
EM.2	White	Clin Champs	Clinical champions/change-makers
EM.3	White	Coll Moment	Collective momentum around improvement
EM.4	White	ProfSoc Affil	Activation of professional and social affiliations and networks
EM.5	White	QMission	Quality as a mission/calling
EM.6	White	EmotInvlv	Emotional involvement in the organization
EM.7	White	Imprv Campaigns	Mounting improvement campaigns
Physical and Technical Processes			
PT.1	Pink	Phys Function	Functional design of built environment
PT.2	Pink	Phys Aesth	Aesthetic design of built environment
PT.3	Pink	Techn-Design Lship	Technology and physical design leadership
PT.4	Pink	Phys-Tech Location	Location of physical and technological systems
PT.5	Pink	ICT Supp	Use of information and communication technology supportive of QI
PT.6	Pink	ClinTechn Supp	Use of clinical/medical technology supportive of QI
Inner and Outer Context			
IC1.1	Grey	OrgSize	Size and scale
IC1.2	Grey	OrgStruc	Organizational structure
IC1.3	Grey	OrgPerf	Organizational performance
OC1.4	Black	Pol-Regulatory Environments	Political and regulatory environments
OC1.5	Black	Mrkt-Resource Environments	Market and resource environments
OC1.6	Black	Soc-Cultural Environments	Social, cultural and professional environments
OC1.7	Black	Technological Environments	Available medical and information technologies

References

Notes to Preface and acknowledgements

1 Bate SP. Whatever happened to organizational anthropology?: a review of the field of organizational ethnography and anthropological studies. *Human Relations*. 1997; **50**: 1147–75.
2 Ramachandran VS, Blakeslee S. *Phantoms in the Brain*. New York: Harper Collins; 1998.
3 Siggelkow N. Persuasion with case studies. *Academy of Management Journal*. 2007; **50**(1): 20–4.
4 Calvino I. *Invisible Cities*. London: Vintage; 1997 [trans. W Weaver].

Notes to About the authors

1 Scott WR, Ruef M, Mendel P, *et al*. *Institutional Change and Healthcare Organizations: from professional dominance to managed care*. Chicago: University of Chicago Press; 2000.
2 Greenhalgh TG, Robert G, Bate P, *et al*. *Diffusion of Innovations in Health Service Organizations: a systematic literature review*. Oxford: Blackwell; 2005.

Notes to Chapter 1

1 IOM (Institute of Medicine). *To Err is Human: building a safer healthcare system*. In: Kohn LT, Corrigan, Donaldson MS, editors. Washington, DC: The National Academies Press; 1999.
2 IOM (Institute of Medicine). *Crossing the Quality Chasm: a new health system for the twenty-first century*. Washington, DC: The National Academies Press; 2001.
3 IOM (Institute of Medicine). *Priority Areas for National Action: transforming Healthcare Quality*. Washington, DC: The National Academies Press; 2003.
4 WHO (World Health Organization). *The World Health Report 2000 – Health Systems: improving performance*. Geneva: World Health Organization; 2000.
5 OECD (Organization for Economic Co-operation and Development). *Towards High-Performing Health Systems: the OECD Health Project*. Paris: OECD; 2004.
6 McGlynn EA. There is no perfect health system. *Health Affairs*. 2004; **23**(3): 100–2.
7 Davis K. Toward a high performance health system: the Commonwealth Fund's new commission. *Health Affairs*. 2005; **24**(5): 1356–60.
8 Berwick D. Will is the way to win the patient safety war. *Health Service Journal*. 2007; **117**(6044): 18–19.
9 McGlynn EA, Asch SM, Adams J, *et al*. The quality of healthcare delivered to adults in the United States. *New England Journal of Medicine*. 2003; **348**(26): 2635–45.
10 Ferlie EB, Shortell SM. Improving the quality of healthcare in the United Kingdom and the United States: a framework for change. *Milbank Quarterly*. 2001; **79**(2): 281–315.
11 Wagner C, Gulácsi L, Takacs E, *et al*. The implementation of quality management systems in hospitals: a comparison between three countries. *BMC Health Services Research*. 2006; **6**(Apr 11): 50.
12 Bate SP, Robert G, McLeod H. *Report on the 'Breakthrough' Collaborative Approach to Quality and Service Improvement within Four Regions of the NHS: a research based investigation of the Orthopaedic Services Collaborative within the Eastern, South & West, South East and Trent regions*. Research Report no. 42. Birmingham: Health Services Management Centre, University of Birmingham; 2002.
13 Ham C, Kipping R, McLeod H. Redesigning work processes in healthcare: lessons from the National Health Service. *Milbank Quarterly*. 2003; **81**(3): 415–39.
14 Shortell SM, O'Brien JL, Carman JM, *et al*. Assessing the impact of continuous quality improvement / total quality management: concept versus implementation. *Health Services Research*. 1995; **30**(2): 377–401.
15 Weiner BJ, Alexander JA, Shortell SM, *et al*. Quality improvement implementation and hospital performance on quality indicators. *Health Services Research*. 2005; **41**(2): 307–34.
16 Pearson ML, Wu SY, Schaefer J, *et al*. A method for assessing the implementation of the Chronic Care Model in quality improvement collaboratives. *Health Services Research*. 2005; **40**(4): 978–96.
17 Hussey PS, Anderson GF, Osborn R, *et al*. How does the quality of care compare in five countries? *Health Affairs*. 2004; **23**(3): 89–99.

18 Blendon RJ, Schoen C, DesRoches C, *et al.* Common concerns amid diverse systems: healthcare experiences in five countries. *Health Affairs.* 2003 (May/June): 106–21.

19 Blendon RJ, Schoen C, Donelan K, *et al.* Physicians' views on quality of care: a five-country comparison. *Health Affairs.* 2001 (May/June): 233–43.

20 Kelley E, Hurst J. *Healthcare Quality Indicators Project: initial indicators report.* OECD Health Working Papers No. 22. Paris: OECD; 2006.

21 OECD (Organization for Economic Co-operation and Development). *Health at a Glance – OECD Indicators 2005.* Paris: OECD; 2005.

22 Jönsson B, Wilking N. A global comparison regarding patient access to cancer drugs. *Annals of Oncology.* 2007; **18**(Suppl 3): iii1–iii77.

23 Jarman B. *Adjusted Hospital Death Rates in the United Kingdom and the United States.* Slide presentation, December 2002.

24 Adler P, Kwon S, Signer JMK. *The 'Six West' Problem: professionals and the intraorganizational diffusion of innovations with reference to the case of hospitals.* Unpublished manuscript.

25 McEwan I. *Saturday.* London: Vintage; 2006.

26 Blendon RJ, Schoen C, DesRoches C, *et al.* Inequities in healthcare: a five-country survey. *Health Affairs.* 2002; **21**(3): 182–91.

27 Schoen C, Doty MM. Inequities in access to medical care in five countries: findings from the 2001 Commonwealth Fund International Health Policy Survey. *Health Policy.* 2004; **67**(3): 309–22.

28 Aynsley-Green A. *Children, Child Health and Society: does every child really matter?* 12th Queen Elizabeth the Queen Mother Lecture. London: The Nuffield Trust; 2006.

29 Berwick DM. A user's manual for the IOM's 'Quality Chasm' report. *Health Affairs.* 2002; **21**(3): 80–90.

30 Becher EC, Chassin MR. Improving the quality of healthcare: who will lead? *Health Affairs.* 2001; **20**(5): 164–79.

31 Detert JR, Schroeder RG, Mauriel JJ. A framework for linking culture and improvement initiatives in organizations. *Academy of Management Review.* 2000; **25**(4): 850–63.

32 Shortell SM, Marsteller JA, Lin M, *et al.* The role of perceived team effectiveness in improving chronic illness care. *Medical Care.* 2004; **42**(11): 1040–8.

33 Lin M, Marsteller J, Shortell SM, *et al.* Motivating change to improve quality of care: results from a national evaluation of quality improvement collaboratives. *Healthcare Management Review.* 2005; **30**(2): 139–56.

34 IHI (Institute for Healthcare Improvement). *Improvement Stories.* http://www.ihi.org/IHI/Topics/Improvement/ImprovementMethods/ImprovementStories/, accessed 23 April 2007.

35 McCarthy D, Staton E. Case study: a transformational change process to improve patient safety at Ascension Health. *Quality Matters.* New York: Commonwealth Fund; 2006. http://www.cmwf.org/publications/publications_show.htm?doc_id=339493, accessed 23 April 2007.

36 Yates GR, Bernd DL, Sayles SM, *et al.* Building and sustaining a systemwide culture of safety. *Joint Commission Journal on Quality and Patient Safety.* 2005; **31**(12): 684–9.

37 Frankel A, Gandhi TK, Bates DW. Improving patient safety across a large integrated healthcare delivery system. *International Journal for Quality in Healthcare.* 2003; **15**(Suppl 1): i31–i40.

38 Odwazny R, Hasler S, Abrams R, *et al.* Organizational and cultural changes for providing safe patient care. *Quality Management in Healthcare.* 2005; **14**(3): 132–43.

39 McCarthy D, Blumenthal D. Stories from the sharp end: case studies in safety improvement. *Milbank Quarterly.* 2006; **84**(1): 165–200.

40 Bradley EH, Webster TR, Baker D, *et al.* Sustaining the innovation: a case study of disseminating the Hospital Elder Life Program. *Journal of the American Geriatrics Society.* 2005; **53**(9): 1455–61.

41 Pettigrew AM. *The Awakening Giant: continuity and change in Imperial Chemical Industries.* Oxford: Blackwell; 1985.

42 Micklethwait J, Wooldridge A. *The Witch Doctors.* New York: Times Books; 1996.

43 Weick KE, Quinn R. Organizational change and development. *Annual Review of Psychology.* 1999; **50**: 361–86.

44 Sandelands L, Drazin R. On the language of organization theory. *Organization Studies.* 1989; **10**(4): 457–8.

45 Øvretveit J, Staines A. Sustained improvement?: findings from an independent case study of the Jönköping quality programme. *Quality Management in Healthcare.* 2007; **16**(1): 68–83.

46 Greenhalgh T, Robert G, Bate P, *et al.* *Diffusion of Innovations in Health Service Organizations: a systematic literature review.* Oxford: Blackwell; 2005.

47 Mohr LB. *Explaining Organizational Behavior.* San Francisco: Jossey Bass; 1982.

48 Pettigrew AM, Woodman, RW, Cameron K. Studying organizational change and development: challenges for future research. *Academy of Management Journal.* 2001; **44**(4): 697–713.

49 Siggelkow N. Persuasion with case studies. *Academy of Management Journal.* 2007; **50**(1): 20–4.

50 Weick KE. *Sensemaking in Organizations.* Thousand Oaks, CA: Sage Publications; 1995.

51 Cacioppe R, Edwards M. Seeking the holy grail of organizational development. *Leadership and Organization Development Journal.* 2005; **26**(2): 86–105.

52 Dawson P. *Organizational Change: a processual approach.* London: Chapman; 1994.

53 Whelan-Berry KS, Gordon JR, Hinings CR. Strengthening organizational change processes: recommendations and implications from a multilevel analysis. *Journal of Applied Behavioral Science.* 2003; **39**(2): 186–207.

54 Langley A. Strategies for theorising from process data. *Academy of Management Review.* 1999; **24**(4): 691–710.

55 Leatherman S, Sutherland K. *The Quest for Quality in the NHS: a chartbook of quality of care in the NHS.* Oxford: The Nuffield Trust/Radcliffe Publishing; 2005.

56 Batalden PB, Godfrey MM, Nelson EC. *Quality by Design: a clinical micro-system approach.* New York: Wiley; 2007.

57 Batalden PB, Nelson EC, Mohr JJ, *et al.* Micro-systems in healthcare: part 5. How leaders are leading. *Joint Commission Journal on Quality and Safety.* 2003; **29**(6): 297–308.

58 Donaldson MS, Mohr JJ. *Exploring Innovation and Quality Improvement in Healthcare Micro-Systems: a cross-case analysis.* A technical report for the Institute of Medicine Committee on the Quality of Healthcare in America. Submitted to the Robert Wood Johnson Foundation, RWJF Grant Number 36222. Washington, DC: Institute of Medicine; 2000.

59 House R, Rousseau DM, Thomas-Hunt M. The meso paradigm: a framework for the integration of micro and macro organizational behavior. *Research in Organizational Behavior.* 1995; **17**: 71–114.

60 Glaser BG, Strauss AL. *The Discovery of Grounded Theory: strategies for qualitative research.* Chicago: Aldine; 1967.

61 Weick KE. The generative properties of richness. *Academy of Management Journal.* 2007; **50**(1): 14–19.

62 Barley SR. Technology as an occasion for structuring: evidence from observations of CT scanners and the social order of radiology departments. *Administrative Science Quarterly;* 1986; **31**: 78–108.

63 Eisenhardt KM. Building theories from case study research. *Academy of Management Review.* 1989; **14**(4): 532–50.

64 Yin RK. *Case Study Research: design and methods.* London: Sage; 2003.

65 Greenhalgh T, Robert G, Macfarlane F, *et al.* Storylines of research: a meta-narrative perspective on systematic review. *Social Science and Medicine.* 2005; **61**(2): 417–30.

66 Britten N, Campbell R, Pope C, *et al.* Using meta-ethnography to synthesize qualitative research: a worked example. *Journal of Health Services Research and Policy.* 2002; **7**(4): 209–15.

67 Campbell R, Pound P, Pope C, *et al.* Evaluating meta-ethnography: a synthesis of qualitative research on lay experiences of diabetes and diabetes care. *Social Science and Medicine.* 2003; **56**(4): 671–84.

68 Paterson BL, Thorne SE, Canam C, *et al. Meta Study of Qualitative Health Research: a practical guide to meta analysis and syntheses.* Thousand Oaks, CA: Sage; 2001.

69 Cortazzi M. Narrative analysis in ethnography. In: Atkinson P, Coffey A, Delmont S, editors. *Handbook of Ethnography.* London: Sage; 2001.

70 Counte MA, Meurer S. Issues in the assessment of continuous quality improvement implementation in healthcare organizations. *International Journal for Quality in Healthcare.* 2001; **13**: 197–207.

71 Pentland BT. Building process theory with narrative: from description to explanation. *Academy of Management Review.* 1999; **24**(4): 711–24.

72 Eisenhardt KM, Graebner ME. Theory building from cases: opportunities and challenges. *Academy of Management Journal.* 2007; **50**(1): 25–32.

Notes to Chapter 2

1 Rogers EM. *Diffusion in Innovations.* 5th ed. New York: Free Press; 2003.

2 Rogers EM, Bhowmik DK. Homophily-heterophily: relational concepts for communication research. *Public Opinion Quarterly.* 1970; **34**: 523.

3 Weick KE. *Making Sense of the Organization.* Oxford: Blackwell; 2001.

4 Weick KE, Quinn RE. Organizational change and development. *Annual Review of Psychology.* 1999; **50**: 361–86.

5 Berwick DM. Improvement, trust, and the healthcare workforce. *Quality and Safety in Healthcare.* 2003; **12**(6): 448–52.

6 Bate SP, Robert G. *Bringing User Experience to Healthcare Improvement: the concepts, methods and practices of experience-based design.* Oxford: Radcliffe Publishing; 2007.

7 Kohn LT, Corrigan JM, Donaldson MS. *To Err is Human: building a safer health system.* Washington, DC: The National Academies Press; 1999.

8 Institute of Medicine. *Crossing the Quality Chasm: a new health system for the twenty-first century.* Washington, DC: National Academy Press; 2001.

9 Bate SP. *Strategies for Cultural Change.* Oxford: Butterworth Heinemann; 1994.

10 Pine BJ, Gilmore JH. *The Experience Economy: work is theatre and every business a stage.* Boston, MA: Harvard Business School Press; 1999.

11 Fitzgerald T. Can change in organizational culture really be managed? *Organization Dynamics.* 1988; Autumn: 5–15.

12 Harris SG. A schema-based perspective on organizational culture. Paper presented to Annual Meeting of the Academy of Management, Washington, DC, 1990.

13 Mack A, Rock I. *Inattentional Blindness.* Cambridge, MA: MIT Press; 1998.

14 Most SB, Simons DJ, Scholl BJ, *et al.* Sustained inattentional blindness: the role of location in the detection of unexpected dynamic events. *Psyche: An Interdisciplinary Journal of Research on Consciousness.* 2000; **6**(14). psyche. cs.monash.edu.au/v6/psyche-6-14-most.html.

15 Weick KE, Sutcliffe KM. *Managing the Unexpected: assuring high performance in an age of complexity*. San Francisco, CA: Jossey-Bass; 2001.

16 Langer E. *The Power of Mindful Learning*. Reading, MA: Addison-Wesley; 1997.

17 Batalden PB, Nelson EC, Mohr JJ, *et al*. Micro-systems in healthcare: part 5. How leaders are leading. *Joint Commission Journal on Quality and Safety*. 2003; **29**(6): 297–308.

18 Godfrey MM, Nelson EC, Wasson JH, *et al*. Micro-systems in healthcare: part 3. Planning patient-centered services. *Joint Commission Journal on Quality and Safety*. 2003; **29**(4): 159–70.

19 Weick KE. Puzzles in organizational learning: an exercise in disciplined imagination. *British Journal of Management*. 2002; **13**: S7–S15.

20 Wenger E, Snyder WM. Communities of practice: the organizational frontier. *Harvard Business Review*. 2000; Jan/Feb: 139.

21 Lave J, Wenger E. *Situated Learning: legitimate peripheral participation*. Cambridge: Cambridge University Press; 1991.

22 Judge WQ, Fryxell GE, Dooley RS. The new task of R&D management: creating goal-directed communities for innovation. *California Management Review*. 1997; **39**(3): 72–85.

23 Borei JM. Chaos to community: one company's journey toward transformation. *World Business Academic Perspectives*. 1992; **6**(2): 77–83.

24 Peck MS. *The Different Drum*. New York: Simon and Schuster; 1987.

25 Pettigrew AM. *The Awakening Giant: continuity and change in ICI*. Oxford: Blackwell; 1985.

26 Pettigrew AM. Contextualist research: a natural way to link theory and practice. In: Lawler EE, editor. *Doing Research That is Useful in Theory and Practice*. San Francisco: Jossey-Bass; 1985.

27 Pettigrew AM, Ferlie E, McKee L. *Shaping Strategic Change: making change in large organizations: the case of the NHS*. London: Sage; 1992.

28 Bevan H, Plsek P. The epic journey towards health systems transformation: lessons from a decade or more of improvement work in the NHS-England. Plenary presentation to the 3rd Annual Asia–Pacific Forum on Quality in Healthcare, Auckland, New Zealand; 2003.

29 Mitleton-Kelly E. Complexity research – approaches and methods: the LSE Complexity Group integrated methodology. In: Keskinen A, Aaltonen M, Mitleton-Kelly E, editors. *Organizational Complexity*. Finland Futures Research Centre, Scientific Papers 1/2003. Helsinki: TUTU Publications; 2003.

30 House R, Rousseau DM, Thomas-Hunt M. The meso paradigm: a framework for the integration of micro and macro organizational behavior. *Research in Organizational Behavior*. 1995; **17**: 71–114.

31 Pettigrew AM, Fenton E. *Innovating New Forms of Organizing*. London: Sage; 2000.

32 Ruigrok W, Pettigrew AM, Whittington R, *et al*., editors. *Innovative Forms of Organizing: international perspectives*. London: Sage; 2003.

33 Miller D. Toward a new contingency approach: the search for organizational gestalts. *Journal of Management Studies*. 1981; **18**: 1–26.

34 Miller D. Configurations of strategy and structure: towards a synthesis. *Strategic Management Journal*. 1986; **7**: 233–49.

35 Miller D. The genesis of configuration. *Academy of Management Review*. 1987; **12**: 686–701.

36 Thompson JA, Bunderson JS. Violations of principle: ideological currency in the psychological contract. *Academy of Management Review*. 2003; **28**(4): 571–86.

37 Pasmore WA. *Creating Strategic Change: designing the flexible, high-performing organization*. Chichester: Wiley; 1994.

38 Ancona D, Chong C. *Entrainment: cycles and synergy in organizational behavior*. Cambridge, MA: Sloan School of Management, MIT; 1991.

39 Donaldson MS, Mohr JJ. *Exploring Innovation and Quality Improvement in Healthcare Micro-systems: a cross-case analysis*. A technical report for the Institute of Medicine Committee on the Quality of Healthcare in America. Submitted to the Robert Wood Johnson Foundation, RWJF Grant Number 36222. Washington, DC: Institute of Medicine; 2000.

40 Nelson EC, Batalden PB, Huber TP, *et al*. Micro-systems in healthcare: part 1. Learning from high-performing frontline clinical units. *Joint Commission Journal on Quality Improvement*. 2002; **28**(9): 472–93.

41 Nelson EC, Batalden PB, Huber TP, *et al*. Micro-systems in healthcare: part 2. Creating a rich information environment. *Joint Commission Journal on Quality and Safety*. 2003; **29**(1): 5–15.

42 Kabat-Zinn J. *Coming to Our Senses*. www.uctv.tv/library-popup.asp?showID=9375 (accessed March 2007).

43 Christianson MK, Sutcliffe KM. Creating collective mindfulness. Paper presented to the 2005 Academy of Management Annual Meeting, Honolulu, HI.

44 Langer EJ. *Mindfulness*. Reading, MA: Addison-Wesley; 1989.

45 Langer EJ, Moldoveanu M. The construct of mindfulness. *Journal of Social Issues*. 2000; **56**: 1–9.

46 Weick KE, Roberts KH. Collective mind in organizations: heedful interrelating on flight decks. *Administrative Science Quarterly*. 1993; **38**(3): 357–81.

47 Weick KE, Sutcliffe KM, Obstfeld D. Organizing for high reliability: processes of collective mindfulness. *Research in Organizational Behavior*. 1999; **21**(81): 81–123.

48 Weick KE, Sutcliffe KM. Hospitals as cultures of entrapment: a re-analysis of the Bristol Royal Infirmary. *California Management Review*. 2003; **45**(2): 73–84.

Notes to Chapter 3

1 Hatch MJ, Schultz M. Scaling the Tower of Babel: relational differences between identity, image and culture in organizations. In: Schultz M, Hatch MJ, Larsen MH, editors. *The Expressive Organization: linking identity, reputation and the corporate brand.* Oxford: Oxford University Press; 2000.

2 Hatch MJ, Schulz M. The dynamics of organizational identity. In: Hatch MJ, Schulz M, editors. *Organizational Identity: a reader.* Oxford: Oxford University Press; 2004.

3 Albert S, Whetten D. Organizational identity. In: Cummings LL, Staw BM, editors. *Research in Organizational Behavior.* 1985; **7**: 263–95.

4 Dutton JE, Dukerich JM, Harquail CV. Organizational images and member identification. *Administrative Science Quarterly.* 1994; **39**: 239–63.

5 Gioia DA, Schultz M, Corley KG. Organizational identity, image, and adaptive instability. *Academy of Management Review.* 2000; **25**(1): 63–81.

6 Gioia DA, Chittipeddi K. Sensemaking and sensegiving in strategic change initiation. *Administrative Science Quarterly.* 1991; **41**: 370–403.

7 Isabella L. Evolving interpretations as a change unfolds: how managers construe key organizational events. *Academy of Management Journal.* 1990; **33**: 7–41.

8 Dukerich JM, Carter SM. Distorted images and reputation repair. In: Schultz M, Hatch MJ, Larsen MH, editors. *The Expressive Organization: linking identity, reputation and the corporate brand.* Oxford: Oxford University Press; 2000.

9 Brown AD, Starkey K. Organizational identity and learning: a psychodynamic perspective. *Academy of Management Review.* 2000; **25**(1): 102–20.

10 Spender J-C, Grinyer PH. Organizational renewal: top management's role in a loosely coupled system. *Human Relations.* 1995; **48**: 909–26.

11 van Riel CBM. Corporate communication orchestrated by a sustainable corporate story. In: Schultz M, Hatch MJ, Larsen MH, editors. *The Expressive Organization: linking identity, reputation and the corporate brand.* Oxford: Oxford University Press; 2000.

12 Whetten DA, Godfrey PC, editors. *Identity in Organizations: building theory through conversations.* Sage: London; 1998.

13 RD&E (Royal Devon and Exeter Healthcare NHS Trust). *Governance Annual Report 2002/2003.* Presented to the Trust Board 25 June 2003.

14 Commission for Health Improvement. *Report of a Clinical Governance Review at Royal Devon and Exeter Healthcare Trust.* London: Commission for Health Improvement; 2001.

15 Cartwright D, Zander A. *Group Dynamics – Research and Theory.* Evanston, Il: Row Peterson; 1968.

16 Bate SP. The impact of organizational culture on approaches to organizational problem-solving. *Organization Studies.* 1984; **5**(1): 43–66.

17 Albert S. The definition and metadefinition of identity. In: Whetten DA, Godfrey PC, editors. *Identity in Organizations: building theory through conversations.* London: Sage; 1998.

18 Carroll CE. The strategic use of the past and future in organizational change. *Journal of Organizational Change Management.* 2002; **15**(6): 556–62.

19 Ashforth BE, Mael, F. Social identity theory and the organization. *Academy of Management Review.* 1989; **14**(1): 20–39.

20 Brown ME. Identification and some conditions of organizational involvement. *Administrative Science Quarterly.* 1969; **14**: 346–55.

21 Ansoff HI. Strategic issue management. *Strategic Management Journal.* 1980; **1**(2): 131–48.

22 Dutton J, Ashford S. Selling issues to top management. *Academy of Management Review.* 1993; **18**(3): 397–428.

23 Dutton JE, Ashford SJ, O'Neill RM, *et al.* Moves that matter: issue selling and organizational change. *Academy of Management Review.* 2001; **44**: 716–36.

24 Scott WR. Conflicting levels of rationality: regulators, managers and professionals in the medical care sector. *Journal of Health Administration Education.* 1985; **3**(Part 2): 113–31.

25 Thompson JD. *Organizations in Action.* New York: McGraw-Hill; 1967.

26 Dukerich JM, Golden BR, Shortell SM. Beauty is in the eye of the beholder: the impact of organizational identification, identity and image on the cooperative behavior of physicians. *Administrative Science Quarterly.* 2002; **47**: 507–33.

27 Zald MN, Morrill C, Rao, H. The impact of social movements on organizations: environment and responses. In: Davis GF, McAdam D, Scott WR, *et al.*, editors. *Social Movements and Organization Theory.* New York: Cambridge University Press; 2005.

28 Coyle-Shapiro JA-M, Morrow P. Individual and organizational antecedents of TQM adoption: a comparison of relative effects and implications for organizational change. Paper presented at Annual Meeting of the Academy of Management, Washington DC, August 2001.

29 Hall DT, Schneider B, Nygren HT. Personal factors in organizational identification. *Administrative Science Quarterly.* 1970; **15**: 176–90.

30 O'Reilly C, Chatman J. Organizational commitment and psychological attachment: the effects of compliance, identification, and internalization on prosocial behavior. *Journal of Applied Psychology.* 1986; **71**: 492–9.

31 Fireman B, Gamson WA. Utilitarian logic in the resource mobilisation perspective. In: Zald MN, McCarthy JD, editors. *The Dynamics of Social Movements*. Cambridge, MA: Winthrop; 1979.

32 Bate SP, Robert G. Knowledge management and communities of practice in the private sector: lessons for modernising the National Health Service in England and Wales. *Public Administration*. 2002; **80**(4): 643–63.

33 Dukerich JM, Kramer R, Parks JM. The dark side of organizational identification. In: Whetten DA, Godfrey PC, editors. *Identity in Organizations: building theory through conversations*. London: Sage; 1998.

34 Pratt MG, Rafaeli A. Organizational dress as a symbol of multilayered social identities. *Academy of Management Journal*. 1997; **40**: 862–98.

35 Pratt MG, Foreman PO. Classifying managerial responses to multiple organizational identities. *Academy of Management Review*. 2000; **25**(1): 18–42.

36 Van de Ven AH, Bunderson S, Lofstrom S. Multiple organizational identities in healthcare. Paper presented at Annual Meeting of the Academy of Management, Boston, 1997.

37 Gioia DA. From individual to organizational identity. In: Whetten DA, Godfrey PC, editors. *Identity in Organizations: building theory through conversations*. London: Sage; 1998.

38 Albert S, Ashforth BE, Dutton JE. Organizational identity and identification: charting new waters and building new bridges. *Academy of Management Review*. 2000; **25**(1): 13–17.

Notes to Chapter 4

1 Berwick DM. Disseminating innovations in healthcare. *Journal of the American Medical Association*. 2003; **289**(15): 1969–75.

2 Levitt B, March JG. Organizational learning. *Annual Review of Sociology*. 1988; **14**: 319–40.

3 Argyris C, Schön DA. *Organizational Learning II: theory, method, and practice*. Reading, MA: Addison-Wesley; 1996.

4 Argyris C. *Reasoning, Learning and Action: individual and organizational*. San Francisco: Jossey-Bass; 1982.

5 March JG. Exploration and exploitation in organizational learning. *Organization Science*. 1991; **2**: 71–87.

6 Gupta AK, Smith KG, Shalley CE. The interplay between exploration and exploitation. *Academy of Management Journal*. 2006; **49**(4): 693–708.

7 He ZL, Wong PK. Exploration vs. exploitation: an empirical test of the ambidexterity hypothesis. *Organization Science*. 2004; **15**(4): 481–94.

8 Eveland JD. Diffusion, technology transfer and implementation. *Knowledge: Creation, Diffusion, Utilisation*. 1986; **8**: 303–22.

9 Greenhalgh TG, Robert G, Bate P, *et al*. *Diffusion of Innovations in Health Service Organizations: a systematic literature review*. Oxford: Blackwell; 2005.

10 Hannan MT, Carroll G. An introduction to organizational ecology. In: Carroll GR, Hannan MT, editors. *Organizations in Industry: strategy, structure, and selection*. New York: Oxford University Press; 1995.

11 Scott WR. *Organizations: rational, natural, and open systems*. 4th ed. Upper Saddle River, NJ: Prentice Hall; 1998.

12 Scott WR, Cole RE. Introduction. In: Cole RW, Scott WR, editors. *The Quality Movement and Organization Theory*. Thousand Oaks, CA: Sage; 2000.

13 Abrahamson E. Management fashion. *Academy of Management Review*. 1996; **21**: 254–85.

14 Weick KE. *Sensemaking in Organizations*. Thousand Oaks, CA: Sage; 1995.

15 Lillirank P. The transfer of management innovations from Japan. *Organization Studies*. 1995; **16**: 971–89.

16 Czarniawska B, Sevon G, editors. *Translating Organizational Change*. Berlin: Walter de Gruyter; 1996.

17 Strang D, Soule SA. Diffusion in organizations and social movements: from hybrid corn to poison pills. *Annual Review of Sociology*. 1998; **24**: 265–90.

18 Brunsson N, Olsen JP. *The Reforming Organization*. London: Routledge; 1993.

19 Abrahamson E, Fairchild G. Management fashions: lifecycles, triggers, and collective learning processes. *Administrative Science Quarterly*. 1999; **44**(4): 708–40.

20 Meyer JW, Rowan B. Institutionalized organizations: formal structure as myth and ceremony. In: Powell WW, DiMaggio PJ, editors. *The New Institutionalism in Organizational Analysis*. Chicago: University of Chicago Press; 1991. (Originally published in *American Journal of Sociology*. 1977; **83**: 340–63).

21 Scott WR. *Institutions and Organizations*. 2nd ed. Thousand Oaks, CA: Sage; 2001.

22 Westphal JD, Gulati R, Shortell SM. Customisation or conformity?: an institutional and network perspective on the content and consequences of TQM adoption. *Administrative Science Quarterly*. 1997; **42**: 366–94.

23 Carruthers BG, Uzzi B. Economic sociology in the new millennium. *Contemporary Sociology*. 2000; **29**(3): 486–94.

24 Lévi-Strauss C. *The Savage Mind*. Chicago: University of Chicago Press; 1966.

25 Cedars-Sinai. *Historical Perspective*. Los Angeles: Cedars-Sinai Health System; 1999.

26 Cedars-Sinai. *Fact Sheet*. Los Angeles: Cedars-Sinai Health System; 1999.

27 Stinchcombe AL. Social structure and organizations. In: March JG, editor. *Handbook of Organizations*. Chicago: Rand McNally; 1965.

28 Baron JN, Hannan MT, Burton MD. Building the iron cage: determinants of managerial intensity in the early years of organizations. *American Sociological Review*. 1999; **64**(4): 527–47.

29 Hatch MJ, Schultz M. Relations between organizational culture, identity and image. *European Journal of Marketing.* 1997; **31**(5/6): 356–65.
30 Hatch MJ, Schultz M. Scaling the Tower of Babel: relational differences between identity, image and culture in organizations. In: Schultz M, Hatch MJ, Larsen MH, editors. *The Expressive Organization: linking identity, reputation and the corporate brand.* Oxford: Oxford University Press; 2000.
31 Cedars-Sinai. *Top the Charts.* Los Angeles: Cedars-Sinai Health System; 2000.
32 Cedars-Sinai. *About Us.* Los Angeles: Cedars-Sinai Health System; 2002.
33 Scott WR, Ruef M, Mendel P, *et al. Institutional Change and Healthcare Organizations: from professional dominance to managed care.* Chicago: University of Chicago Press; 2000.
34 Montgomery K. A prospective look at the specialty of medical management. *Work and Occupations,* 1990; **17**: 178–97.
35 Aldrich H, Herker D. Boundary spanning roles and organizational structure. *Academy of Management Review.* 1977; **2**(2): 217–30.
36 Leifer R, Delbecq A. Organizational/environmental interchange: a model of boundary spanning activity. *Academy of Management Review.* 1978; **3**(1): 40–50.
37 Bate SP. The role of stories and storytelling in organizational change efforts: the anthropology of an intervention within a hospital. *Intervention: Journal of Culture, Organization and Management.* 2004; **1**(1): 27–43.
38 IOM (Institute of Medicine). *To Err is Human: building a safer health system.* Washington, DC: National Academy Press; 1999.
39 IOM (Institute of Medicine). *Crossing the Quality Chasm: a new health system for the 21st century.* Washington, DC: National Academy Press; 2001.
40 Abrahamson E. Avoiding repetitive change syndrome. *MIT Sloan Management Review.* 2004; **45**(2): 93–5.
41 Cole RE. *Strategies for Learning: small group activities in American, Japanese and Swedish Industry.* Berkeley: University of California Press; 1989.
42 Cole RE. *Managing Quality Fads: how American business learned to play the quality game.* New York: Oxford University Press; 1999.
43 Bate SP, Robert G. Knowledge management and communities of practice in the private sector: lessons for modernizing the National Health Service in England and Wales. *Public Administration.* 2002; **80**(4): 643–63.
44 Berwick DM. Improvement, trust, and the healthcare workforce. *Quality and Safety in Healthcare.* 2003; **12**(6): 448–52.
45 Brown JS, Duguid P. Organizational learning and communities of practice: toward a unified view of working, learning, and innovation. *Organization Science.* 1991; **2**(1): 40–57.
46 Wenger E. *Communities of Practice.* Cambridge: Cambridge University Press; 1998.
47 Lave J, Wenger E. *Situated Learning: legitimate peripheral participation.* Cambridge: Cambridge University Press; 1991.
48 Wenger E, Snyder WM. Communities of practice: the organizational frontier. *Harvard Business Review.* 2000; 78(1): 139.
49 Pettigrew AM, McKee L. *Shaping Strategic Change: making change in large organizations.* London: Sage; 1992.
50 Barnsley JL, Lemieux-Charles L, McKinney MM. Integrating learning into integrated delivery systems. *Healthcare Management Review.* 1998; **23**(1): 18–28.
51 Greenhalgh T, Robert G, MacFarlane F, *et al.* Diffusion of innovations in service organizations: systematic review and recommendations. *Milbank Quarterly.* 2004; **82**(4): 581–629.
52 Pfeffer J, Salancik GR. Organizational decision-making as a political process: the case of a university budget. *Administrative Science Quarterly.* 1974; **19**(2): 135–51.
53 Hackman JR, Wageman R. Total Quality Management: empirical, conceptual, and practical issues. *Administrative Science Quarterly.* 1995; **40**: 309–42.
54 Whetten DA, Godfrey P, editors. *Identity in Organizations: developing theory through conversations.* Thousand Oaks, CA: Sage; 1998.
55 Dutton JE, Dukerich JM. Keeping an eye on the mirror: image and identity in organizational adaptation. *Academy of Management Journal.* 1991; **34**: 517–54.
56 Deal TE, Kennedy AA. *Corporate Cultures.* New York: Perseus; 2000.
57 Zammuto RF, Krakower JY. Quantitative and qualitative studies of organizational culture. *Research in Organizational Change and Development.* 1991; **5**: 83–114.
58 Deming WE. *Out of the Crisis.* Cambridge, MA: Massachusetts Institute of Technology, Center for Advanced Engineering Study; 1986.
59 Roehm HA, Castellano JF. The Deming view of a business. *Quality Progress.* 1997; **30**(2): 39–45.

Notes to Chapter 5

1 Gronn P. Distributed leadership as a unit of analysis. *Leadership Quarterly.* 2002; **13**: 423–51.
2 Ferlie EB, Shortell S. Improving the quality of healthcare in the United Kingdom and the United States: a framework for change. *Milbank Quarterly.* 2001; **79**(2): 281–315.
3 Denis J-L, Lamothe L, Langley A. The dynamics of collective leadership and strategic change in pluralistic organizations. *Academy of Management Journal.* 2001; **44**(4): 809–37.

4 Bate SP. *Strategies for Cultural Change*. Oxford: Butterworth-Heinmann; 1994.

5 Pettigrew A. Andrew Pettigrew on executives and strategy. *European Management Journal*. 2002; **20**(1): 20–34.

6 Gibb CA. Leadership. In: Lindzey G, Aronson E, editors. *Handbook of Social Psychology*. Reading, MA: Addison-Wesley; 1954.

7 Quinn J. *The Intelligent Enterprise*. New York: Free Press; 1992.

8 Nelson EC, Batalden PD, Huber TP, *et al.* Micro-systems in healthcare: part 1. Learning from high performing frontline clinical units. *Joint Commission Journal of Quality Improvement*. 2002; **28**(9): 472–93.

9 Klazinga N, Delnoij D, Kulu-Glasgow I. Measuring up: improving health systems performance in OECD countries – can a tulip become a rose? Presentation at OECD, 2001. http://www.oecd.org/dataoecd/48/32/1959887.pdf.

10 Okma KGH. *Healthcare, Health Policies, and Healthcare Reforms in the Netherlands*. The Hague: International Publication Series Health, Welfare and Sports, No. 7; 2001.

11 Juran Institute. *Healthcare improvement*. http://www.juran.com/lower.cfm?article_id=28 (accessed 10 March 2005).

12 RdGG (Reinier de Graaf Groep). *Realization of Pursuing Perfection: from 'ever better' to perfection: Phase 2*. Delft; RdGG; 2002.

13 Stahr H. Developing a culture of quality within the United Kingdom healthcare system. *International Journal of Healthcare Quality Assurance*. 2001; **14**(4): 174–80.

14 ISO (International Organization for Standardization). *ISO 9000 / ISO 14000*. http://www.iso.org/iso/en/iso9000-14000/index.html (accessed 26 August 2005).

15 INK (Instituut Nederlandse Kwaliteit / Netherlands Quality Institute). www.ink.nl (accessed 8 August 2005).

16 NIAZ (Nederlands Instituut voor Accreditatie van Ziekenhuizen / Netherlands Institute for Accreditation of Hospitals). http://www.niaz.nl (accessed 8 August 2005).

17 RdGG (Reinier de Graaf Groep). *Annual Quality Report* [Kwaliteitsjaarverslag]. Delft: RdGG; 2003.

18 IOM (Institute of Medicine). *Crossing the Quality Chasm: a new health system for the 21st century*. Washington, DC: National Academy Press; 2001.

19 Schein EH. *Organizational Culture and Leadership*. San Francisco: Jossey-Bass; 1992.

20 RdGG (Reinier de Graaf Groep) and Kwaliteitsinstituut voor de Gezondheidszorg CBO. *Pursuing Perfection: raising the bar for healthcare performance*. Utrecht: CBO; 2005

21 Bredenhoff E, Schuring S, Caljouw R. Zorg in focus: op zoek naar routine in het zorgproces. *Medisch Contact*. 2004; **59**(34): 1304–8.

22 RdGG (Reinier de Graaf Groep). http://www.rdgg.nl (accessed 10 March 2005).

23 Hodgson RC, Levinson DJ, Zaleznik A. *The Executive Role Constellation*. Boston: Harvard Business School Press; 1965.

24 Kotter JP. *Leading Change*. Boston: Harvard Business School; 1996.

25 Detert J, Schroeder RG, Mauriel JJ. A framework for linking culture and improvement initiatives in organizations. *Academy of Management Review*. 2000; **25**(4): 850–63.

26 Weber V, Joshi M. Effecting and leading change in healthcare organizations. *Joint Commission Journal of Quality Improvement*. 2000; **26**(7): 388–99.

27 Llewellan S. Two-way windows: clinicians as medical managers. *Organization Studies*. 2001; **22**(4): 593–623.

28 Mohr JJ, Batalden PB. Improving safety on the front lines: the role of clinical managers. *Quality and Safety in Healthcare*. 2002; **11**(1): 41–50.

29 Garside P. Organizational context for quality. *Quality in Healthcare*. 1998; **7**: S8–S15.

30 RdGG (Reinier de Graaf Groep). *Annual Quality Report* [Kwaliteitsjaarverslag]. Delft: RdGG; 2001.

31 Krantz J. Lessons from the field: an essay on the crisis of leadership in contemporary organizations. *Journal of Applied Behavioral Science*. 1990; **26**(1): 49–64.

Notes to Chapter 6

1 Trist EL, Bamforth KW. Some social and psychological consequences of long-wall methods of coal getting. *Human Relations*. 1951; **4**: 3–38.

2 Emery FE, Trist EL. Sociotechnical systems. In: Emery FE, editor. *Systems Thinking*. London: Penguin Books; 1969.

3 Trist E. *The Evolution of Socio-Technical Systems: a conceptual framework and an action research programme*. Ontario: Ontario Quality of Working Life Centre; 1981.

4 Trist E. The sociotechnical perspective: the evolution of sociotechnical systems as a conceptual framework and as an action research program. In: Van de Ven AH, Joyce WF, editors. *Perspectives on Organization Design and Behavior*. New York: Wiley-Interscience; 1981.

5 Pasmore WA. Social science transformed: the socio-technical perspective. *Human Relations*. 1995; **48**(1): 1–22.

6 Fox WM. Sociotechnical system principles and guidelines: past and present. *Journal of Applied Behavioral Science*. 1995; **31**(1): 91–105.

7 Beekun RI. Assessing the effectiveness of sociotechnical interventions: antidote or fad? *Human Relations*. 1989; **42**(10): 877–97.

8 Cherns A. The principles of sociotechnical design. *Human Relations*. 1976; **9**(8): 783–92.

9 Cherns A. Principles of sociotechnical design revisited. *Human Relations.* 1987; **40**(3): 153–62.

10 Torraco RJ. Work design theory: a review and critique with implications for human resource development. *Human Resource Development Quarterly.* 2005; **16**(1): 85–109.

11 Stoelwinder JU, Clayton PS. Hospital organization development: changing the focus from 'better management' to 'better patient care'. *Journal of Applied Behavioral Science.* 1978; **14**(3): 400–14.

12 Pasmore W, Petee J, Bastian R. Sociotechnical systems in healthcare: a field experiment. *Journal of Applied Behavioral Science.* 1986; **22**(3): 329–39.

13 Tonges MC. Work designs: sociotechnical systems for patient care delivery. *Nursing Management.* 1992; **23**(1): 27–32.

14 Chisholm RF, Ziegenfuss JT. A review of applications of the sociotechnical systems approach to healthcare organizations. *Journal of Applied Behavioral Science.* 1986; **22**(3): 315–27.

15 Weisbord MR. Why organization development hasn't worked (so far) in medical centers. *Healthcare Management Review.* 1976; **1**(2): 17–38.

16 Begun JW, Zimmerman B, Dooley KJ. Healthcare organizations as complex adaptive systems. In: Mick SS, Wyttenbach ME, editors. *Advances in Healthcare Organization Theory.* San Francisco: Jossey-Bass; 2003.

17 McDaniel RR. A view from complexity science. *Frontiers of Health Service Management.* 1999; **16**(1): 44–8; 49–50.

18 Niepce W, Molleman E. Work design issues in Lean Production from a sociotechnical systems perspective: Neo-Taylorism or the next step in sociotechnical design. *Human Relations.* 1998; **51**(3): 259–87.

19 Liu G, Shah R, Schroeder RG. Linking work design to mass customisation: a sociotechnical systems perspective. *Decision Sciences.* 2006; **37**(4): 519–45.

20 Persico J, McLean GN. The evolving merger of socio-technical systems and quality improvement theories. *Human Systems Management.* 1994; **13**(1): 11–18.

21 Stinchcombe A. Social structure and organizations. In: March JG, editor. *Handbook of Organizations.* Chicago: Rand McNally; 1965.

22 Bazzoli GJ, Chan B, Shortell SM, *et al.* The financial performance of hospitals belonging to health networks and systems. *Inquiry.* 2000; **37**(3): 234–52.

23 Shortell SM, Gillies RR, Anderson DA. The new world of managed care: creating organized delivery systems. *Health Affairs.* 1994; **13**(5): 46–64.

24 Burns LR, Gimm G, Nicholson S. The financial performance of integrated health organizations. *Journal of Healthcare Management.* 2005; **50**(3): 191–212.

25 Cheng JLC, Kesner IF. Organizational slack and response to environmental shifts: the impact of resource allocation patterns. *Journal of Management.* 1997; **23**: 1–18.

26 Greenhalgh T, Robert G, Bate P, *et al. Diffusion of Innovations in Health Service Organizations: a systematic literature review.* Oxford: Blackwell; 2005.

27 Bourgeois LJ III. On the measurement of organizational slack. *Academy of Management Review.* 1981; **6**: 29–39.

28 Lawson MB. In praise of slack: time is of the essence. *Academy of Management Executive.* 2001; **15**(3): 125–35.

29 Rogers E. *Diffusion of Innovations.* New York: Free Press; 1995.

30 Pava C. Redesigning sociotechnical systems design: concepts and methods for the 1990s. *Journal of Applied Behavioral Science.* 1986; **22**: 202–21.

31 AHA (American Hospital Association). *Fast Facts on US Hospitals* [updated 20 October 2006]. AHA Resource Center: Chicago; 2006.

Notes to Chapter 7

1 Feldman MS, Khademian AM. Empowerment and cascading vitality. In: Cameron KS, Dutton JE, Quinn RE, editors. *Positive Organizational Scholarship: foundations of a new discipline.* Berrett-Koehler: San Francisco; 2003.

2 Koberg CS, Boss W, Senjam JC, *et al.* Antecedents and outcomes of empowerment: empirical evidence from the healthcare industry. *Group and Organization Management.* 1999; **34**(1): 71–91.

3 Connor DR. *Leading at the Edge of Chaos: how to create the nimble organization.* San Francisco: John Wiley; 1998.

4 Blanchard KH, Carlos JP, Randolph WA. *The Empowerment Barometer and Action Plan.* Escondido, CA: Blanchard Training and Development; 1995.

5 Conger JA. Motivate performance through empowering. In: Locke EA, editor. *The Blackwell Handbook of Principles of Organizational Behavior.* Oxford: Blackwell Publishing; 2004.

6 Quinn RE, Spreitzer GM. The road to empowerment: seven questions every leader should consider. *Organizational Dynamics.* 1997; **26**(2): 37–49.

7 Conger JA, Kanungo RN. The empowerment process: integrating theory and practice. *Academy of Management Review.* 1988; **13**(3): 471–82.

8 McClelland DC. *Power: the inner experience.* New York: Harper; 1975.

9 Quinn RE. *Deep Change: discovering the leader within.* San Francisco: Jossey-Bass; 1996.

10 Seibert SE, Silver SR, Randolph WA. Taking empowerment to the next level: a multiple-level model of empowerment, performance and satisfaction. *Academy of Management Journal*. 2004; **47**(3): 332–49.

11 Spreitzer G. Psychological empowerment in the workplace: dimensions, measurement and validation. *Academy of Management Journal*. 1995; **38**(5): 1442–65.

12 Spreitzer G. Social structural antecedents of workplace empowerment. *Academy of Management Journal*. 1996; **39**(2): 483–504.

13 Adler PS, Kwon S-W, Singer JMK. *The 'Six-West' Problem: professionals and the intraorganizational diffusion of innovations, with particular reference to the case of hospitals*. Working paper 3–15. Marshall School of Business, University of Southern California; 2003. Full text available at: http://www.marshall.usc.edu/web/MOR.cfm?doc id=5561.

14 Spreitzer GM, Doneson D. Musings on the past and future of employee empowerment. In: Cummings T, editor. *Handbook of Organizational Development*. Thousand Oaks, CA: Sage; 2005.

15 Liden RC, Arad S. A power perspective of empowerment and work groups: implications for human resources management research. *Research in Personnel and Human Resources Management*. 1996; **14**: 205–51.

16 Randolph WA. Navigating the journey to empowerment. *Organizational Dynamics*. 1995; **24**(4): 19–32.

17 Manz CC, Sims HP Jr. *SuperLeadership: leading others to lead themselves*. New York: Prentice-Hall Press; 1989.

18 Weiss JW. *Organizational Behavior and Change*. St Paul, MN: West; 1996.

19 McDonald R. Individual identity and organizational control: empowerment and modernisation in a primary care trust. *Sociology of Health and Illness*. 2004; **26**(7): 925–50.

20 Bate SP. *Strategies for Cultural Change*. Oxford: Butterworth-Heinemann; 1995.

21 Commission for Health Improvement. *Report of a Clinical Governance Review at Peterborough Hospitals NHS Trust*. London: The Stationery Office; 2002.

22 Cook J, Wall T. New work and attitude measures of trust, organizational commitment, and personal needs fulfilment. *Journal of Occupational Psychology*. 1980; **53**: 39–52.

23 Firth-Cozens J. Organizational trust: the keystone to patient safety. *Quality and Safety in Healthcare*. 2004; **13**: 56–61.

24 Wall T, Jackson P, Davids K. Operator work design and robotics systems performance: a serendipitous field study. *Journal of Applied Psychology*. 1992; **77**: 353–62.

25 Prasad A. Understanding workplace empowerment as inclusion. *Journal of Applied Behavioral Science*. 2001; **37**(1): 51–69.

26 Hammer M, Champy J. *Re-engineering the Corporation: a manifesto for business revolution*. New York: Harper Business; 1993.

27 Probert D, Stevenson B, Tang NKH, *et al*. The introduction of patient process re-engineering in the Peterborough Hospitals NHS Trust. *Journal of Management in Medicine*. 1999; **13**(5): 308–24.

28 Banks CJ. *The Peterborough Hospitals NHS Trust Transformation Project: are we tinkering at the edges?* MSc dissertation. Sheffield Hallam University; 1999.

29 Locock L. *Maps and Journeys: redesign in the NHS*. Birmingham: Health Services Management Centre, University of Birmingham; 2001.

30 Mintzberg, H. *Power in and Around Organizations*. New Jersey: Prentice Hall; 1983.

31 Quinn JB. *Intelligent Enterprise: a knowledge and service based paradigm for industry*. New York: Free Press; 1992.

32 Child J. *Organization: contemporary principles and practice*. Oxford: Blackwell; 2005.

33 Connor DR. *Managing at the Speed of Change*. New York: Villard Books; 1992.

34 Kanter R. *The Change Masters*. New York: Simon and Schuster; 1983.

35 Greenhalgh T, Robert G, Bate P, *et al*. *Diffusion of Innovations in Health Service Organizations: a systematic literature review*. Oxford: Blackwell; 2005.

36 Dunphy DC, Stace DA. Transformational and coercive strategies for planned organizational change: beyond the OD model. *Organization Studies*. 1988; **9**(3): 317–34.

37 Newell S, Scarborough H, Swan J, *et al*. The importance of process knowledge for cross project learning: evidence from a UK hospital. *Proceedings of the 35th Hawaii International Conference on System Sciences*. Big Island, HI: HICSS; 2002.

38 Wrzesniewski A, Dutton JE. Crafting a job: revisioning employees as active crafters of their work. *Academy of Management Review*. 2001; **25**(2): 179–201.

Notes to Chapter 8

1 Ferlie EB, Shortell SM. Improving the quality of healthcare in the United Kingdom and the United States: a framework for change. *Milbank Quarterly*. 2001; **79**(2): 281–315.

2 Pfeffer J. *The Human Equation*. Boston: Harvard Business School Press; 1998.

3 Ayanian JZ, Guadagnoli E, McNeil BJ, *et al*. Treatment and outcomes of acute myocardial infarction among patients of cardiologists and generalist physicians. *Archives of Internal Medicine*. 1997; **157**(22): 2570–6.

4 Reinertsen JL. Physicians as leaders in the improvement of healthcare systems. *Annals of Internal Medicine*. 1998; **128**(10): 833–8.

5 Appelbaum E, Batt R. *The New American Workplace: transforming work systems in the United States.* Ithaca, NY: ILR Press; 1994.

6 Brown P, Zavestoski S, McCormick S, *et al.* Embodied health movements: new approaches to social movements in health. *Sociology of Health and Illness.* 2004; **26**(1): 50–80.

7 Epstein S. *Impure Science: AIDS, activism, and the politics of knowledge.* Berkeley: University of California; 1996.

8 Davis GF, McAdam D, Scott WR *et al.,* editors. *Social Movements and Organization Theory.* New York: Cambridge University Press; 2005.

9 Bate SP, Robert G, Bevan H. The next phase of healthcare improvement: what can we learn from social movements? *Quality and Safety in Healthcare.* 2004; **13**(1): 62–6.

10 McCarthy JD, Zald MN. Resource mobilization and social movements: a partial theory. *American Journal of Sociology.* 1977; **82**(6): 1212–41.

11 McCarthy JD, Zald MN. The enduring vitality of the resource mobilization theory of social movements. In: Turner JH, editor. *Handbook of Sociological Theory.* New York: Kluwer Academic/Plenum; 2001.

12 Bodenheimer T, Wagner EH, Grumbach K. Improving primary care for patients with chronic illness: the chronic care model, Part 2. *Journal of the American Medical Association.* 2002; **288**(15): 1909–14.

13 Berwick DM. A primer on leading the improvement of systems. *British Medical Journal.* 1996; **312**(7031): 619–22.

14 Langley GJ, Nolan KM, Norman CL, *et al. The Improvement Guide.* San Francisco: Jossey-Bass; 1996.

15 Wilson T, Berwick DM, Cleary PD. What do collaborative improvement projects do?: experience from seven countries. *Joint Commission Journal on Quality and Safety.* 2003; **29**(2): 85–93.

16 della Porta D, Diani M. *Social Movements: an introduction.* Malden, MA: Blackwell; 1999.

17 Scott WR. *Organizations: rational, natural, and open systems.* Upper Saddle River, NJ: Prentice Hall; 2002.

18 Ward DE. *The AmFAR AIDS Handbook: the complete guide to understanding HIV and AIDS.* New York: WW Norton and Company Inc; 1999.

19 Goodwin J, Jasper JM, Poletta F, editors. *Passionate Politics: emotions and social movements.* Chicago: University of Chicago Press; 2001.

20 Bennett L, Ross MW, Sunderland R. The relationship between recognition, rewards and burnout in AIDS caring. *AIDS Care.* 1996; **8**(2): 145–53.

21 Haviland ML, Healton CG, Weinberg GS. Delivering HIV/AIDS services: the professional care provider speaks out. *American Journal of Preventive Medicine.* 1997; **13**(6 Suppl): 12–18.

22 d'Oronzio JC. A human right to healthcare access: returning to the origins of the patients' rights movement. *Cambridge Quarterly of Healthcare Ethics.* 2001; **10**(3): 285–98.

23 Bury M. The sociology of chronic illness. *Sociology of Health and Illness.* 1991; **13**: 451–68.

24 Llewellyn S. Two-way windows: clinicians as medical managers. *Organization Studies.* 2001; **22**(4): 593–623.

25 Greenhalgh T, Robert G, McFarlane F, *et al.* Diffusion of innovations in service organizations: systematic review and recommendations. *Milbank Quarterly.* 2004; **82**(4): 581–629.

26 Katz MH, Cunningham WE, Fleishman JA, *et al.* Effect of case management on unmet needs and utilization of medical care and medications among HIV-infected persons. *Annals of Internal Medicine.* 2001; **135**(8 Pt 1): 557–65.

27 Shortell SM, O'Brien JL, Carman JM, *et al.* Assessing the impact of continuous quality improvement / total quality management: concept versus implementation. *Health Services Research.* 1995; **30**(2): 377–401.

28 Quinn RE, Kimberly JR. *Managing Organizational Transitions.* Homewood, IL: Dow Jones-Irwin; 1984.

29 Kaluzny A, McLaughlin C. Managing transitions: assuring the adoption and impact of TQM. *Quality Review Bulletin.* 1992; **18**(11): 380–4.

30 Wagner EH, Austin BT, Van Korff M. Organizing care for patients with chronic illness. *Milbank Quarterly.* 1996; **74**(4): 511–44.

31 Gifford AL, Sengupta S. Self-management health education for chronic HIV infection. *AIDS Care.* 1999; **11**(1): 115–30.

32 Benford RB, Snow DA. Framing processes and social movements: an overview and assessment. *Annual Review of Sociology.* 2000; **26**: 611–39.

33 McAdam D, McCarthy JD, Zald MN. Introduction: opportunities, mobilizing structures, and framing processes: toward a synthetic, comparative perspective on social movements. In: McAdam D, McCarthy JD, Zald MN, editors. *Comparative Perspectives on Social Movements: political opportunities, mobilizing structures, and cultural framings.* Cambridge: Cambridge University Press; 1996.

34 Øvretveit J, Bate P, Cleary P, *et al.* Quality collaboratives: lessons from research. *Quality and Safety in Healthcare.* 2002; **11**: 345–51.

35 Øvretveit J, Gustafson D. Evaluation of quality improvement programmes. *Quality and Safety in Healthcare.* 2002; **11**(3): 270–5.

36 Petchey R, Williams J, Farnsworth B, *et al.* A tale of two (low prevalence) cities: social movement organizations and the local policy response to HIV/AIDS. *Social Science and Medicine.* 1998; **47**(9): 1197–208.

37 Clemens ES, Minkoff DC. Beyond the Iron Law: rethinking the place of organizations in social movement research. In: Snow DA, Soule SA, Kriesi H, editors. *The Blackwell Companion to Social Movements.* Malden, MA: Blackwell; 2004.

38 Michels R. *Political Parties: a sociological study of the oligarchical tendencies of modern democracy*. New York: Free Press; 1962 [1911].

39 Weick KE. Educational organizations as loosely coupled systems. *Administrative Science Quarterly*. 1976; **21**: 1–19.

40 Orton JD, Weick KE. Loosely coupled systems: a reconceptualization. *Academy of Management Review*. 1990; **15**: 203–23.

41 Denis J.-L, Lamothe L, Langley A. The dynamics of collective leadership and strategic change in pluralistic organizations. *Academy of Management Journal*. 2001; **44**(4): 809–37.

42 Scott WR. Conflicting levels of rationality: regulators, managers and professionals in the medical care sector. *Journal of Health Administration Education*. 1985; **3**(part 2): 113–31.

Notes to Chapter 9

1 Kluckhohn FR, Strodtbeck FL. *Variations in Value Orientations*. New York: Row, Peterson; 1961.

2 Bate SP. The impact of organizational culture on approaches to organizational problem-solving. *Organization Studies*. 1984; **5**(1): 43–66.

3 Øvretveit J, Aslaksen A. *The Quality Journey of Six Norwegian Hospitals: an action evaluation*. Oslo: The Norwegian Medical Association; 1999.

4 Nelson LA. A case study in organizational change: implications for theory. *The Learning Organization*. 2003; **10**: 18–30.

5 Gouldner A. *Patterns of Industrial Bureaucracy*. New York: Free Press; 1954.

6 Powell WW, Di Maggio PJ. *The New Institutionalism in Organizational Analysis*. Chicago: University of Chicago Press; 1991.

7 Meyer JW, Rowan B. Institutionalized organizations: formal structure as myth and ceremony. In: Powell WW, DiMaggio PJ, editors. *The New Institutionalism in Organizational Analysis*. Chicago: University of Chicago Press; 1991.

8 Scott WR. *Institutions and Organizations*, 2nd ed. Thousands Oaks, CA: Sage; 2001.

9 Scott WR, Ruef M, Mendel P, *et al. Institutional Change and Healthcare Organizations: from professional dominance to managed care*. Chicago: University of Chicago Press; 2000.

10 Smelser N. *Theory of Collective Behavior*. London: Routledge and Kegan Paul; 1962.

11 McAdam, D, McCarthy JD, Zald MN. Introduction: opportunities, mobilizing structures, and framing processes – toward a synthetic, comparative perspective on social movements. In: McAdam D, McCarthy JD, Zald MN, editors. *Comparative Perspectives on Social Movements: political opportunities, mobilizing structures, and cultural framings*. Cambridge: Cambridge University Press; 1996.

12 Pettigrew A, Ferlie E, McKee L. *Shaping Strategic Change*. London: Sage; 1992.

13 Institute of Medicine. *To Err is Human: building a safer health system*. Washington, DC: National Academy Press; 2000.

14 Institute of Medicine. *Crossing the Quality Chasm: a new health system for the 21st century*, Washington, DC: National Academy Press; 2001.

15 de Caluwé L, Vermaak H. *Learning to Change: a guide for organizational change agents*. London: Sage; 2003.

16 Bate SP, Robert G, Bevan H. The next phase of healthcare improvement: what can we learn from social movements? *Quality and Safety in Healthcare*. 2004; **13**(1): 62–6.

17 Kelman S. *Unleashing Change: a study of renewal in government*. Washington, DC: Brookings Institution Press; 2005.

18 Stensakar IG, Langley A. Change management matters?: a political perspective on change processes and outcomes. Paper prepared for Academy of Management Conference, January 2005.

19 Bate SP. *Strategies for Cultural Change*. Oxford: Butterworth-Heinemann; 1994.

20 Kotter JP. *Leading Change*. Boston, MA: Harvard Business School Press; 1996.

21 Kotter JP. *The Heart of Change: real-life stories of how people change their organizations*. Boston, MA: Harvard Business School Press; 2002.

22 Weick KE. The significance of corporate culture. In: Frost PJ, Moore LF, Louis MR, *et al.*, editors. *Organizational Culture*. Beverly Hills, CA: Sage; 1985.

23 Wilkins AL. *Developing Corporate Character. how to successfully change an organization without destroying it*. San Francisco, CA: Jossey-Bass; 1989.

24 Bate SP, Robert G. *Bringing User Experience to Healthcare Improvement: the concepts, methods and practices of experience-based design*. Oxford: Radcliffe Publishing; 2007.

Notes to Chapter 10

1 Meyer JA, Silow-Carroll S, Kutyla T, *et al. Hospital Quality: ingredients for success – overview and lessons learnt*. New York: The Commonwealth Fund; 2004.

2 Whelan-Berry KS, Gordon JR, Hinings CR. Strengthening organizational change processes: recommendations and implications from a multilevel analysis. *Journal of Applied Behavioral Science*. 2003; **39**(2): 186–207.

3 Strickland F. *The Dynamics of Change*. London: Routledge; 1998.

4 Morgan G. *Images of Organization*. London: Sage; 1986.

5 The first Organization Studies summer workshop on 'Theorizing process in organizational research'. *Organization Studies*. 2005; **26**(1): 157–9.

6 Sandelands L, Drazin, R. On the language of organization theory. *Organization Studies*. 1989; **10/4**: 457–8.

7 McGlynn EA, Asch SM, Adams J, *et al*. The quality of healthcare delivered to adults in the United States. *New England Journal of Medicine*, 2003; **348**(26): 2635–45.

8 Anderson RA, Crabtree BF, Steele DJ, *et al*. Case study research: the view from complexity sciences. *Qualitative Health Research*. 2005; **15**(5): 669–85.

9 Corning PA. *The Synergism Hypothesis: a theory of progressive evolution*. New York: McGraw Hill; 1983.

10 Corning PA. Synergy and self-organization in the evolution of complex systems. *Systems Research*. 1995; **12**(2): 89–121.

11 Pettigrew AM, Woodman, RW, Cameron K. Studying organizational change and development: challenges for future research. *Academy of Management Journal*. 2001; **44**(4): 697–713.

12 Helms Mills J. *Making Sense of Organizational Change*. London: Routledge; 2003.

13 Greenhalgh T, Robert G, Bate SP, *et al*. *Diffusion of Innovations in Health Service Organizations*. Oxford: Blackwell; 2005.

14 Kelman S. *Unleashing Change: a study of renewal in government*. Washington, DC: Brookings Institution Press; 2005.

15 Masuch M. Vicious circles in organizations. *Administrative Science Quarterly*. 1985; **30**: 14–33.

16 Perlow LA, Gittell JH, Katz N. Contextualising patterns of work group interaction: towards a nested theory of structuration. *Organization Science*. 2004; **15**(5): 520–36.

17 Langley A. Strategies for theorizing from process data. *Academy of Management Review*. 1999; **24**(4): 691–710.

18 Luke DA, Harris JK. Network analysis in public health: history, methods, and applications. *Annual Review of Public Health*. 2007; **28**: 69–73.

19 Scott J. *Social Network Analysis: a handbook*. 2nd edition. London: Sage; 2000.

20 Wasserman S, Faust K. *Social Network Analysis: methods and applications*. Cambridge: Cambridge University Press; 1994.

21 Ryan G. 'What do sequential behavioral patterns suggest about the medical decision-making process?': modelling home case management of acute illnesses in a rural Cameroonian village. *Social Science and Medicine*. 1998; **46**(2): 209–25.

22 Meredith LS, Mendel P, Pearson M, *et al*. Implementation and maintenance of quality improvement for treating depression in primary care. *Psychiatric Services*. 2006; **57**: 48–55.

23 Miles MB, Huberman AM. *Qualitative Data Analysis*. Newbury Park, CA: Sage; 1994.

24 Langley A, Truax J. A process study of new technology adoption in smaller manufacturing firms. *Journal of Management Studies*. 1994; **31**: 619–52.

25 Borgatti SP, Everett, MG, Freeman LC. *Ucinet 6 for Windows: software for social network analysis* (Version 6.29). Boston: Analytic Technologies; 2002.

26 Borgatti, SP. 2002. *NetDraw: network visualization software* (Version 1.0.0.21). Boston: Analytic Technologies; 2002.

27 de Nooy W, Mrvar A, Batageli V. *Exploratory Social Network Analysis with Pajek*. New York: Cambridge University Press; 2005.

28 Weick KE. *The Social Psychology of Organizing*. Reading, MA: Addison-Wesley; 1979.

29 van Aken JE. Design science and organization development interventions. *Journal of Applied Behavioral Sciences*. 2007; **43**(1): 67–88.

30 Adler PS, Riley P, Kwon S-K, *et al*. Performance improvement capability: keys to accelerating performance improvement in hospitals. *California Management Review*. 2003; **45**(2): 12–33.

31 Kanter RM. *The Change Masters*. New York: Simon and Schuster; 1983.

32 Beckhard R, Pritchard W. *Changing the Essence: the art of creating and leading fundamental change in organizations*. San Francisco, CA: Jossey-Bass; 1992.

33 Senge P. *The Fifth Discipline*. New York: Doubleday; 1990.

34 Watson JG, Korukonda AR. The TQM jungle: a dialectical analysis. *International Journal of Quality and Reliability Management*. 1995; **12**(9): 100–9.

35 Bate SP, Khan R, Pye A. Towards a culturally sensitive approach to organization structuring: where organization design meets organization development. *Organization Science*. 2000: 11(2): 197–211.

36 Chaudry B, Wang J, Wu S, *et al*. Systematic review: impact of health information technology on quality, efficiency, and costs of medical care. *Annals of Internal Medicine*. 2006; **144**: E12–E22.

37 Lorenzi NM, Riley RT, Blyth AJC, *et al*. Antecedents of the people and organizational aspects of medical informatics: review of the literature. *Journal of the American Medical Informatics Association*. 1997; **4**: 79–93.

38 Aarts J, Peel V, Wright G. Organizational issues in health informatics: a model approach. *International Journal of Medical Informatics*. 1998; **52**: 235–42.

39 Poulymenakou A, Holmes A. A contingency framework for the investigation of information systems failure. *European Journal of Information Systems*. 1996; **5**: 34–46.

40 Bruch H, Ghoshal S. Unleashing organizational energy. *MIT Sloan Management Review.* 2003; **45**(1): 45–51.
41 Eisenhardt KM. Building theories from case study research. *Academy of Management Review.* 1989; **14**(4): 532–50.

Notes to Chapter 11

1 Bate SP. The role of stories and storytelling in organizational change efforts. *Intervention Research: International Journal on Culture, Organization and Management.* 2004; **1**(1): 27–42.
2 Bate SP. The role of stories and storytelling in organizational change efforts: a field study of an emerging community of practice within the UK National Health Service. In: Hurwitz B, Greenhalgh T, Skultans V, editors. *Narrative Research in Health and Illness.* London: BMJ Publications; 2004.
3 Marshak RJ. Managing the metaphors of change. *Organizational Dynamics.* 1993; **22**(1): 44–56.
4 Inns D. Organization development as a journey. In: Oswick C, Grant D, editors. *Organization Development: metaphorical explorations.* London: Pitman; 1996.
5 Pettigrew AM. Success and failure in corporate transformation initiatives. In: Galliers RD, Baets WRJ, editors. *Information Technology and Organizational Transformation: innovation for the 21st century organization.* Wiley: Chichester; 1998.
6 Weick KE. The generative properties of richness. *Academy of Management Journal.* 2007; **50**(1): 14–19.
7 Whelan-Berry KS, Gordon JR, Hinings CR. Strengthening organizational change processes: recommendations and implications from a multilevel analysis. *Journal of Applied Behavioral Science.* 2003; **39**(2): 186–207.
8 Pirsig RM. *Zen and the Art of Motorcycle Maintenance.* London: Vintage; 1974.
9 Detert JR, Schroeder RG, Mauriel JJ. A framework for linking culture and improvement initiatives in organizations. *Academy of Management Review.* 2000: **25**(4); 850–63.
10 Kanter RM, Stein BA, Jick TD. *The Challenge of Organizational Change: how people experience it and manage it.* New York: The Free Press; 1992.
11 Weick KE. *Making Sense of the Organization.* Oxford: Blackwell; 2001.
12 Waterman RH. *The Renewal Factor.* London: Bantam; 1987.
13 Collins J. *Good to Great: why some companies make the leap . . . and others don't.* New York: HarperBusiness; 2001.
14 Collins J. The 10 greatest CEOs of all time. *Future.* July 21 2003.
15 Schaffer RH, Thomson HA. Successful change programs begin with results. *Harvard Business Review*, January/February 1992: 80–89.
16 Schaffer RH, McCreight MK. Build your own change model. *Business Horizons.* **47**(3): 33–8.
17 Fay B. Critical realism? *Journal for the Theory of Social Behavior.* 1990; **20**: 33–41.
18 McGlynn EA, Asch SM, Adams J, *et al.* The quality of healthcare delivered to adults in the United States. *New England Journal of Medicine.* 2003; **348**(26): 2635–45.
19 Eisenhardt KM. Building theories from case study research. *Academy of Management Review.* 1989; **14**(4): 532–50.
20 Huy QN. Emotional capability, emotional intelligence and radical change. *Academy of Management Review.* 1999; **24**(2): 325–45.
21 Mohr JJ, Batalden PB. Improving safety on the front lines: the role of clinical micro-systems. *Quality and Safety in Healthcare.* 2002; **11**: 45–50.
22 Nelson EC, Batalden PB, Huber TP, *et al.* Micro-systems in healthcare: part 1. Learning from high-performing frontline clinical units. *The Joint Commission.* 2002; September: 472–91.
23 Dawson P, Buchanan D. The way it really happened: competing narratives in the political process of technological change. *Human Relations.* 2005; **58**: 845–65.
24 House R, Rousseau DM, Thomas-Hunt M. The meso-paradigm: a framework for the integration of micro and macro organizational behavior. *Research in Organizational Behavior*, 1995; **17**: 71–114.
25 Bartunek J, Borgatti S. Front and backstage processes of an organizational restructuring effort. *Journal of Applied Behavioral Science.* 2003; **39**(3): 243–58.
26 Langley A. Strategies for theorizing from process data. *Academy of Management Review.* 1999; **24**(4): 691–710.
27 Thorngate W. Possible limits on a science of social behavior. In: Strickland JH, Aboud FE, Gergen KJ, editors. *Social Psychology in Transition.* New York: Plenum; 1976.
28 Weick KE. *The Social Psychology of Organizing.* Reading, MA: Addison-Wesley; 1979.

Index

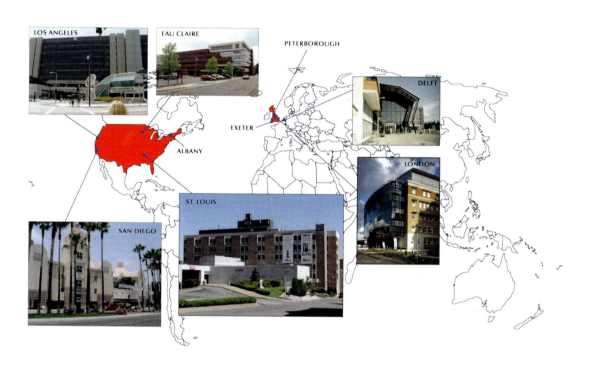

FIGURE A Map of case study sites

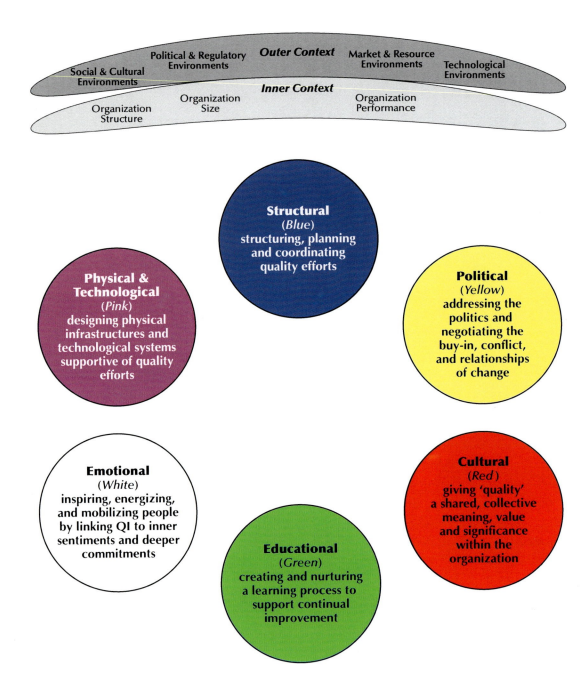

FIGURE 9.1 Organizing for quality in healthcare: the six universal challenges

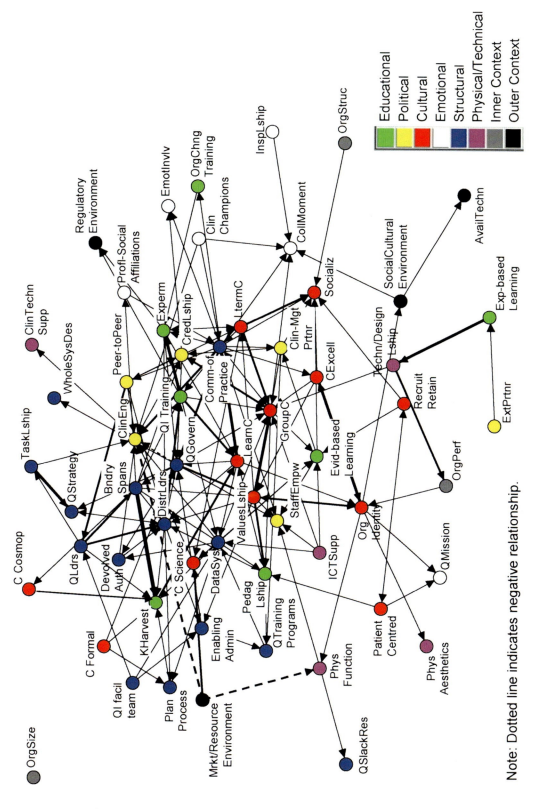

FIGURE 10.1 Cedars-Sinai 'detailed' sub-process map

Note: Dotted line indicates negative relationship.

Educational
Political
Cultural
Emotional
Structural
Physical/Technical
Inner Context
Outer Context

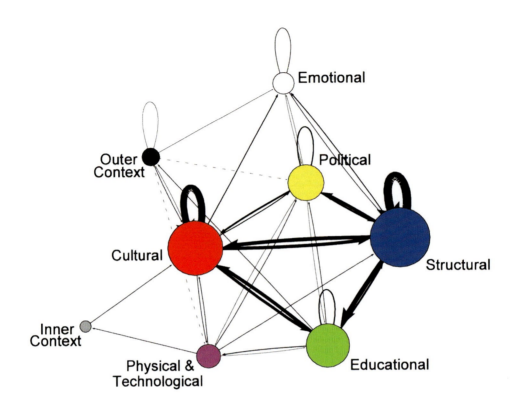

Process	Total Sub-Process Ties (#)	W/in process (%)	IN-ties (%)	OUT-ties (%)	Most Central Sub-Processes
Structural	100	31%	24%	45%	Communities-of-Practice, Quality governance systems, Distributed leadership, Boundary-spanner roles, Data and monitoring systems
Cultural	85	28%	40%	32%	Group culture, Values/symbolic leadership, Culture of learning, Organizational identity
Educational	54	7%	52%	41%	QI training, Knowledge harvesting
Political	37	11%	54%	35%	
Emotional	13	15%	62%	23%	
Physical & Technical	16	0%	44%	56%	
Outer Context	9	11%	33%	56%	
Inner Context	4	0%	50%	50%	

FIGURE 10.2 Cedars-Sinai 'high level' process map

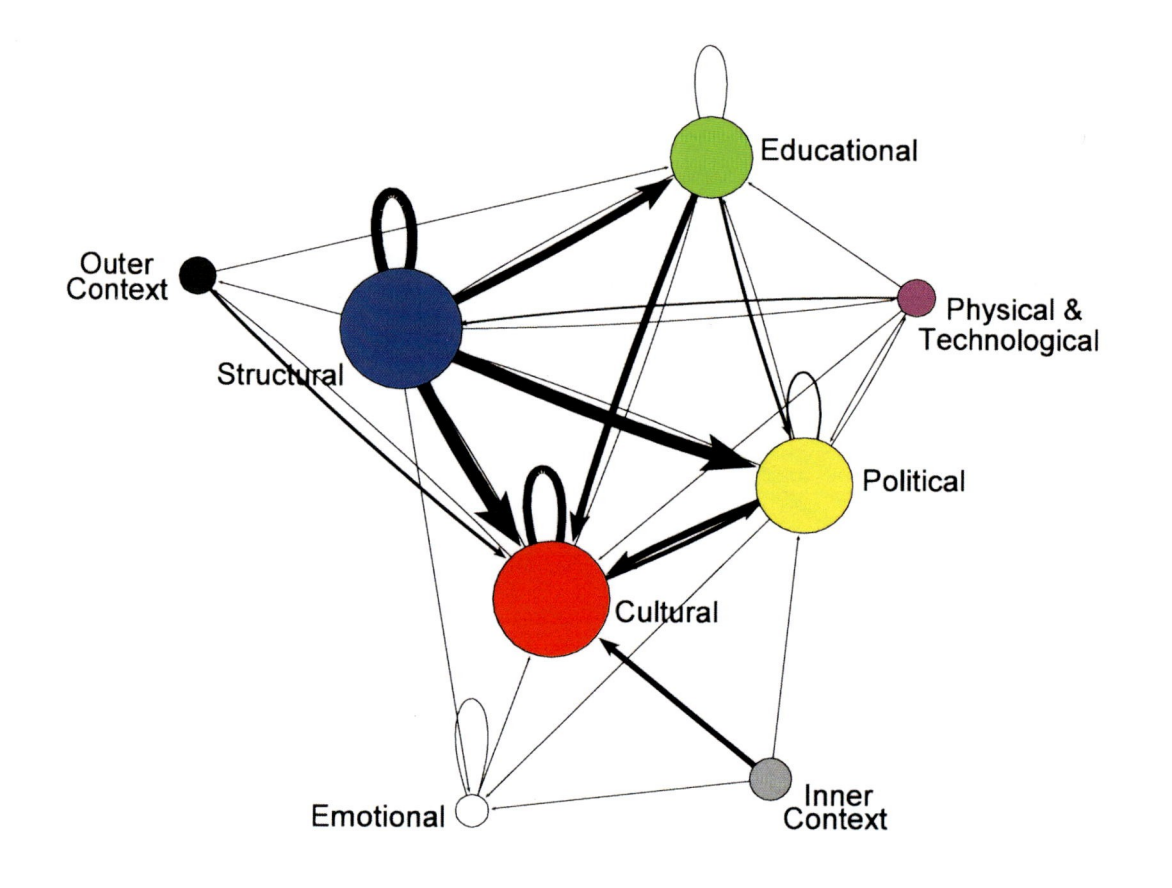

Process	Total Sub-Process Ties (#)	W/in process (%)	IN-ties (%)	OUT-ties (%)	Most Central Sub-Processes
Structural	83	19%	8%	72%	QI facilitating team, Decentralized authority system
Cultural	77	16%	73%	12%	Culture of empowerment, Group culture
Political	52	6%	63%	31%	Empowering staff
Educational	38	5%	50%	45%	Experimental & pilots
Inner Context	10	0%	0%	100%	
Outer Context	8	0%	38%	63%	
Physical & Technical	8	0%	25%	75%	
Emotional	6	17%	67%	17%	

FIGURE 10.3 Peterborough 'high level' process map

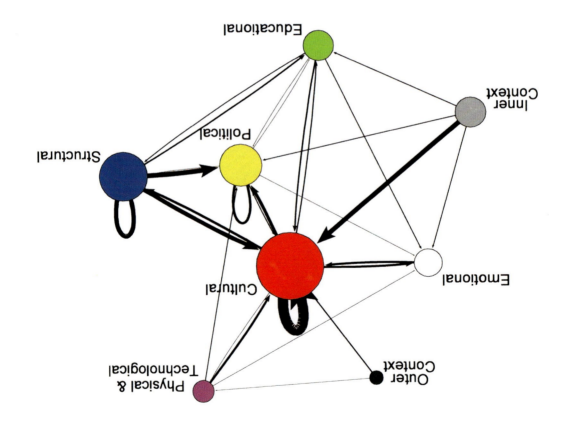

Process	Total Sub-Process Ties (#)	W/in process (%)	IN-ties (%)	OUT-ties (%)	Most Central Sub-Processes
Cultural	93	30%	46%	24%	Organizational identity, Group culture
Structural	49	24%	18%	57%	
Political	36	17%	69%	14%	
Educational	19	0%	53%	47%	
Inner Context	19	0%	0%	100%	
Emotional	16	0%	69%	31%	
Physical & Technical	10	0%	20%	80%	
Outer Context	4	0%	0%	100%	

FIGURE 10.4 Royal Devon and Exeter 'high level' process map

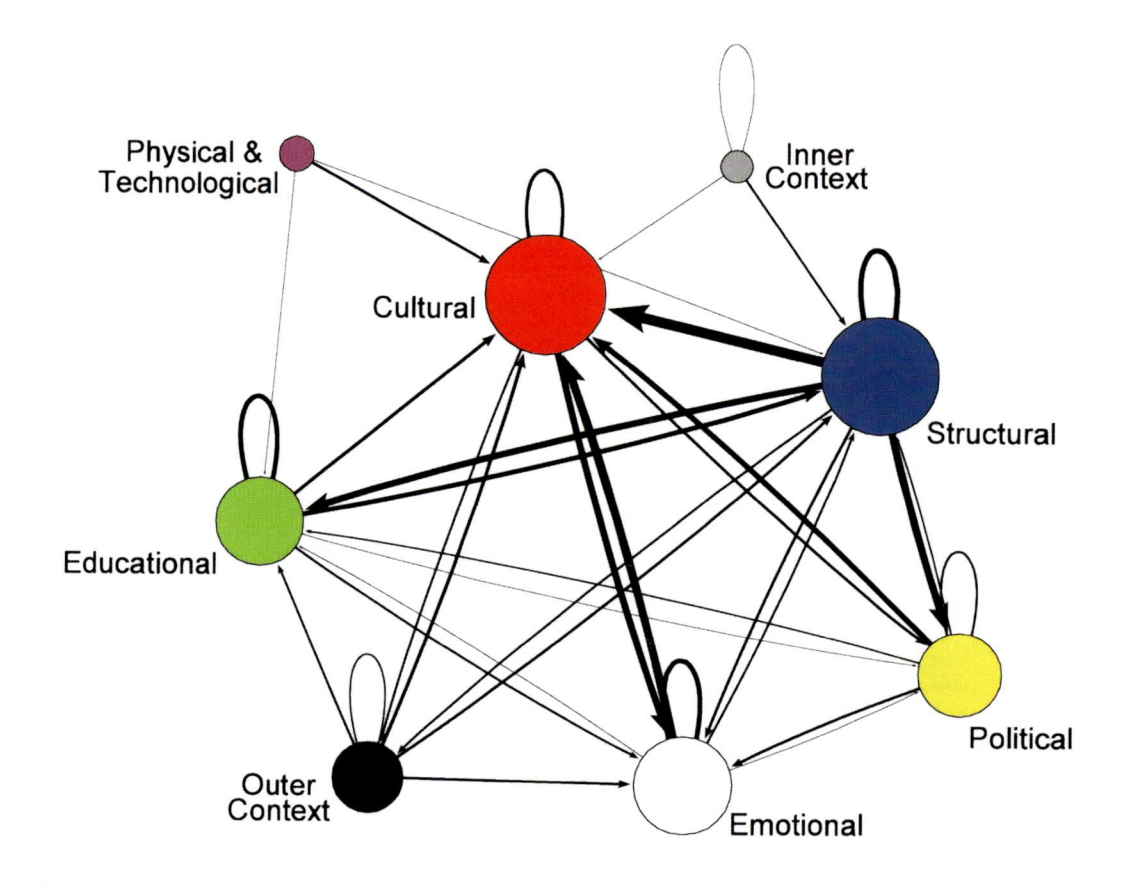

Process	Total Sub-Process Ties (#)	W/in process (%)	IN-ties (%)	OUT-ties (%)	Most Central Sub-Processes
Cultural	68	7%	69%	24%	Patient-centered ethic, Culture of excellence
Structural	66	11%	29%	61%	Task-centered leadership, Organizational slack
Emotional	46	13%	52%	35%	Collective momentum
Educational	37	16%	43%	41%	QI training
Political	33	9%	15%	45%	External partnering
Outer Context	24	8%	67%	25%	Social and cultural environments
Physical & Technical	6	0%	0%	100%	
Inner Context	5	20%	0%	80%	

FIGURE 10.5 Albany 'high level' process map

Organizational case study	Most central sub-processes
Cedars-Sinai	Communities-of-Practice; Group culture; Quality governance systems; Distributed leadership; Values/symbolic leadership; Boundary-spanner roles; Culture of learning; QI training; Data and monitoring systems; Knowledge harvesting; Organizational identity
Peterborough	QI facilitating team; Culture of empowerment; Group culture; Empowering staff; Experimentation & pilots; Decentralized authority system
Royal Devon and Exeter	Organizational identity; Group culture
Albany	Task-centered leadership; QI training; Organizational slack; Patient-centered ethic; Collective momentum; External partnering; Culture of excellence; Social and cultural environments

FIGURE 10.6 Most central sub-processes across four case studies